# Contemporary Topics in Immunobiology
# Volume 9

# Contemporary Topics in Immunobiology



---

# Contemporary Topics in Immunobiology

# Volume 9

## Self / Non-self Discrimination

Edited by

John J. Marchalonis
*Frederick Cancer Research Center*
*Frederick, Maryland*

and

Nicholas Cohen
*University of Rochester*
*Rochester, New York*



PLENUM PRESS • NEW YORK AND LONDON

The Library of Congress cataloged the first volume in this series as follows:

Contemporary topics in immunobiology. v. 1-
1972–
New York, Plenum Press.
v. illus. 24cm. annual.

1. Immunology–Periodicals.
QR180.C632 574.2'9'05 79-179761
ISSN 0093–4054

Library of Congress Catalog Card 79-179761
ISBN 0-306-40263-7


A Division of Plenum Publishing Corporation
227 West 17th Street, New York, N.Y. 10011



Printed in the United States of America

F. Macfarlane Burnet first used the phrase "self/non-self discrimination" in 1940. His concepts have provided a challenge to two generations of immunologists. It is with great pleasure that we dedicate this volume to Sir Mac on the occasion of his 80th birthday.

J. J. Marchalonis
N. Cohen
M. G. Hanna, Jr.

## *Contributors*


| | |
|---|---|
| Thomas C. Cheng | *Institute for Pathobiology*<br>*Center for Health Sciences*<br>*Lehigh University*<br>*Bethlehem, Pennsylvania 18015* |
| Michael J. Chorney | *Institute for Pathobiology*<br>*Center for Health Sciences*<br>*Lehigh University*<br>*Bethlehem, Pennsylvania 18015* |
| Adrienne E. Clarke | *School of Botany*<br>*University of Melbourne*<br>*Parkville, Victoria 3052, Australia* |
| Nicholas Cohen | *Department of Microbiology*<br>*Division of Immunology*<br>*University of Rochester*<br>*School of Medicine and Dentistry*<br>*Rochester, New York 14642* |
| Jack D. Cowan | *Department of Biophysics and Theoretical Biology*<br>*and the College*<br>*University of Chicago*<br>*Chicago, Illinois 60637* |
| Michael Edidin | *Department of Biology*<br>*The Johns Hopkins University*<br>*Baltimore, Maryland 21218* |
| B. F. Edwards | *Department of Biology*<br>*Reed College*<br>*Portland, Oregon 97202* |
| Charles A. Janeway, Jr. | *Department of Pathology*<br>*Immunology Division*<br>*Yale University School of Medicine*<br>*New Haven, Connecticut 06510* |
| R. Bruce Knox | *School of Botany*<br>*University of Melbourne*<br>*Parkville, Victoria 3052, Australia* |

| | |
|---|---|
| Heinz Köhler | *La Rabida–University of Chicago Institute*<br>*Chicago, Illinois 60649* and<br>*Departments of Pathology and Biochemistry*<br>*University of Chicago*<br>*Chicago, Illinois 60637* |
| Stephen P. Lerman | *Department of Pathology*<br>*New York University School of Medicine*<br>*New York, New York 10016* |
| John J. Marchalonis | *Cancer Biology Program*<br>*NCI Frederick Cancer Research Center*<br>*Frederick, Maryland 21701* |
| Daniel Meruelo | *Irvington House Institute*<br>*Department of Pathology*<br>*New York University Medical Center*<br>*New York, New York 10016* |
| Michael A. Palladino | *Department of Pathology*<br>*New York University School of Medicine*<br>*New York, New York 10016* |
| Donald A. Rowley | *La Rabida–University of Chicago Institute*<br>*Chicago, Illinois 60649* and<br>*Departments of Pathology and Pediatrics*<br>*University of Chicago*<br>*Chicago, Illinois 60637* |
| L. N. Ruben | *Department of Biology*<br>*Reed College*<br>*Portland, Oregon 97202* |
| G. Jeanette Thorbecke | *Department of Pathology*<br>*New York University School of Medicine*<br>*New York, New York 10016* |
| Gregory W. Warr | *Cancer Biology Program*<br>*NCI Frederick Cancer Research Center*<br>*Frederick, Maryland 21701* |

## *Preface*

The problem that virtually all cells have in discriminating between "self" and "non-self" molecules and cells has been considered at great length in immunobiology. However, cells that clearly are incapable of carrying out mammalian-type immune functions can exhibit exquisite specificity in their capacity to discriminate among syngeneic, allogeneic, and xenogeneic cells. In this volume of *Contemporary Topics in Immunobiology* we have chosen to consider the general problem of self/non-self discrimination as it is manifest in recognition reactions of plants and invertebrates and in the evolutionary development of the immune response of vertebrates. A broad, many-faceted approach is taken toward fundamental issues in immunobiology in order to develop innovative concepts of receptor function as well as to delineate traditional views.

The capacity of plants to discriminate between self and non-self is addressed in Chapter 1 by R. B. Knox and Adrienne E. Clarke. These authors provide examples of cell–cell recognition in plants that parallel those occurring in invertebrates and vertebrates. In general, tolerance (acceptance) of grafts is restricted to plants within closely related genera. Recognition is mediated by callus cells, which proliferate at wound surfaces in higher plants, and there is a correlation between cell and tissue type and antigenic markers detectable with the use of mammalian antibodies. Certain flowering plants exhibit precise discrimination in fertilization, when pollen must be from the same species, but fertilization occurs only if the pollen is genetically non-self. Self-incompatibility provides an excellent model for study of the genetic and molecular basis of recognition in plants because a specific recognition, or *S*-gene, system has been described and an antigenic glycoprotein has been implicated as the *S*-gene product. The authors discuss cell–cell recognition in plants in the context of concepts derived in cell biology and cellular immunology.

M. J. Chorney and T. C. Cheng in Chapter 2 consider cellular recognition reactions in invertebrates. They focus upon three questions: (1) Do invertebrates show specificity in the recognition of antigen? (2) What is the molecular basis for this interaction? (3) Does a phylogenetic lineage of immunoreactive complexity exist, which eventually leads to the complex vertebrate immune response?

They discuss phagocytic-cell reactions and humoral factors such as agglutinins and consider the possible roles of lectins and putative precursors of immunoglobulins and major-histocompatibility-complex (MHC) products in the elaboration of specific cell recognition by invertebrate cells.

L. N. Ruben and B. F. Edwards (Chapter 3) and G. Jeanette Thorbecke, M. A. Palladino, and S. P. Lerman (Chapter 4) address the evidence for the existence and function of cell–cell cooperation in specific immune responses of nonmammalian vertebrates. Ruben and Edwards provide an extensive review of data pertinent to the existence of primary and secondary lymphoid organs and lymphoid heterogeneity in lower vertebrates (cyclostomes, fishes, amphibians, and reptiles). They propose that collaborative cellular interactions in humoral immunity may have been a fundamental feature of vertebrate evolution, and that the appearance of such interactions did not await the evolutionary emergence of the bone marrow or bursa of Fabricius as hematopoietic sources. They present evidence supporting the provocative concept that complexity of T-cell function increases with evolution within each vertebrate class and suggest that the primitive lymphocytes in evolution might resemble mammalian B cells rather than T cells. Thorbecke *et al.* give a detailed, scholarly review and present new evidence relating to lymphoid-cell cooperation in immune responses of the chicken, a species that has been used effectively in recent studies of T and B cells. These authors provide clear evidence that T cells have the capacity to exhibit a fine degree of molecular recognition specificity, and they further define the complexity of T–B and T–macrophage interaction in this avian species.

The importance of the MHC in many immunological phenomena has led to research into the evolutionary history of this gene complex. N. Cohen (Chapter 5) analyzes recent immunological and immunogenetic studies with cold-blooded vertebrates and suggests that MHC phylogeny may be a saga of convergent evolution of Class-II-region genes (i.e., *I*-region homologous). Functional markers characteristic of this region in mice indicate the presence of the MHC in advanced fishes and anuran amphibians and its absence in primitive fishes, primitive amphibians, and some, if not all, reptiles. Salamanders have been the most extensively studied group of vertebrates that apparently lack the complete homologue of the MHC. Although a mixed-lymphocyte-reaction (MLR) locus has been provisionally identified in salamanders, it is not a major-histocompatibility (class-I) locus and it is not functionally linked to a predominant *H* locus. Moreover, the salamander system described by Cohen is of considerable interest to those attempting to ascertain theoretically the function of the MHC, because the putative MLR locus is minimally polymorphic, possessing only two codominant alleles.

G. W. Warr (Chapter 6) confronts the evidence for the existence of immunoglobulins on the surface of lymphocytes of vertebrate species ranging from teleost fishes to mammals. He marshals clear evidence supporting the presence of immunoglobulin polypeptide determinants on T- and B-like lymphocytes of representatives of all classes of vertebrates studied, and proposes that immunoglobulin, or a structurally related molecule, serves as the receptor for primary binding of antigen by all lymphocytes in all vertebrates. Monomeric IgM, or a closely related immunoglobulin, appears to be universally present as an antigen receptor on lymphocytes of the B-cell series. In addition, a second major class of B-lymphocyte surface immunoglobulin (IgD) has been described in primates and some rodents. T cells bear immunoglobulinlike receptors whose heavy chains are likely to be of a new and unique class, and the association of light chains with these molecules is a controversial issue.

The preceding chapters document the evolutionary generality (within the vertebrates) of cell–cell cooperation, the importance of the MHC, and the universality of immunoglobulin in antigen recognition. C. A. Janeway, Jr., (Chapter 7) concentrates on well-studied rodent models and addresses the complexity of T-cell populations and the function of distinct T-cell subsets in positive and negative (suppressive) T–T, T–B, and T–macrophage interactions. He emphasizes the importance of the MHC for specific recognition of antigen by T cells and offers a provocative hypothesis that accounts for the requirement for products of immunoglobulin genes ($V_H$) and MHC genes in self/non-self discrimination by T cells. He hypothesizes that T cells carry at least two kinds of specific receptors, one for MHC antigens and one for non-MHC antigens. Both of these receptors are predicted to bear $V_H$-encoded and distinct idiotypic determinants.

D. A. Rowley, H. Köhler, and J. A. Cowan (Chapter 8) approach the problem of immunoregulation at its highest level of complexity. They develop the concept of an "immunologic network" in which the intensity and quality of immune responses arise from a complex regulatory system consisting of molecules and cells specifically connected by the complementarity of receptors for antigen and receptors for receptors. The network is modulated by multiple positive and negative feedback loops.

D. Meruelo and M. Edidin (Chapter 9) offer a novel approach to the biological function of the MHC by clarifying and unifying all of the processes and interactions that appear to be regulated or modified by the MHC. Besides the involvement of the MHC in the genetic control of immune responses, the MHC exerts some genetic influence over a variety of traits not currently considered to have an immunological basis. These include the following: levels of plasma testosterone, weights of steroid-sensitive organs, mating behavior, developmental effects, e.g., cleft palate, levels of cAMP, binding of hormones to cell membranes, and cell to cell adhesion. Meruelo and Edidin build upon these observations to develop a broadly based concept of MHC function alternative to those proposed on the basis of immunological studies (for example, see Chapter 7). They suggest that the products of the MHC, especially serologically detectable molecules, function at the cell surface to modify or moderate the interaction of specific cell receptors (which are not themselves MHC products) with ligands or other cells, thereby enhancing or diminishing the degree of ligand–receptor interaction. They emphasize that the MHC effects would be expected to be of a quantitative, rather than all-or-none, nature, and that modification of binding by MHC-encoded molecules would be expected to vary with the chemistry of the substances bound and the *in situ* arrangement of the receptors and MHC products involved. These authors, moreover, propose that polymorphism of the MHC is generated (at least partially) when viruses, chiefly oncogenic viruses, integrate into the mammalian genome at or near the MHC region.

J. J. Marchalonis (Chapter 10) addresses general problems confronted in biochemical and biophysical studies of molecular interactions and the recognition specificity of surface receptors. He stresses the fundamental theoretical and practical distinction between specific primary recognition (i.e., binding of ligand by surface receptors) and immune activation and differentiation. Primary binding of ligand is a diffusion-controlled process that is governed by the laws of thermodynamics. It is a rapid process, which is dependent upon affinity of the receptors and does not show *H*-linked restriction. Specific immune differentiation, by contrast, has primary binding as its initial event but requires metabolic energy, takes minutes, hours, or days to occur, and shows *H*-linked restriction. Marchalonis proposes that primary antigen recognition by T and B cells is carried out by immunoglobulin V-region structures, but that subsequent events of activation and differentiation, e.g., cell–cell interaction, show MHC-influenced regulation, a concept consistent with that developed by Meruelo and Edidin (Chapter 9). Specific cell-surface receptors possibly functioning on diverse cell types, e.g., lectins, immunoglobulins, and MHC products, are compared on the basis of available structural data. Recent data reviewed include peptide characterization of the heavy chain of T-cell immunoglobulin and its comparison with B-cell products. The use of spin-labeled probes in the study of an early event that follows primary binding of ligand by lymphocyte redistribution of membrane lipids and receptors is described.

This volume, thus, addresses self/non-self discrimination, a central problem in immunobiology, from a number of conceptual viewpoints. We believe that this approach has allowed a clear statement of certain basic questions of immunologically and nonimmunologically mediated cell recognition, and has generated novel and testable solutions to some of the quandaries of immunobiology and cell biology. We thank the authors for their stimulating and informative contributions.

John J. Marchalonis
Nicholas Cohen

## *Contents*

*Chapter 8*

**An Immunologic Network**

*Donald A. Rowley, Heinz Köhler, and Jack D. Cowan*

*Chapter 1*

# *Discrimination of Self and Non-self in Plants*

**R. Bruce Knox and Adrienne E. Clarke**

*School of Botany*
*University of Melbourne*
*Parkville, Victoria 3052, Australia*

## I. INTRODUCTION

The plant, like the animal, survives and reproduces itself in a potentially hostile environment. Like the animal, it has developed recognition systems that enable it to respond to external challenges and to select appropriate gametes from the variety presented to it. The defense mechanisms that the plant has evolved for coexistence with a spectrum of potential fungal and microbial pathogens appear to involve interaction between an extracellular component of the pathogen and an unknown receptor, presumably on the surface of the host plant. The interaction may initiate the production of a range of plant antibiotics (for review see Albersheim and Anderson-Prouty, 1975; Strobel, 1974; Deverall, 1977; Friend and Threlfall, 1976). This field is currently the subject of much interest and speculation.

Another expression of the ability of the plant to discriminate self from non-self is seen in the capacity of plant stems to accept or reject grafts; in general, as in the animal systems, self grafts are accepted and non-self grafts are rejected. The information available on this subject is considered in the first part of this review.

A fundamental event in the life of a plant occurs during sexual reproduction, in which there is mutual recognition between compatible mating partners, an event that is essential to the continuity of plant life (Burnet, 1971; Heslop-Harrison, 1975*a*,*b*; Linskens, 1976; and Clarke and Know, 1978). This is one plant cell recognition system that is genetically well defined and where some information regarding the nature of the interacting cell surfaces is now available. This subject is considered in detail in the present review. In unicellular lower plants, the requirements for cell recognition are more limited and a +/− system of mating interactions is well known. Because preparations of single cell types are available in these systems, much progress has been made in understanding the molecular expression of the recognition systems. This area has recently been reviewed (van den Ende, 1976) and the present review is restricted to the recognition systems of multicellular vascular plants. The mutual coexistence of genetically distinct progeny within the parental tissue and the existence of differentiated cell types within a single tissue or organ in plants as well as in animals are other examples of the capacity of different cells for recognition and cooperative interaction.

## II. BIOLOGY OF RECOGNITION SYSTEMS IN VASCULAR PLANTS

### A. Some Case Histories of Somatic Interactions

#### *1. Stem Transplantation*

Plant stems can be cut and grafted onto the stems of the same or closely related species; under suitable conditions the graft will take and vascular connections will form to perfect the connection. The process is initially dependent on the wound response, which is evoked immediately after the stem is severed and results in extensive metabolic and biochemical changes in the cells adjacent to the wound, including "wound respiration," increased RNA and protein synthesis, intensification of phosphate uptake and oxidative phosphorylation, and increased phospholipid synthesis (Laties, 1975), together with the appearance of the wall polysaccharide callose (Currier, 1957; Stone and Clarke, 1980). Such changes finally lead to the proliferation of adjacent whole cells that divide in a periclinal plane, parallel to the edge of the cut surface, giving rise to callus cells that provide the initial adhesion between the grafted stems.

The processes involved in herbaceous stem grafts have been elegantly demonstrated by Lindsay *et al.* (1974) and Yeoman and Brown (1976), who used a technique providing quantitative estimates of the strength of the graft union at various periods after making the graft. Self grafts developed some cohesive strength within a few hours, the degree of cohesion increasing during the first 3 to 4 days, the primary binding period (Fig. 1). After day 4, there is a spectacular rise in cohesion, attributed to formation of the secondary binding complex, including the onset of vascular differentiation and lignification. Using the same system, Yeoman and Brown (1976) report that double grafts were equally successful on a single plant: in these, a portion of stem is placed between the two pieces of self stem to be grafted, so that two unions are formed. Polarity is important, as grafts in which the intercalated stem was inverted at grafting

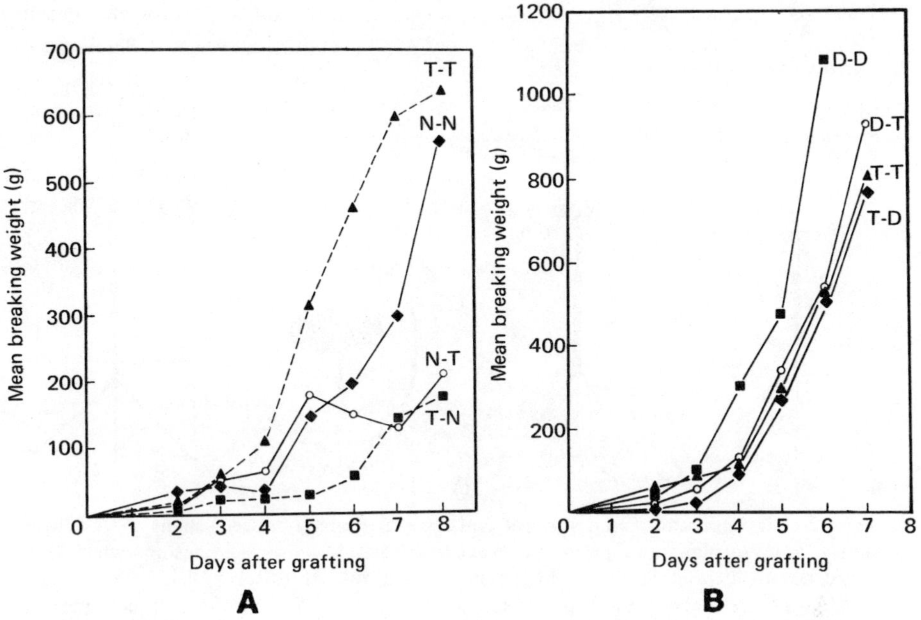


Figure 1. (A) A comparison of the increase in breaking weight of self grafts of *Lycopersicum* (T-T) and *Datura* (D-D) with heterografts of these two species (T-D and D-T). Each point is the mean of at least six values. The heterografts of *Datura* with *Lycopersicum* yield viable plants that can be grown successfully for extended periods of time. The stock and scion of the combination exhibit vascular continuity within four days of graft initiation. (B) A comparison of the increase in breaking weight of self grafts of *Lycopersicum* (T-T) and *Nicandra* (N-N) with heterografts of these two species (N-T and T-N). Each point is the mean of at least 5 values. The heterografts of *Nicandra* with tomato never achieve vascular continuity between stock and scion and can only be maintained, even on a temporary basis, by keeping them in an environment in which the humidity is very high (above 80%). From Yeoman and Brown (1976).

were unsuccessful. Also, if the graft was broken between 1 and 3 days after initial grafting, and immediately replaced, subsequent cohesive strength was achieved at a higher rate than in the original graft. Yeoman and Brown (1976) interpret this response as indicating that the different components of the cohesive complex had been activated or synthesized already, so that the lag period in synthesis was reduced. Whether this is, in fact, evidence of a memory in the transplantation response cannot yet be determined, as the data are incomplete.

Heterografts with other related plant genera may exhibit quite a different response. Grafts with *Nicandra physaloides* showed reduced cohesion, developing callus tissue at the site of union, but they failed to differentiate vascular connections, and the grafts failed (Fig. 1). However, heterografts with the thorn apple, *Datura stramonium*, were almost as successful as homografts

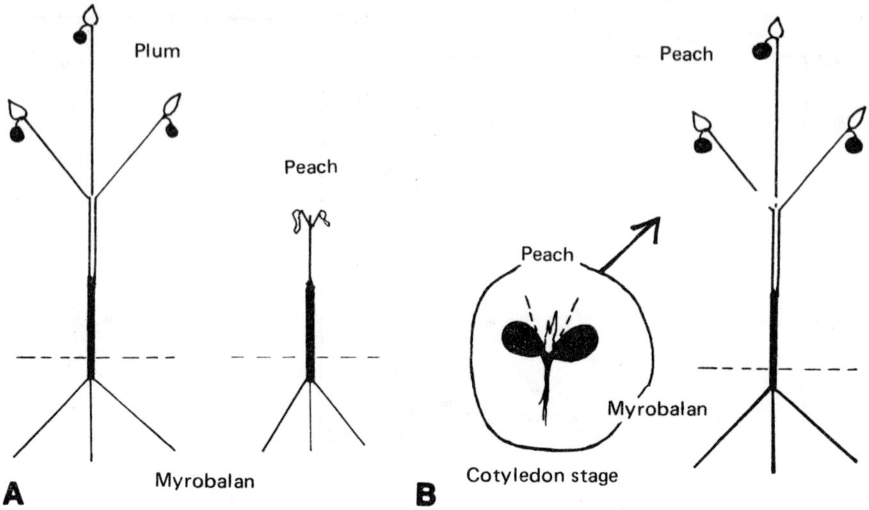


Figure 2. Diagrammatic presentation of grafting experiments between stems of wild cherry plum (cv. myrobalan) and plum and peach cultivars. A shows relationships when grafts carried out with standard 2-year-old rootstock of myrobalan (black in diagram) grafted to stems of plum (successful) or peach (unsuccessful); B shows results of peach grafts to myrobalan carried out at seedling cotyledon stage (successful). Data of Herrero and Tabuence (1969).

(Fig. 1). Reactions in all cases were completely reciprocal. These results provide the basis of an experimental system in which the nature of the recognition events of somatic-cell interactions could be explored.

Evidence concerning the development of the recognition response in woody plants has been provided by Herrero and Tabuenca (1969). They found that grafts of peach stems on stocks of wild cherry plum, cv. myrobalan, failed if made on adult (2-years-old) material (Fig. 2). However, successful grafts were obtained if made at the seedling cotyledon stage. Presumably the recognition system involved in graft rejection is not expressed at such an early stage in development.

### 2. *Chimeras and Graft Hybrids*

Certain plants in cultivation exist as mosaics of two different species or cultivars, termed chimeras. Charles Darwin in his book *Animals and Plants under Domestication* in 1875 recognized them as graft hybrids, for example, *Citrus* "Bizzaria orange" and *Laburnum adami.* Both exhibited characters that were intermediate between other known species or cultivars and produced occasional buds that closely resembled the supposed parental types, and both were propagated entirely by vegetative grafts. The hypothesis that these were of sexual hybrid origin was dismissed by Winkler (1907), who demonstrated that they arose as chimeras. He made stem grafts between *Solanum lycopersicum* and *S. nigrum.* He propagated shoots that arose from the callus at the graft union, and found that they possessed intermediate characters that were the result of the coexistence of sectors of parental tissues within the apical meristem. Almost half the apex had cells of the characteristic shape and cytological features of *S. lycopersicum*, while the remainder closely resembled *S. nigrum.*

Bauer (1909) conducted breeding experiments and cytological observations of *Pelargonium* plants that possessed different patterns of green-and-white-mottled leaves, and later showed that these originated from chimeras. The variation in leaf color resulted from heritable differences in the plastids of the outer three layers of cells of the apical meristem. The cells of these layers could contain green or white plastids or even a mixture of the two, and increased by anticlinal cell division to give concentric layers with normal or mutant plastid types, which would subsequently be expressed during leaf development. Chimeras in flower and fruit color have also been described, and are often characterized by a striped appearance. Today, interspecific chimeras are known in a wide range of horticultural plants (see review by Tilney-Bassett, 1963) but the partners are generally restricted to closely related species. This indicates that the cells of closely related species and cultivars can not only tolerate each other but also participate together in organogenesis without rejection.

In the Soviet Union and Eastern Europe, graft hybrids have been widely used as sources of new variation in agricultural and horticultural crops, following the extensive work of Michurin (1950). Not all the results can readily be explained in terms of chimera formation; for example, Glavinic (1956) in Yugoslavia grafted two cultivars of tomato, *Lycopersicum esculentum:* seedling shoots of cv. golden trophy onto mature stems of cv. Kartofelisni. The grafts succeeded, and produced flowers that were self-pollinated. Among the progeny were plants with leaf and fruit characters of the parental stock cv. Kartofelisni.

An excellent example of graft hybrid formation has been established in tomato breeding programs. Normally *L. esculentum* and *L. peruvianum* will not hybridize, nor are hybrid seeds set if the two species are grafted and the flowers produced on the graft are pollinated with pollen from the opposite grafting partner. However, if grafting is performed at the seedling cotyledon stage (see Fig. 2) within about 10 days of seedling germination, successful seed production is obtained (Nirk, 1959). This hybridization program has been used successfully to introduce genes for disease resistance from *L. peruvianum* into commercial tomato stocks.

Although the practical applications of these techniques have been exploited, the underlying biological mechanism remains unexplained. It is possible that the flowering shoots arose from chimeras at the graft union, and that the cells producing the gametes were from mosaics of both cultivars. Pandey (1976) has proposed that graft hybrids could arise by transformation, chromosome fragments of the cut cells from one partner at the graft union being incorporated into the nuclei of whole cells of the other. A further possible explanation arises from a number of recent immunobiological experiments with plant tissues that have demonstrated the existence of a characteristic suite of determinants that specify plant cells according to their tissue, organ, or species (see Section III.A). It has been shown that the expression of these determinants changes from embryonic to adult plant tissue in corn, *Zea mays* (Khavkin *et al.*, 1978*b*). There is also a wider expression of antigenic determinants in callus cells than in their parental cells (Raff *et al.*, 1979; Khavkin *et al.*, 1978*a*). It is these callus cells that arise at the cut ends of grafted stems, and may mediate interchange of information at the graft union (see Section A.3). The expression of determinants in the graft may also be altered as a result of graft union at the embryonic stage, and this process may be subject to hormonal influence from the rootstock.

### *3. Callus Cells*

Circumstantial evidence concerning the factors responsible for tissue and cell specificity has come from experiments with cells in tissue culture. Explants from organs such as stems and roots, when taken into sterile culture on solid media, undergo cell proliferation to produce masses of callus cells that can be subcultured and maintained in a state of active division in a nutrient medium containing synthetic hormones. The callus mass that forms can be subcultured into liquid medium to produce aggregates of cells in a suspension culture.

The cultured callus cells are obviously morphologically different from the parent tissue. There is circumstantial evidence to suggest that they also have different properties and presumably different determinants from the cells that gave rise to them. There is also some evidence to suggest that callus cells from different sources have many common characteristics (Raff *et al.*, 1978, 1979; Khavkin *et al.*, 1978*a*). A variety of explanations for these observations have been given: lack of genetic uniformity in callus tissue, differences in metabolic pathways that vary in different growth media (Butcher and Connolly, 1971), or permanent genetic change in the callus tissue arising from loss or addition of chromosomes and the development of somatic mutations (Heinz and Mee, 1971; Tommerup and Ingram, 1971). In view of the events of cellular differentiation involved in callus formation, it is likely that the callus cell is a cell type in its own right, different both in morphology and in determinants from other plant cells, including those from which it is derived. This would explain the observed differences in isozymes, protein electrophoretic patterns, and antigens between callus cells and intact tissue (see review by Clarke and Know, 1978), and also the similarities between callus tissues derived from different organs of the same plant (see Section III.A). It would seem reasonable to expect that, like animal cells in culture, some surface antigenic determinants are lost and new determinants appear. For example, blood-group A and B antigens are lost from fibroblasts after only a few cell divisions in culture (Chessin *et al.*, 1965). However, the possibility that the cells still carry determinants characteristic of the parent tissue remains open.

Adjacent inoculations of self callus cells will grow confluently in culture (Gautheret, 1945), as will callus from different genera within the same family, for example, *Salix* and *Populus.* Cells from different families, for example, *Acer* and *Sambucus*, induced mutual rejection responses within a few hours, with adjacent cell clumps undergoing a necrotic reaction. Intergeneric responses have been further investigated by Ball (1969), who detected three different responses: (1) Cells did not grow together; (2) cells grew together but were separated by a "wound zone" of dark-brown material, for example, between cells of *Nicotiana* and *Dahlia*, and between *Zinnia* and *Lobelia*; and (3) cells grew confluently through initiation of new cell division, as, for example, when *Chenopodium* and *Amaranthus* or *Nicotiana* and *Daucus* calluses were mixed. Ball (1971) further found that if one callus was placed above another, growth of both calluses continued, and various labeled tracers in the agar medium, for example, [$^3$H]leucine, accumulated in both calluses, suggesting that even where there are no direct cellular links, such as plasmodesmata, through the walls, some transfer of small metabolites occurred.

Little is known of the degree of cellular contact or metabolite exchange within callus cultures. Plasmodesmata are not frequent in Jerusalem artichoke callus cell walls (Bagshaw, 1969), but it seems likely that most metabolites are secreted from the cells through the cell wall and diffuse into the medium. A variety of substances are secreted into callus culture fluids. Some of these are identical with wall components (McNeil *et al.*, 1979) and a variety of other cellular components–including proteins, glycoproteins, enzymes, and potential toxins and antibiotics–could possibly be involved in the intact tissue in the recognition of self and maintenance of cellular integrity.

Studies of the interactions of callus cells of woody plants have demonstrated these cells' involvement in the acceptance or rejection of stem grafts. Fujii and Nito (1972) induced callus formation in stem explants of seven fruit cultivars grown on nutrient agar, then examined their interactions for evidence of fusion after 3 weeks' incubation in the dark at 25°C. They identified four conditions: (1) Adjacent callus cells failed to grow together, and the upper clump of cells died when grown on top of another clump (Score 0); (2) adjacent callus cells showed slight penetration but clumps easily separated when grown one above the other, and both grew (Score 1); (3) clumps grew together, but could be separated by applied force (Score 2); and (4) clumps showed complete fusion, and could not be separated by force (Score 3). The results are summarized in Table I. Scores approached zero in interactions between calluses belonging to different families, suggesting either nonrecognition or some kind of rejection. Scores were slightly higher in interactions between genera within the same fam-

**Table I. Interactions between Clumps of Callus Cells Derived from Stems of Seven Tree Fruits[a]**

| Interactions between callus cells[b] | Mean score[c] A | Mean score[c] B |
|---|---|---|
| 1. Self | 3.0 | 3.0 |
| 2. Different species of *Malus* | 3.0 | 2.0 |
| 3. Different genera within Rosaceae | 1.8 | 1.0 |
| 4. Different families | 1.2 | 0.9 |

[a]Extracted from data of Fujii and Nito (1972).
[b]Apple (*Malus pumila, M. prunifolia*), pear (*Pyrus serotina*), peach (*Prunus persica*), all of the family Rosaceae; and persimmon (*Diospyros kaki*), chestnut (*Castanea crenata*), and grape (*Vitis vinifera*), belonging to different families.
[c]Column A shows mean score from cells grown side by side; B from clumps grown one above the other. Scored 0 for no interaction, 3 for complete fusion (see text).

ily, Rosaceae, and were highest with values approaching those of self between different species within one genus, *Malus.* In these cases, the boundary between the two pieces of callus is not evident on microscopic examination, suggesting mutual recognition and tolerance. An unusual response in a distantly related pair, persimmon and chestnut, was observed where the tissues grew tightly together, but a distinct brown zone was still evident when the tissue was sectioned. These results indicate that callus cells have some ability to discriminate between self and non-self.

#### 4. *Differentiation Programs in Tobacco Tissue*

A system for experimentally manipulating differentiation programs of plant cells without the intervention of callus cells has been developed. Essentially, a dermal strip is placed on nutrient agar with constant auxin and cytokinin levels. By altering the concentration and nature of the added sugars, the tissue can be induced to differentiate directly into buds, flowers, or roots (Tran Thanh Van, 1977). This implicates receptors for the various sugars, possibly lectins, at the dermal cell surfaces. Cell-surface lectins have also been implicated in the control of differentiation in animal tissues (Nowak *et al.*, 1977).

### B. Some Case Histories of Sexual Interactions

One of the most striking examples of the ability of plants to discriminate between self and non-self is found in the male–female recognition system leading to fertilization. The male gametes are contained in the pollen grains, while the female egg cell is found in the ovule, which lies deep within the pistil. The mechanism by which the pollen is received and allowed to germinate at the female receptive surface, the stigma, provides a cell-recognition system that has been characterized in genetic, morphological, biochemical, and immunological terms.

### *1. Pollination in Cycads and the Maidenhair Tree, Ginkgo*

*Ginkgo biloba* is a gymnosperm of considerable evolutionary antiquity, and resembles the cycads in possessing both male and female trees and motile male gametes. In other gymnosperms and flowering plants, the male gametes are non-motile, transported to the egg within the pollen tube. In cycads, a pollen tube is produced when the pollen germinates within the pollen chamber (Fig. 3), but it simply acts as an anchor. The ripe male gametes are released to swim freely in a pool of fluid bathing the egg-containing structures, the archegonia. Here, recognition of compatible mating partners occurs, presumably at the surface of the egg.

The female megaspore has a patterned outer surface (Fig. 3), structurally resembling the exine wall of flowering plant pollen, and it is also coated with proteins and glycoproteins derived from surrounding parental tissue (Pettitt,

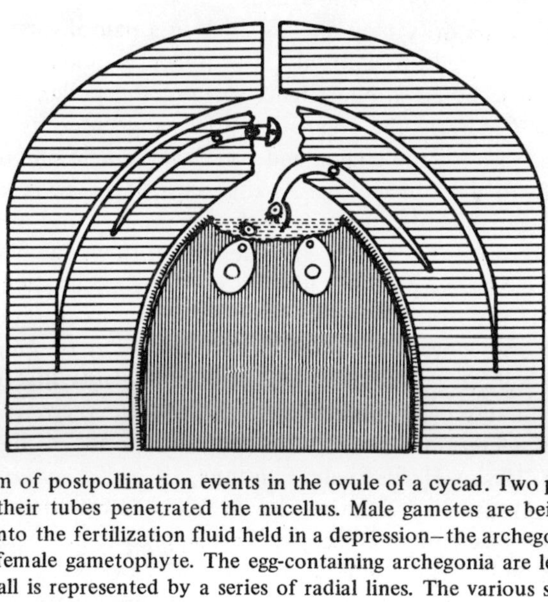

Figure 3. Diagram of postpollination events in the ovule of a cycad. Two pollen grains have germinated and their tubes penetrated the nucellus. Male gametes are being released from the lower grain into the fertilization fluid held in a depression–the archegonial chamber–at the apex of the female gametophyte. The egg-containing archegonia are left unshaded and the megaspore wall is represented by a series of radial lines. The various structures are not drawn to scale. From Pettitt (1977).

1977). These include the enzyme esterase, a concanavalin-A-binding glycoprotein fraction, and a hemagglutinin. This surface secretion is believed to form the fluid constituting the archegonial pool. Foreign pollen of other gymnosperm genera, such as conifers, successfully germinates in the pollen chamber of *Ginkgo*, and its tubes penetrate the nucellus, demonstrating that the recognition of foreign pollen does not occur at this site in the ovule (Lee, 1955), but presumably occurs at a subsequent stage in the archegonial pool.

Hydrolytic enzymes have also been detected at the germinal pores of cycad and *Ginkgo* pollen (Pettitt, 1977) in similar wall sites to those occurring in *Pinus* and flowering plants (Knox and Heslop-Harrison, 1970), and they presumably function in pollen-tube penetration and growth.

In these primitive vascular plants there is little evidence for specificity in the initial stages of pollination. Discrimination occurs when the motile sperms contact the egg surface or secretion.

### *2. Pollen–Stigma Interactions in Gladiolus and Crocus*

The flowering plants, or angiosperms, are more highly evolved than the gymnosperms, and have a correspondingly more advanced system for discrimination between self and non-self in the fertilization process. The major difference is the involvement of the pollen tube in the progression of the recognition sequence, compared with the direct contact of naked sperm with the female surface and secretions of *Ginkgo* and cycads.

Pollen grains at maturity may already contain a pair of sperm cells, or these may be produced by cell division only after pollen germination on a receptive stigma surface. If accepted at the stigma surface, the pollen tube bearing the sperm cells must penetrate the stigmatic cuticle and enter the wall system of the transmitting tissue of the stigma and style, where it is supported nutritionally in its growth to the embryo sac. At this stage, the sperms are released, one to fertilize the egg, the other to fuse with the primary endosperm nucleus in the double-fertilization event that is characteristic of flowering plants.

The stigma shows adaptations for the mode of pollination. Those plants whose pollen is transported from anther to stigma by air currents, for example, grasses, have stigmas covering a large surface area that is sometimes entirely coated with an adhesive substance, whereas those plants that rely on animal vectors such as insects often have a wet type of stigma, covered with a mucilaginous pool of secretion that traps the pollen adhering to the fur of insects (see review by Y. Heslop-Harrison and Shivanna, 1977).

The mutual events of pollination can be followed by direct observation by light or scanning electron microscopy. This approach has been elegantly exploited by Heslop-Harrison and co-workers (see review by Heslop-Harrison, 1975). The subsequent events within the pistil require other methods, the most commonly used involving the staining of the pollen tubes with aniline blue and

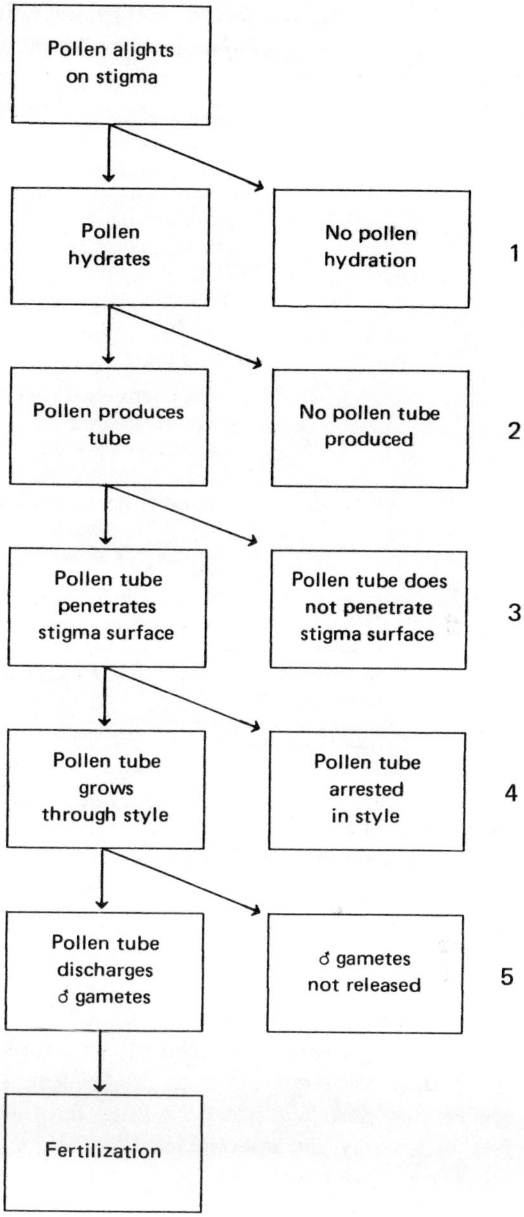


Figure 4. Sequence of events leading to fertilization in flowering plants, based on information from recent experimental work. The sequence for a compatible pollination is shown in left, and the various cutoff points leading to incompatibility on right (barriers 1–5).

observation by fluorescent microscopy (Linskens and Esser, 1957).

In two systems, *Crocus* and *Gladiolus* (family Iridaceae), which are self-fertile and have easily accessible stigmas and anthers, the major events of polli-

**Table II. Barriers to Intergeneric Pollination in *Crocus* and *Gladiolus* of the Family Iridaceae**[a]

| Barrier[b] of pollen arrest | Pollen applied: A. Stigma of *Crocus chrysanthus* cv. | Pollen applied: B. Stigma of *Gladiolus gandavensis* cv. |
|---|---|---|
| 1 | ***Iris daufordiae***[c]<br>*Camellia japonica*<br>*Cestrum psittacinum*<br>*Scilla sibirica* | ***Iris***<br>*Dryandra*<br>*Gloriosa rotschildiana*<br>*Lolium perenne*<br>*Narcissus poeticus*<br>*Prunus avium* |
| 3 | ***Freesia refracta***<br>*Brassica balearica*<br>*Cassandra calyculata*<br>*Coronilla valentinum*<br>*Erysimum capitatum*<br>*Hibbertia tetrandra*<br>*Senecio grandifolia* | ***Crocosmia aurea***<br>*Aquilegia vulgaris*<br>*Papaver icelandicum* |
| 4 | ***Schizostylis coccinea***<br>*Arabis cyprea* | |

[a]Compilation from data of Y. Heslop-Harrison (1977) for *Crocus* and Knox *et al.* (1976) and unpublished for *Gladiolus*.
[b]Barrier numbers refer to Fig. 4.
[c]Pollen genera/species listed in bold type belong to same family as the female stigma; others belong to different families.

nation have been delineated. The recognition events can be considered as a sequential series (Heslop-Harrison, 1975*a*, Knox *et al.*, 1976) each having an option in which the interaction can be terminated (Fig. 4 and Table II). Hydration and swelling of compatible pollen is usually one of the first events occurring soon after touchdown on the stigma surface. Foreign pollen may fail to hydrate (Fig. 5A), as seen in the response of *Gladiolus* stigmas to pollen of *Gloriosa* (family Liliaceae); or it may successfully pass this barrier only to be halted at a later stage. A specific attachment of compatible pollen to the stigma surface has been demonstrated in *Brassica* (Roggen, 1972). Pollen from closely related species may germinate, but the tubes fail to penetrate the stigma surface (Fig. 5B), as seen by the response of *Gladiolus* stigmas to pollen of *Crocosmia*, another genus in the same family.

Not all interspecific matings are arrested as early as is indicated for *Gladiolus* and *Crocus* in Table II. Lewis and Crowe (1958) record interspecific matings between different families in which pollen tubes grew successfully through the style to the ovule, and they document the unilateral nature of many of these

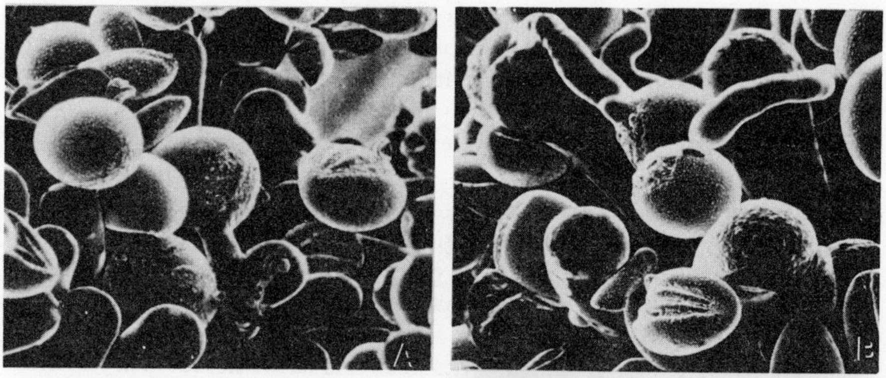


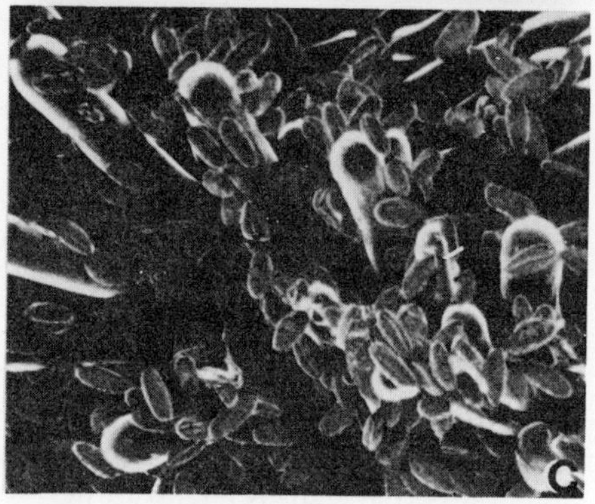


Figure 5. Scanning electron micrographs of living *Gladiolus* stigma 2 h after pollination with: A, compatible *Gladiolus* pollen (× 225); B, *Crocosmia aurea* pollen (× 320); and C, *Gloriosa rotschildiana* pollen (× 150). All reproduced at 70%. From Knox *et al.* (1976).

matings. For example, pollen of *Solanum* spp. (family Solanaceae) is inhibited in the styles of *Antirrhinum* spp. (family Scrophulariaceae), whereas in the reciprocal mating, pollen tubes of *Antirrhinum* readily grew down into the ovary of *Solanum.* The site of arrest in interspecific incompatibility characteristically parallels that of self-incompatibility (see Sections 3 and 4, and de Nettancourt, 1977).

Direct observation allows definition of the morphological events of pollination but gives little indication of their molecular basis. The nature of the interacting pollen-wall and stigma-surface components has been investigated by Heslop-Harrison and co-workers using a combination of cytochemical and electrophoretic techniques, and their findings have recently been extensively reviewed (Heslop-Harrison, 1975*a*, 1976). Both interacting surfaces contain complex mixtures of enzymically and antigenically active proteins, glycoproteins, lipids, carbohydrates, and pigments. In the *Gladiolus* and *Crocus* pollen walls, these components are stored in both the intine and exine layers. The components of the intine are synthesized by the haploid pollen protoplast

(Knox, 1971; Knox and Heslop-Harrison, 1970); those of the exine are transferred from the diploid parental cells of the tapetum (Knox *et al.*, 1975). The stigma surface contains a secretion that may have a dry, adhesive appearance [as in *Gladiolus* (Knox *et al.*, 1976)], or be stored in wall cavities [as in *Crocus* (Y. Heslop-Harrison, 1977)], or form a pool of exudate (see review by Heslop-Harrison and Shivanna, 1977).

Modification of the stigma surface markedly affects the pollination process. After short-term exposure to proteolytic enzymes, stigmas of *Crocus* still have living papillae, as judged by retention of cytoplasmic streaming, but in subsequent compatible pollinations, the pollen tubes germinate but are unable to attach themselves to the papillae and fail to penetrate the stigma cuticle (Y. Heslop-Harrison, 1977). A similar series of events has been recorded for *Agrostemma* (J. and Y. Heslop-Harrison, 1975*b*). Binding of the lectin Con A to the surface of *Gladiolus* stigmas has a similar consequence for normally compatible *Gladiolus* pollen. Pollen-tube growth appeared to be stimulated by the presence of the lectin on the stigma surface (cf. Southworth, 1975), and many grains developed more than one pollen tube (Fig. 6). Binding of Con A to *Gladiolus* stigmas can be inhibited by specific monosaccharides (Knox *et al.*, 1976), suggesting that it exerts its effect by binding to surface components essential for pollination. These data, together with the results of manipulated pollinations in which the pollen or stigma were treated with various organic solvents prior to pollination (see Clarke and Knox, 1978, for review), all suggest that communication between the intact pollen and stigma surfaces is essential for the recognition events that lead to fertilization.

### 3. *Response to Self- and Foreign Pollination in Sunflower and Cosmos*

The pollination systems of *Gladiolus* and *Crocus* are self-compatible, successful seedset occurring following either self- or cross-pollination. However, about two-thirds of the families of flowering plants exhibit some kind of self-incompatibility in which self-pollination is prevented, thus favoring outbreeding within the species. In such cases, although pollination does not lead to fertilization, the self pollen is recognized at the stigma surface, it germinates, and the pollen tube may grow to an extent specific for each system. At some stage the subsequent events of fertilization (see Fig. 4) are prevented, and this cessation can be correlated with the deposition of the polysaccharide callose that appears to occlude the pollen tubes, providing a cytochemically detectable and active manifestation of the rejection response (Heslop-Harrison *et al.*, 1974, 1976).

Experimental pollinations with sunflower, *Helianthus annuus*, and *Cosmos bipinnatus*, both members of the tribe Heliantheae of the family Compositae, have provided valuable evidence on the nature of rejection and of the role of

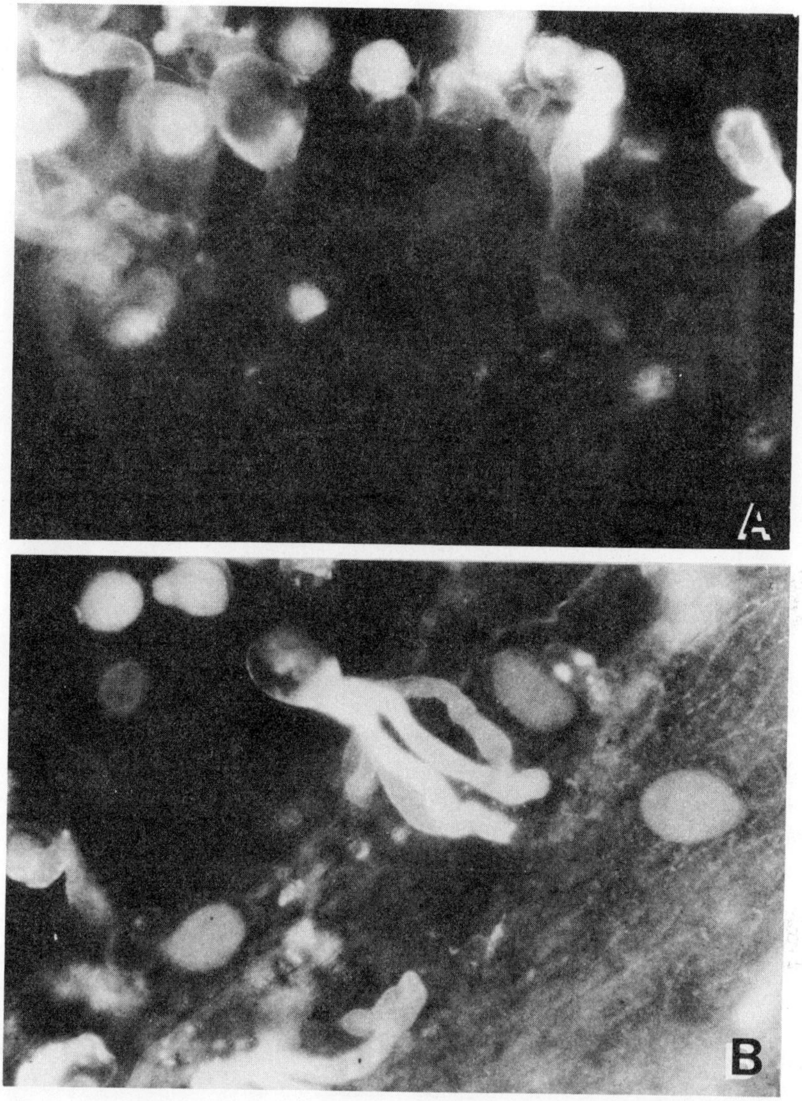


Figure 6. Control of pollination in *Gladiolus*, revealed by fluorescence microscopy after staining whole mounts of pollinated stigmas with aniline blue, which stains the polysaccharide callose in the pollen grain and pollen tubes, indicating pollen-tube behavior. A, Normal stigma surface. Pollen tubes penetrate the surface and grow towards the style (base of photograph). B, Stigma surface after con A treatment, as described in text. Pollen tubes grow over surface, often producing two tubes, without apparent penetration (× 250).

pollen-recognition substances in the reactions. Both genera have a sporophytic form of self-incompatibility. In *Cosmos*, the system is determined by *S* genes and the pollen grains show the parental phenotype at the stigma, rather than expressing their own haploid genotype (Crowe, 1954). In sunflower, two gene loci may be involved (Habura, 1957; Shchori, 1969). Following self-pollination in both systems, the pollen tubes are produced, but they are inhibited on the stigma surface. Callose is produced, occluding both pollen tubes and stigmatic papillae during the self-interaction. This active rejection response can be detected within 15 min in *Cosmos* (Howlett *et al.*, 1975). In compatible matings, much less callose is produced and it takes the form of plugs that seal off the growing tip containing the living cytoplasm.

In sunflower, the callose rejection response also occurs following matings with pollen of other genera within the family Compositae (Vithanage and Knox, 1977), but not with genera from the other families tested. Stored dead pollen of genera such as ragweed, *Ambrosia trifida*, or *Aster* could still induce an effective stigma response. These experiments suggest that the elicitor is rapidly diffusible and probably located in the pollen walls, as in the crucifers (see Section 4).

Earlier experiments on interspecific recognition mechanisms and manipulated pollinations in Populus (Knox *et al.*, 1972) implicated pollen-wall proteins and glycoproteins in stigma recognition. Similar experiments have implicated pollen-wall proteins as recognition substances in *Cosmos*. *Cosmos*-pollen mixes consisting of live self pollen (incompatible) and gamma-irradiated killed pollen from a compatible genotype gave significant self-seedset in experiments in which self pollen alone hardly set any seeds (Table III), and no effects were obtained with killed self pollen in the mixes (Howlett *et al.*, 1975). Seedset obtained was about 20% of the compatible rate. The effect could also be produced if the killed compatible pollen was replaced with an extract of the wall-protein fraction from compatible pollen, which was applied to the stigmas prior to selfing, whereas it is important to note that the corresponding protein fraction from self pollen did not affect seedset (Table III). One interpretation of these results is that a factor present in the extract interacts with the stigma to permit acceptance of self pollen; alternatively, the self pollen may itself be altered by the presence of the compatible fraction. The extracts were derived from the pollen walls and did not contain cytoplasmic components. It is interesting that heated extracts (60°C, 10 min) that still contain several antigenic proteins are equally effective in allowing successful self-pollination.

These data provide some evidence for the role of pollen-wall components as recognition substances. Although proteins and glycoproteins have been implicated as the elicitors, it is possible that the active fraction may be carbohydrate or low-molecular-weight material associated with the other fractions during purification.

**Table III. Experimental Evidence for the Role of Pollen-Wall Proteins of *Cosmos bipinnatus* in Pollen–Stigma Recognition[a]**

| Stigma treatment[b] | % Seedset[c] |
|---|---|
| 1. *Compatible* pollen | 100 |
| 2. Killed[d] *self* + *compatible* pollen | 84 |
| 3. *Self* pollen | 2 |
| 4.1. Killed[d] *self* + *self* pollen | 4 |
| 4.2. *Self* diffusate[e] + *self* pollen | 3 |
| 5.1. Killed[d] *compatible* pollen | 9 |
| 5.2. *Compatible* diffusate | 8 |
| 6.1. Killed[d] *compatible* + *self* pollen | 27 |
| 6.2. *Compatible* diffusate + *self* pollen | 12 |
| 6.3. Heated *compatible* diffusate (10 min, 60°C) + *self* pollen | 15 |

[a] Data from Howlett *et al.* (1975), pooled from 5 experiments.
[b] *C. bipinnatus* is self-incompatible, but self-pollination can be stimulated by various pollen mixes and treatment of stigmas with pollen proteins.
[c] Differences between seedset in treatments 3–4 and 6 are statistically significant ($p < 0.02$).
[d] 100 kR gamma irradiation.
[e] Diffusates are short-term extracts of living pollen precipitated with $(NH_4)_2SO_4$ at 0.9 saturation and purified by Sephadex-G25 chromatography, and applied at a concentration of 1 mg/ml for 2 min before live pollen.

### *4. Response to Self-Pollination in Crucifers*

Several genera of Cruciferae possess a well-defined sporophytic self-incompatibility system, which is manifested by pollen-tube inhibition on the stigma surface (Christ, 1959), accompanied by callose deposition in both pollen tubes and stigmatic papillae (Dickinson and Lewis, 1973*a*,*b*; Heslop-Harrison *et al.*, 1974). Both groups have demonstrated that the stigma callose response to self pollen is elicited by pollen-wall fractions derived from the exine cavities. These fractions are synthesized by the diploid parental cells of the tapetum. This means that the pollen grains are effectively coated with parentally specified components providing a ready means for expression of the parental phenotype at the pollen surface, as suggested by Heslop-Harrison (1968).

Experimental evidence for the role of pollen-surface components in eliciting callose deposition has been obtained by Dickinson and Lewis (1973*a*,*b*). Exine material was collected by centrifuging surface material from dry pollen directly into Millipore filter disks, which were then applied to the surface of unpollinated stigma papillae of self and compatible genotypes. Callose was induced in self but not in compatible stigmas. Heslop-Harrison *et al.* (1974) showed that the callose rejection response could be elicited in self stigmas by pollen prints on agar films and by short-term surface diffusates. Attempts to fractionate the pollen diffusate by thin-layer gel filtration, followed by the application of unpollinated stigmas to the gel surface, revealed that the active component present was associated with the protein fraction of molecular weight 10,000-25,000. Further work is needed to characterize precisely the eliciting component.

### 5. *Response to Self in Gametophytic Self-Incompatibility Systems*

In gametophytic systems of self-incompatibility, the expression of the *S* gene is determined by the genotype of the individual pollen grain at the stigma surface or in the style. Pollen-tube inhibition can occur at a variety of sites, from within the stigma to the embryo sac itself. We will now consider evidence from experiments with three different gametophytic systems: *Oenothera*, *Petunia* and *Lycopersicum*, and *Lilium.*

The evening primrose, *Oenothera organensis*, shows self-pollen inhibition within the stigma (Emerson, 1940). This was confirmed by grafting experiments: when the stigma is removed, there is no inhibition of self-pollen tubes in the style (Bali and Hecht, 1965). Immersion of stigmas in hot water, 5 min at 50°C, also overcame the incompatibility response (Kumar and Hecht, 1965). The fate of the pollen is apparently determined after it alights on the wet stigma surface, when the grains contact a surface layer of mucilaginous material, produced by the breakdown of the stigma-surface cells (Dickinson and Lawson, 1975). Such stigmatic inhibition is unusual in gametophytic systems, with the exception of grasses in which pollen tubes are inhibited shortly after entry into the stigma (Hayman, 1956). In *Oenothera*, the self-pollen tubes become occluded with callose, while differences have also been detected in components staining with periodic acid–Schiff reaction between the self and compatible pollen–tube protoplasts (Dickinson and Lawson, 1975).

Pollen-tube arrest within the transmitting tissue of the style occurs in *Petunia hybrida* (van der Pluijm and Linskens, 1966) and in the wild tomato, *Lycopersicum peruvianum* (de Nettancourt *et al.*, 1973). Arrest of self tubes is accompanied by marked thickening and swelling of the tips, which become occluded with callose and in many instances appeared to burst, as if in premature discharge of the male gametes. In *Lycopersicum*, Cresti *et al.* (1976) have shown that the mucilaginous walls of the transmitting tissue rapidly accumulated protein at maturity, presumably providing for nutrition of the tubes or for interaction with them. De Nettancourt *et al.* (1974) observed a concentric type of endoplasmic reticulum in the pollen-tube cytoplasm of self tubes, which they consider to reflect inhibition of protein synthesis. This hypothesis has been supported by Cresti *et al.* (1977), who showed that *Lycopersicum peruvianum* pollen exposed to lethal doses of gamma irradiation produces pollen tubes that are arrested in compatible pistils the same distance down the style as untreated self tubes under similar conditions (one-third to half the length of the style). They also demonstrated the characteristic concentric type of endoplasmic reticulum found in self tubes. Both *Petunia* and *Lycopersicum* have a wet stigma, but its role in the self-incompatibility response has not been defined.

Self-incompatibility in the lillies *Lilium longiflorum* and *L. henryi* is markedly different from the other two systems. Here, pollen grains germinate on the wet stigma surface and the tube grows down over the surface directly into a mucilage-coated stylar canal, where self-pollen-tube growth is inhibited. No tissue penetration occurs in the style canal prior to inhibition. The stigma has been shown from the grafting experiments to have no primary role in self-incompatibility (Dickinson and Lawson, 1975) and the response can be eliminated by exposing the styles to gamma irradiation or hot-water treatment. Neither pollen washes nor pollen mixes of live self with killed compatible pollen have a demonstrable effect on the response (Fett *et al.*, 1976), which suggests that the reaction is determined by interaction between the pollen tube and the style surface or secreted mucilage.

## III. IMMUNOBIOLOGY OF RECOGNITION SYSTEMS

All the recognition reactions discussed—those associated with grafting and callus-cell interaction and between cells involved in male-female recognition—must ultimately depend on some interaction at the molecular level. It is accepted that analogous reactions between animal cells are mediated by molecular interaction between membrane-associated determinants (Hughes, 1976*a*,*b*). The situation in plant tissues is different in that the plasma membrane is overlaid with a rigid cellulosic cell wall, and in surface cells a thick cuticle often covers the wall and poses another potential barrier between the plasma membrane and the external milieu. Within a particular tissue, the plasma membranes of the component cells often have some continuity via the plasmodesmata. The role of these connections as channels of communication and the possible means for transfer of information between plant cells in contact have been considered by Gunning and Robards (1976) and Clarke and Knox (1978). The study of the molecular basis of plant-cell recognition is just beginning and to date has been based mainly on attempts to demonstrate different plant-cell specificities by examining antigenic determinants.

### A. Antigenic Determinants of Somatic Cells and Protoplasts

The determinants of somatic plant cells may be expressed at the plasma-membrane surface. This has been investigated by preparing isolated protoplasts. Preparation involves incubation of the cells with preparations of cell-wall-degrading enzymes, and wall removal is generally monitored cytochemically by the disappearance of wall polysaccharide material staining with fluorescent brightener dyes (Nagata and Takebe, 1970). Under these conditions, gross removal of the cell wall is achieved, but the extent to which any saccharide determinants on the plasma membrane may have been degraded by treatment with the mixed glycosidase preparation cannot be predicted. Thus it is not possible to say whether the differences in surface properties of different plant protoplasts detected in immunological experiments reflect the presence of species-specific surface antigens or whether they reflect varying degrees of enzymic degradation of antigenic determinants common to all plant protoplasts —or even a combination of both possibilities. If, for example, a complex carbohydrate membrane determinant with an immunodominant terminal saccharide unit were revealed during the enzymic removal of the cell wall, further treatment with the glycosidase mixture might hydrolyze the terminal glycosidic linkage and reveal the penultimate saccharide, which would then become the dominant sugar of a new determinant. Prolonged treatment might be expected to reveal a sequence of different determinants, perhaps in a way similar to that in which different determinants in the ABO blood group system are revealed by sequential enzymic removal of terminal saccharides (Watkins, 1972, Clamp *et al.*, 1978).

Most of the work with protoplasts has been directed at obtaining close contact between protoplasts in order to facilitate cell fusion and hybridization. As a by-product of this research, some information on the immunological determinants on protoplast surfaces has become available. Agglutination experiments with protoplasts from *Vicia*, soybean, and bromegrass by their homologous and heterologous antisera have demonstrated that there was considerable cross-reactivity as each of the protoplast preparations was agglutinated by each of the antisera, but not by normal rabbit serum (Hartmann *et al.*, 1973). Some specificity was demonstrated, as the titers for the homologous agglutination reactions were in general higher than those of the heterologous agglutination. It is interesting that the monocotyledon *Bromus* and the dicotyledon *Vicia* cross-reacted extensively, suggesting the presence of surface antigens common to the protoplasts. Neither antibody treatment (Hartmann *et al.*, 1973) nor Con A binding to protoplasts (Williamson *et al.*, 1976) affected their growth or division, or the regeneration of the cell wall during subsequent culture. Presumably the antigenic determinants of the protoplast surface are not directly involved in control of wall formation. These protoplasts, like animal cells, were also liable to complement-induced lysis after antibody treatment.

The existence of both species- and organ-specific antigens as well as determinants common to a range of plant organs has been demonstrated by immunodiffusion in tobacco plants (Boutenko and Volodarsky, 1968); in corn roots (Misharin *et al.*, 1974, Khavkin *et al.*, 1978*b*); and in *Gladiolus* leaves, corms, and petals (Clarke *et al.*, 1977). The relationships between parental antigens from leaves, stems, pistils, and anthers and their derived callus cells and protoplasts have been examined by similar methods in the sweet cherry, *Prunus avium* (Raff *et al.*, 1979). For example, a specific antigen of the cherry leaf also occurred in leaf callus, while other leaf antigens were held in common with other organs. In addition, the callus cells possessed their own specific antigens that were not expressed in the parental organs. Evidence that the antigens were located at the plasma membrane and in the periphery of the cytoplasm was obtained by immunofluorescence. Plasma-membrane location of the antigens was confirmed using a protoplast-rosetting technique (Raff *et al.*, 1979).

Immunobiological methods are being developed in attempts to type plant tissues, organs, cultivars, and species on the basis of their antigenic determinants. For example, antisera to leaf extracts have been successfully used to discriminate between three cultivars of *Populus nigra* and a hybrid with *P. deltoides* (Sterba, 1975). In addition, Boyarskii (1972) found that antiserum against a pest (*Eriophyes ribis* Nal.) of the blackcurrant, *Ribes sanguineum*, will cross-react with antigens from pest-susceptible but not pest-resistant cultivars. The sharing of antigens by host and parasite has been reviewed by Deverall (1977).

## B. The Search for the *S*-Gene Product of Self-Incompatibility

In interactions between cells of flowering plants, the only defined genetic system is the *S* gene of incompatibility. Since 1929, when East postulated that the *S*-gene product might resemble an animal antigen, attempts have been made to examine the *S*-gene product by immunobiological methods. Most of the work has been carried out with either pollen or stigma preparations, and to date it has given only a correlation between antigenic specificity and *S*-allele specificity; the *S*-gene product remains to be isolated and characterized.

### *1. The S Antigen of Pollen*

In 1952, Lewis began a long series of experiments aimed at detecting the gene product of the *S*-allele system in *Oenothera organensis.* He argued, following East (1929), that since each *S* allele produces a different and highly specific reaction, there is likely to be a pollen antigen that reacts with a complementary stylar substance with the same specificity. He had available nine clones of *O. organensis*, all of which are heterozygous for pairs of combinations of 4 different alleles. The antigen extract was prepared from ether-washed pollen by a combined freeze–thawing maceration method using long-term extracts that would contain both pollen-wall and cytoplasmic proteins and glycoproteins and raised rabbit antisera to the preparation.

Antisera titers and specificity were tested by a microprecipitin ring test.

Maximum titer in homologous tests was 1280, while it was only 200 for heterologous tests with antisera raised against other *S*-specific genotypes. Antisera absorbed with other S-antigen preparations were tested against their homologous antigens or against those in which only one common *S* allele was present (Table IV). Tests against their homologous antigens gave high titers, with progressively lower titers as the relationship became distant. Maximum titers compared favorably with the heterologous reactions obtained with the original unabsorbed sera, indicating that the majority of precipitins present were directed to common antigenic components.

Two different plants, presumably with different genetic backgrounds, appear to have been used as a source of $S_3S_6$ antigens, so covering the possibility that *S*-allele specificity is expressed in plants with widely different backgrounds. There seems little doubt that these pioneering experiments effectively demonstrated the correlation between antigen specificity and *S* genotype in pollen of *Oenothera.*

Analogous results were later obtained by Linskins (1960), who used precipitin ring tests to investigate *S*-allele specificity in both pollen and styles of *Petunia hybrida.* Again, the highest titers were obtained in homologous reactions. This is interpreted as evidence of the presence of S-specific antigens in both pollen and styles. The correlation extended to cross-reactions between pollen antisera and stigma antigens, and vice versa, suggesting that the antigens of pollen and style are immunologically closely related, if not identical. The antisera used are of high specificity, but of lower titer than those used by Lewis (1952), and Linskens did not attempt absorption experiments. These exciting preliminary results have not been followed up by more thorough testing against the same *S* genotypes in other genetic backgrounds.

The techniques of immunodiffusion and immunoelectrophoresis became widely used in the 1960s, enabling a qualitative picture of the number of pollen antigens and their immunological relationships to be obtained. Lewis and co-

**Table IV. Correlation between Antigen Specificity and *S* Alleles of Pollen of *Oenothera organensis*, as Determined by Precipitin Ring Tests[a]**

| | | Maximum titer against pollen antigens: | | | | | |
|---|---|---|---|---|---|---|---|
| *S* allele tested | Absorption AS/AA | $S_2S_6$ | $S_3S_4$ | $S_3S_6$ | $S_3S_6$ | $S_4S_6$ | $S_2S_3$ |
| 1. $S_2$ and $S_6$ | $S_2S_6/S_3S_4$ | 200 | 5 | 100 | 100 | 100 | 200 |
| 2. $S_2$ | $S_2S_6/S_3S_6$ | 25 | NT | 5 | 2 | 5 | 25 |
| 3. $S_3$ and $S_4$ | $S_3S_4/S_2S_6$ | 5 | 100 | 50 | 50 | 100 | NT |
| 4. $S_4$ | $S_3S_4/S_3S_6$ | 2 | 5 | 5 | 5 | 5 | 50 |

[a]Data from Lewis (1952) shows maximum titers obtained against absorbed antisera when tested against antigen extracts with indicated *S*-allele specifications. AS, antiserum; AA, absorbing antigen; NT, not tested.

workers used these methods to substantiate further the correlation between S-antigen specificity and the presence of specific *S* alleles in *Oenothera* pollen. The putative S antigen was claimed to constitute at least 20% of total pollen protein, and it diffused from the pollen into isotonic medium within 30 min (Makinen and Lewis, 1962), which suggests that the antigen is located in the intine layer, where release is slower (Knox *et al.*, 1975). Perhaps the most convincing demonstration of antiserum specificity is given by radial immunodiffusion tests using antisera to homozygous $S_6$ pollen. The narrowest precipitate surrounded the well containing $S_2S_3$ extract, with greater amounts surrounding $S_3S_6$ and $S_4S_6$ wells (approximately 50 and 75% of homologous $S_6S_6$ reaction respectively). In later studies, Lewis *et al.* (1967) took plates of agar containing $S_6$-pollen antisera and showed that individual pollen grains produced precipitates when sprinkled on the gel. No reaction was obtained with pollen from $S_2S_3$ anthers, while 53 and 62% of pollen from $S_3S_6$ anthers formed precipitates in two experiments, which is close to the expectation of 50%, whereas pollen from homologous $S_6S_6$ anthers gave 81, 91, and 100% in three experiments.

### 2. *The S Antigen of Stigmas*

Evidence of the presence of an antigen with *S*-allele specificity in the stigma of the cabbage, *Brassica oleracea* var. *capitata*, has been obtained by Nasrallah, Wallace, and co-workers at Cornell University. The S-specific antigen has been qualitatively characterized by immunoadsorption, immunoelectrophoresis, and polyacrylamide-gel electrophoresis, but as with the pollen S antigen, it remains to be isolated and its nature determined.

Antisera were raised against homogenates of pistils with specific *S* alleles. Three different *S* genotypes were tested. Three bands were obtained by immunodiffusion (Nasrallah and Wallace, 1967*a*,*b*), 2 of which were common to pistils with different *S* genotypes, while the third and most intense band was considered to be specific for each *S* genotype. However, the finding that these three bands could be further resolved by immunoelectrophoresis into a total of nine bands makes this interpretation equivocal. The transfer of the putative S antigens to both $F_1$ and $F_2$ generations after the plant had been crossed with another genotype can be followed immunologically (Nasrallah *et al.*, 1970, 1972). S antigens have also been detected in stigmas of kale and Brussels sprout (Landova and Landa, 1973, Sedgley, 1974*a*,*b*; Kucera and Polak, 1975). These are varieties of *Brassica oleracea*, and share a similar spectrum of *S* alleles.

The *Brassica* stigma antigens are freely diffusible from whole stigmas (Nasrallah and Wallace 1967*a*,*b*) and do not appear until 3 days before anthesis, at which time self-incompatibility can be demonstrated. Prior to this period, bud pollination with self pollen will yield selfed progeny.

The only information about the nature of the putative S antigen is indirect and has been derived from electrophoretic techniques. The *Brassica* S antigen has a high isoelectric point (Nasrallah *et al.*, 1970; Nishio and Hinata, 1977) and its carbohydrate content has been demonstrated by its susceptibility to periodate oxidation and its affinity with the lectin concanavalin A (Nishio and Hinata, 1978).

### *3. The S Antigen in Perspective*

During the past 50 years there has been continuing speculation on the nature of the *S*-gene product and its interactions in the pollen and stigma to control self-incompatibility, and several hypotheses and models have been advanced (see reviews by Heslop-Harrison, 1975; Lewis, 1976; Linskens, 1976; de Nettancourt, 1977). Lewis (1965) advanced two widely accepted alternatives: that the interactions depend on the binding of mutually complementary and stereospecific receptors on pollen and stigma, or that identical molecules from the two partners interact to produce an inhibitory complex. Despite this, no experimental evidence for the molecular basis of the interactions has been published.

Some evidence indicating the presence of common antigens in pollen and stigmas has been obtained (Linskens, 1960). However, whether or not these would combine during pollination and whether the combination would initiate the rejection response are not resolved. Recently, the antigenic basis of cellular identity in plants has been explored: There seem to be antigenic components typical of the organs of an individual plant and others that are common to different organs and tissues. It is relevant that some of the pollen and stigma antigens are also present in vegetative organs and yet retain demonstrable tissue specificity after immunoabsorption (Clarke *et al.*, 1977). Preliminary experiments with the sweet cherry, *Prunus avium*, which has a gametophytic self-incompatibility system, indicate that some apparent S-antigen specificity is expressed in somatic tissue (Raff *et al.*, 1977).

It has been proposed (Clarke and Knox, 1978) that the *S* gene may be a multigene family like those controlling immunoglobulin or ribosome biosynthesis (Hood *et al.*, 1975). This would mean that the products of different *S* alleles would be closely related, so that the different S antigens would be expected to show some degree of immunological identity. The data reviewed above, especially those for *Brassica* stigmas, indicate that the S antigen is specific for each genotype (Nasrallah *et al.*, 1967*a*,*b*). However, it is possible to reinterpret these data (Nasrallah *et al.*, 1967*b*; Figs. 1-3 and 5-7) as revealing the existence of partially identical antigens in the different *S* genotypes. Closely related antigens may not be distinguishable by immunodiffusion, and higher-resolution quantitative methods would be needed to resolve this point.

A surprising feature of many reported studies has been the low titer of the

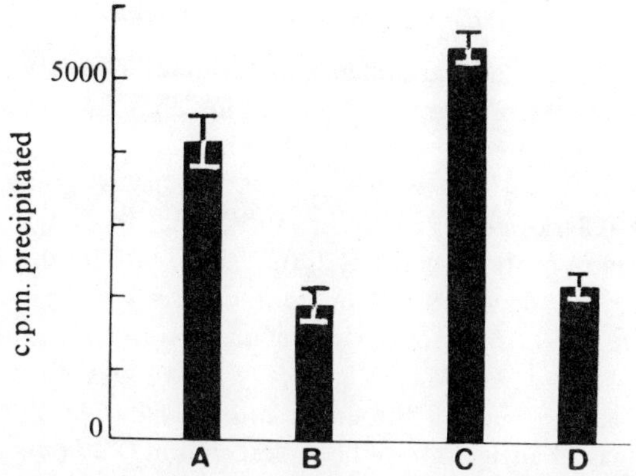


Figure 7. Immune precipitation of [$^{125}$I]pollen and stigma antigens of *Gladiolus* by homologous and heterologous antiserums. A double-antibody precipitating system was used: 200 μl of radioiodinated pollen or stigma extracts ($10^6$ c.p.m.) were added to 100 μl of a 1:20 dilution of rabbit antiserum. The precipitate was developed by addition of 200 μl of a 1:4 dilution of goat antiserum to rabbit IgG, followed by incubation for 1 h at 37°C and 15 h at 4°C. Data given are [$^{125}$I] radioactivities associated with precipitates that were washed twice by centrifugation. A, [$^{125}$I] pollen + antipollen serum; B, [$^{125}$I] pollen + antistigma serum; C, [$^{125}$I] stigma + antistigma serum; D, [$^{125}$I] stigma + antipollen serum. From Clarke *et al.* (1977).

antisera raised to specific *S* genotypes after absorption; for example, Nasrallah (1965) injected 12 rabbits with stigma antigens and only 3 gave antisera with demonstrable S-specific antigens, while Sedgley (1974*a*,*b*) injected 11 rabbits and only 4 responded with specific antisera after absorption. Sedgley noted that both her successful antisera and those of Nasrallah *et al.* (1967*a*,*b*) were all prepared against stigmas with *S* alleles high in the dominance series of sporophytic self-incompatibility. The poor and variable antigenicity of the S antigens low in the dominance series might be interpreted in terms of the sequential loss of immunodominant units down the series. The *Brassica S*-gene product appears to be a glycoprotein. If, for example, the ultimate specificity resides with the carbohydrate moiety, the sequential loss of terminal monosaccharide units could give the observed variation. Such sequences of immunodominant sugars are known to occur in the blood-group antigens (Watkins, 1966) and the Ia antigens (McKenzie *et al.*, 1977), and variations in antigenicity of oligosaccharide sequences have been recorded (Robert *et al.*, 1973).

## C. Recognition at the Pollen–Stigma Interface

Some information is available regarding the molecular nature of the interacting cell surfaces in pollination.

### *1. Pollen-Surface Macromolecules*

Short-term diffusates of the pollen grain contain a variety of proteins, glycoproteins, carbohydrates, pigments, and lipids that have been qualitatively demonstrated in a number of systems (Knox *et al.*, 1975; Heslop-Harrison, 1975). Recently, a quantitative analysis of *Gladiolus* pollen diffusates has become available (Clarke *et al.*, 1979) and shows that the major macromolecular components contain protein, carbohydrate, and lipid in the ratio 10:6:0.2. The monosaccharides of glycoprotein components were galactose, mannose, glucose, arabinose, and rhamnose. Uronic acids were not detectable. All the mannose was associated with an antigenically active glycoprotein fraction that bound to con A-sepharose, and the major monosaccharide of the lipid fraction was glucose. At least 9 antigens have been detected in *Gladiolus* pollen diffusates (Knox, 1971; Clarke *et al.*, 1977), and in the molecular weight range of 20,000 to 70,000 (see Fig. 8).

Iwanami (1968) demonstrated by immunoelectrophoresis the presence of more than 15 antigens in pollen of *Coreopsis* and *Zea*, and several were common to pollen of unrelated species. A similar number of antigens have been detected in grass pollens (Augustin, 1959), and these include the allergens, which were later shown to be glycoprotein in nature (Johnson and Marsh, 1965) and to consist of two principal groups of closely related allergens of molecular weight

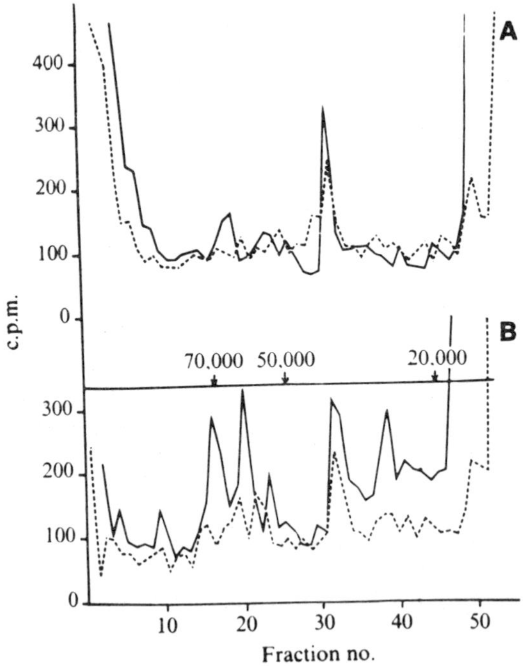


Figure 8. Analysis of [$^{125}$I] stigma (A) and pollen (B) antigens of *Gladiolus* on SDS-polyacrylamide gels after precipitation of homologous antisera (solid line) and heterologous antisera (broken line). Immunoprecipitates were dissociated in 200 μl of Tris buffer, pH 6.8, containing 3% SDS and 5% β-mercaptoethanol, and run on SDS-polyacrylamide gels. The gels were sliced and radioactivity was determined using a Packard autogamma counter. From Clarke *et al.* (1977).

30,000 and 17,000 respectively. King *et al.* (1964) isolated and purified the most potent allergen from ragweed pollen, antigen E, which proved to be a protein of molecular weight 39,000 with 4 subunits (King *et al.*, 1974). Both grass- and ragweed-pollen allergens cross-react extensively with immunologically similar fractions in related pollen; for example, pollen antigens of sunflower and *Cosmos* show reactions of partial identity with ragweed antigen E (Knox, 1973). Some, however, show remarkable specificity for closely related genera only, for example, the heat-labile basic antigen A of grass pollen (Watson and Knox, 1976). Pollen antigens possessing allergenic activity specifically bind to IgE in the sera of allergic patients, and this forms the basis of a test for allergenicity, the radioallergosorbent test (RAST) (for review see Evans, 1975).

Molecules diffusing from grass pollen that has settled on leaf surfaces may have remarkable effects in stimulating the penetration and greatly increased infectivity of pathogenic fungal spores (Preece, 1976). The active component is in the cationic fraction, and it is heat-stable and active at low dilutions of pollen extract. A diffusible, heat-stable fraction from pollen of carrotweed, *Parthenium hysterophorus*, had the remarkable property of inhibiting compatible self-pollen germination on stigmas of quite unrelated flowers of tomato (*Lycopersicum esculentum*), French bean (*Phaseolus vulgaris*), and chili (*Capsicum annuum*) (Char, 1977). The nature of the interaction is not known, though toxins, saponin, for example, are known to be present in pollen of horse chestnut (*Aesculus*) and lime (*Tilia*), and alkaloids are present in pollen of *Hyoscyamus* (for review, see Stanley and Linskens, 1974).

### 2. *Stigma-Surface Macromolecules*

The receptive layer that is secreted onto the stigma surface acts both as an adhesive and for recognition. Although it is a true secretion and does not resemble a bilayered membrane in its ultrastructural appearance (Mattsson *et al.*, 1974; Heslop-Harrison *et al.*, 1975; Y. Heslop-Harrison, 1976; Knox and Clarke, 1978), it can be compared with a membrane in its involvement in a defined recognition reaction.

Clarke *et al.* (1979) have shown that the stigma surface of *Gladiolus* comprises almost equal quantities of protein and carbohydrate, with only trace amounts of lipid. Analysis of the monosaccharide composition revealed that 5 sugars are present: principally galactose and arabinose, with small amounts of glucose, rhamnose, and mannose. Chromatography on con A–sepharose showed that the glycoproteins binding to the lectin contained all the mannose. The remainder, not binding to the lectin, consisted mainly of a weakly antigenic high-molecular-weight arabinogalactan, whose characteristics have recently been reviewed (Clarke and Knox, 1978; Clarke *et al.*, 1979) and which may play a role in recognition or adhesion, or both processes. The lipid fraction contained glucose, showing that it is present as a glycolipid, probably a sterolglucoside.

Several antigens are presnet on the *Gladiolus* stigma surface, with a range of molecular weight from 20,000 to 70,000 (Fig. 8), with the principal antigen of molecular weight 40,000.

### 3. Molecular Basis of Pollen–Stigma Interactions

The proteins and glycoproteins of both pollen and stigma surfaces of *Gladiolus* have been labeled with $^{125}$I and fractionated by SDS-polyacrylamide gel electrophoresis (Knox *et al.*, 1976). This technique revealed a multicomponent pattern that approaches the complexity of the glycoproteins of the lymphocyte membrane (see review by Marchalonis, 1977).

The studies of Linskens (1960, 1966) on *Petunia* revealed the existence of antigens common to pollen and stigma. These initial observations have been extended for *Gladiolus* by examination of immunoprecipitates of $^{125}$I-labeled antigens (Fig. 7) and following fractionation by SDS-polyacrylamide gel electrophoresis (Fig. 8). The patterns show a major antigen in the stigma preparation with a molecular weight of 40,000, which cross-reacts with antisera raised to pollen from the same plant. The reciprocal experiment (Fig. 8) confirms this: The pollen preparation contains more than 7 antigens, of which the antigen of molecular weight 40,000 cross-reacts with antisera raised to the stigma preparation.

After identifying the range of macromolecular components present at the interacting pollen and stigma surfaces, the next logical step is to look for specific-binding interactions between these molecules. Attempts to demonstrate *in vitro* binding of stigma-surface preparations to pollen antigens separated by immunoelectrophoresis failed, because of the general binding capacity of the preparation. This stickiness of the stigma surface has been demonstrated by its ability to bind a number of proteins and glycoproteins (Knox *et al.*, 1976), and the arabinogalactan protein component has been implicated in the general adhesive properties. This general binding obscures tests for specific binding. Even if this difficulty can be overcome and a specific molecular interaction associated with a compatible pollination can be demonstrated, the next step in showing that such a binding initiates a cytoplasmic response poses a number of technical problems that have yet to be solved.

## IV. CONCLUSIONS

Evidence has been presented showing that somatic cells of higher plants have the ability to discriminate between self and non-self. In general, tolerance is limited to plants within closely related genera, although some exceptions are known. It appears that the expression of self is mediated by callus cells that proliferate at the wounded surfaces; however, the existence of different cell types within chimeras indicates the latitude of expression and tolerance of self and non-self in somatic cells. The nature of the determinants is not known, but there is a correlation between cell and tissue type and antigenic specificity. These antigens are apparently membrane-associated and would thus be analogous to the surface determinants of animal cells.

A rejection response to incompatible grafts and to artificially cultured callus-cell clumps in contact can be demonstrated. The pathology of this rejection response in these two systems is not well defined: There may be a local damaging response, or perhaps one tissue simply seals itself off from the other, by, for example, callose deposition. The possibility that even in the absence of circulating cells in a plant there is some capacity for memory in recognition has not been systematically explored. These are all potentially very rewarding fields for investigation.

The only system that has been defined in terms of a specific recognition gene is the *S* gene of self-incompatibility. A major advance has been the finding that the *S*-gene product is antigenic. This immediately throws the question of the nature of the *S*-gene product open to investigation by all the high-resolution techniques of modern immunobiology. So far, a basic glycoprotein has been implicated as the putative *S* antigen, but it has been neither isolated nor characterized. Just how this *S* antigen is involved in the mutual-recognition sequence is not known. It is expressed and operative at the interacting surfaces between mating partners? Is it complementary to a particular receptor in one or the other mating partner? Indeed, is any interaction between the *S*-gene product and another macromolecule effective in initiating a cytoplasmic response? Another question that might be raised is whether self-compatible genotypes give a complete positive interaction while the incompatible genotypes give a defective product resulting in a partial interaction that induces the alternative rejection response. These questions may be approached by judicious manipulation of the polyallelic mutation series of specific *S* genotypes of self-incompatibility.

Several potential candidates for mediating these recognition reactions at the molecular level—the tissue antigens, lectins, arabinogalactan proteins, and arabinoxylans—have been considered in detail elsewhere (Clarke and Knox, 1978). In this review we have stressed the antigenic nature of the plant-cell determinants. It is worth mentioning that lectins are being implicated in an increasing number of recognition reactions in animal systems (Brown and Hunt, 1978) and have been found in both pollen and the female reproductive tissues of plants (Denborough, 1964; Golynskaya *et al.*, 1976; Pettitt, 1977). The role of lectins in plant tissues is still a matter of speculation (Kauss, 1976), and whether or not they are identical with any of the tissue antigens is not known. Another group of molecules of particular interest are the 1,3β-glucans which not only form the basis of "callose" produced during the wounding and rejection responses (Stone and Clarke, 1980), but are also able to elicit the production of antibiotics in both plants and crustaceans (Albersheim and Valent, 1979; Unestam and Söderhall, 1977).

It is now 50 years since East (1929) first pointed out the similarity between the antigen–antibody interaction of vertebrates and self-incompatibility in flowering plants. Today, the antigen–antibody interactions are understood at the molecular level, and we have a framework for understanding the molecular basis of plant-cell recognition.

## ACKNOWLEDGMENTS

It is a pleasure to thank our graduate students for helpful discussion, and the Australian Research Grants Committee, University of Melbourne, and American Society of Zoologists for financial support; Mrs. Susan Harrison for assistance with the bibliography; and Ms. Marg Robertson for excellent secretarial assistance.

## V. REFERENCES

Albersheim, P., and Anderson-Prouty, A. J., 1975, Carbohydrates, proteins, cell surfaces and biochemistry of pathogenesis, *Annu. Rev. Plant Physiol.* **26**:31.

Albersheim, P., and Valent, B. S., 1978, Host–pathogen interactions in plants. Plants when exposed to oligosaccharides of fungal origin defend themselves by accummulating antibiotics, *J. Cell Biol.* **78**:627.

Augustin, R., 1959, Grass-pollen allergens. II. Antigen–antibody precipitation patterns in gels: Their interpretation as a serological problem in relation to skin reactivity, *Immunology* **2**:148.

Bagshaw, V., 1969, Change in Ultrastructure during the Development of Callus Cells, Ph.D. thesis, University of Edinburgh.

Bali, P. N., and Hecht, A., 1965, The genetics of self-incompatibility in *Oenothera rhombipetala*, *Genetica* **36**:159.

Ball, E. A., 1969, Histology of mixed callus cultures, *Bull. Torrey Bot. Club* **96**:52.

Ball, E. A., 1971, Growth of plant tissues upon a substrate of another kind of tissue, *Z. Pflanzenphysiol.* **65**:140.

Baur, E., 1909, Das Wesen und die Erblichkeitsverhältnisse der "Varietates albomarginatae hort" von *Pelargonium zonale*, *Z. Vererbungsl.* **1**:330.

Boutenko, R. G., and Volodarsky, A. D., 1968, Analyse immunochimique de la différenciation cellulaire dans les cultures de tissus de tabac, *Physiol. Veg.* **6**:299.

Boyarskii, B. G., 1972, Methods of producing immunobiological preparations to diagnose currant pests, evaluate varietal resistance and determine the food chains of *Eriophyes ribis* Nal. and *Tetrastichus eriophyes* Taylor, *Dokl. TSKhA*, No. **173**:166 (in Russian).

Brown, J. C., and Hunt, R. C., 1978, Lectins, *Int. Rev. Cytol.* **52**:277.

Burnet, F. M., 1971, "Self-recognition" in colonial marine forms and flowering plants in relation to the evolution of immunity, *Nature* **232**:230.

Butcher, D. N., and Connolly, J. D., 1971, An investigation of factors which influence the production of abnormal terpenoids by callus cultures of *Andrographis paniculata* Nees., *J. Exp. Bot.* **22**:314.

Char, M. B. S., 1977, Pollen allelopathy, *Naturwissenschaften* **64**:489.

Chessin, L. M., Bramson, S., Kuhns, W. J., and Hirschhorn, K., 1965, Studies on the A, B, O(H) blood groups on human cells in culture, *Blood* **25**:944.

Christ, B., 1959, Entwicklungsgeschichtliche und physiologische Untersuchungen über die Selbst-sterilität von *Cardamine pratensis* L., *Z. Bot.* **47**:88.

Clamp, J. R., Allen, A., Gibbons, R. A., and Roberts, G. P., 1978, Structure of gastrointestinal mucus glycoproteins and the viscous and gel forming properties of mucus. *B. Med. Bull.* **34**:28.

Clarke, A. E., and Knox, R. B., 1978, Cell recognition in flowering plants, *Q. Rev. Biol.* **53**:2.

Clarke, A. E., and Stone, B. A., 1979, Form and function of arabinogalactans and arabinogalactan proteins, *Phytochemistry* **18**:521.

Clarke, A. E., Knox, R. B., Harrison, S., Raff, J., and Marchalonis, J. J., 1977, Common antigens and male–female recognition in plants, *Nature* **265**:161.

Clarke, A. E., Gleeson, P., Harrison, S., and Knox, R. B., 1979, Cell recognition in plants: Characterization of pollen and stigma surface determinants. *Proc. Natl. Acad. Sci. USA* **76**:3358.

Cresti, M., Van Went, J. E., Pecini, E., and Willemse, M., 1976, Ultrastructure of the transmitting tissue of the *Lycopersicum peruvianum* style: Development and histochemistry, *Planta* **132**:305.

Cresti, M., Ciampolini, F., Pacini, E., Sree Ramulu, K., Devreux, M., and Laneri, U., 1977, Ultrastructural aspects of pollen tube growth inhibition after gamma irradiation in *Lycopersicum peruvianum*, *Theor. Appl. Genet.* **49**:297.

Crowe, L. K., 1954, Incompatibility in *Cosmos bipinnatus*, *Heredity* **8**:1.

Currier, H. B., 1957, Callose substance in plant cells, *Am. J. Bot.* **44**:478.

Denborough, M. A., 1964, Blood groups and disease, *B. Med. J.* **2**:190.

de Nettancourt, D., 1977, *Incompatibility in Angiosperms*, Springer-Verlag, Berlin and New York.

de Nettancourt, D., Devreux, M., Bozzini, A., Cresti, M., Pacini, E., and Sarfatti, G., 1973, Ultrastructural aspects of self incompatibility mechanisms in *Lycopersicum peruvianum*, *J. Cell Sci.* **12**:403.

de Nettancourt, D., Devreux, M., Laneri, U., Pacini, E., Cresti, M., and Sarfatti, G., 1974, Genetical and ultrastructural aspects of self- and cross-incompatibility in interspecific hybrids between self-compatible *L. esculentum* and self-incompatible *L. peruvianum*, *Theor. Appl. Genet.* **44**:278.

Deverall, B. J., 1977, Defense mechanisms of plants, Cambridge Monographs in Experimental Biology, No. 19, Cambridge University Press.

Dickinson, H. G., and Lawson, J., 1975, Pollen tube growth in the stigma of *Oenothera organensis* following compatible and incompatible intraspecific pollinations, *Proc. R. Soc. London Ser. B.* **188**:327.

Dickinson, H. G., and Lewis, D., 1973*a*, Cytochemical and ultrastructural differences between intraspecific compatible and incompatible pollinations in *Raphanus*, *Proc. R. Soc. Lond. Ser. B.* **183**:21.

Dickinson, H. G., and Lewis, D., 1973*b*, The formation of the tryphine coating the pollen grains of *Raphanus* and its properties relating to the self incompatibility system, *Proc. R. Soc. Lond. Ser. B.* **184**:149.

East, E. M., 1929, Self sterility, *Bibliogr. Genet.* **5**:331.

Emerson, S. H., 1940, Growth of incompatible tubes in *Oenothera organensis*, *Bot. Gaz.* **101**:890.

Evans, R. (ed.), 1975, *Advances in Diagnosis of Allergy: RAST*, Symposia Specialists, Miami, Fla.

Fett, W. F., Paxton, J. D., and Dickinson, D. B., 1976, Studies on the self-incompatibility response of *Lilium longiflorum*, *Am. J. Bot.* **63**:1104.

Friend, J., and Threlfall, D. R. (eds.), 1976, *Biochemical Aspects of Plant–Parasite Relations*, Academic Press, London and New York.

Fujii, T., and Nito, N., 1972, Studies on the compatibility of grafting of fruit trees. I. Callus fusion between rootstock and scion, *J. Jpn. Soc. Hort. Sci.* **41**:1.

Gautheret, R. J., 1945, Une voie nouvelle en biologie végétale, in: *La Culture des Tissus Végétaux*, Gallimard, Paris.

Glavinic, R., 1956, Vegetative hybridization of tomatoes, *Agrobiology* **1956**:86 (in Russian).

Golynskaya, E. L., Bashirova, N. V., and Tomchuk, N. N., 1976, Phytohaemagglutinins from the pistil of *Primula* as possible proteins of generative incompatibility, *Fiziol. Rast.* **23**:88.

Gunning, B. E. S., and Robards, A. W. (eds.), 1976, *Intercellular Communication in Plants: Studies on Plasmodesmata*, Springer-Verlag, Berlin.

Hartmann, J. X., Kao, K. N., Gamborg, O. L., and Miller, R. A., 1973, Immunological methods for the agglutination of protoplasts from cell suspension cultures of different genera, *Planta* **112**:45.

Habura, F. C., 1957, Self and cross fertility in sunflower, *Z. Physiol.* **37**:280.

Hayman, D. L., 1956, The genetic control of incompatibility in *Phalaris coerulescens* Desf., *Aust. J. Biol. Sci.* **9**:321.

Heinz, D. J., and Mee, G. W. P., 1971, Morphological, cytogenetic and enzymatic variation in *Saccharum* species hybrid clones derived from callus tissue, *Am. J. Bot.* **58**:257.

Herrero, J., and Tabuenca, M. C., 1969, Incompatibility between stock and scion. X. Behavior of the peach/myrobolan combination when grafted at the cotyledon stage, *Ann. Aula Dei* **10**:937.

Heslop-Harrison, J., 1968, Ribosome sites and S-gene action, *Nature* **218**:90.

Heslop-Harrison, J., 1975*a*, Incompatibility and the pollen–stigma interaction, *Ann. Rev. Plant Physiol.* **26**:403.

Heslop-Harrison, J., 1975*b*, Physiology of the pollen grain surface, *Proc. R. Soc. London Ser. B.* **190**:275.

Heslop-Harrison, J., 1976, A new look at pollination, *Rep. E. Malling Res. Stn.* **1975**:141.

Heslop-Harrison, J., and Heslop-Harrison, Y., 1975*a*, Fine-structure of the stigmatic papillae of *Crocus*, *Micron* **6**:45.

Heslop-Harrison, J., and Heslop-Harrison, Y., 1975*b*, Enzymic removal of the proteinaceous pellicle of the stigma papilla prevents pollen tube entry in the Caryophyllaceae, *Ann. Bot.* **39**:163.

Heslop-Harrison, J., Knox, R. B., and Heslop-Harrison, Y., 1974, Pollen wall proteins: Exine held fractions associated with the incompatibility response in Cruciferae, *Theoret. Appl. Genet.* **44**:133.

Heslop-Harrison, J., Knox, R. B., Heslop-Harrison, Y., and Mattson, O., 1975, Pollen-wall proteins: Emission and role in incompatibility responses, in: *Biology of the Male Gamete* (J. G. Duckett and P. A. Racey eds.), pp. 181–202, Academic Press, London and New York.

Heslop-Harrison, Y., 1976, Localisation of concanavalin A binding sites on the stigma surface of a grass species, *Micron* **7**:33.

Heslop-Harrison, Y., 1977, The pollen–stigma interaction: Pollen tube penetration in *Crocus*, *Ann. Bot.* **4**:913.

Heslop-Harrison, Y., and Shivanna, K. R., 1977, The receptive surface of the angiosperm stigma, *Ann. Bot.* **41**:1233.

Hood, L., Campbell, J. H., and Elgin, S. C. R., 1975, The organization, expression and evolution of antibody genes and other multi-gene families, *Annu. Rev. Genetics* **9**:305.

Howlett, B. J., Knox, R. B., Paxton, J. D., and Heslop-Harrison, J., 1975, Pollen-wall proteins: Physico-chemical characterization and role in self-incompatibility in *Cosmos bipinnatus*, *Proc. R. Soc. London Ser. B.* **188**:167.

Hughes, C., 1976*a*, Cell surface membranes of animal cells as the sites of recognition of infectious agents and other substances, in: *Specificity in Plant Diseases* (R. K. S. Wood and A. Graniti, eds.), p. 77, Plenum Press, London and New York.

Hughes, C., 1976*b*, *The Plasma Membrane*, Butterworths, London.

Iwanami, Y., 1968, Physiological researches of pollen. 19. Studies on the antigen substances in the pollen grains by immunoelectrophoresis, *J. Yokohama City Univ.*, 184 CC-59, *Biol.* **26**:1.

Johnson, P., and Marsh, D. G., 1965, The isolation and characterization of allergens from the pollen of ryegrass (*Lolium perenne*), *Eur. Polymer J.* **1**:63.

Kauss, H., 1976, The possible physiological role of lectins, in: *Cell Wall Biochemistry Related to Specificity in Host–Plant Pathogen Interactions* (B. Solheim and J. Raa, eds.), pp. 347–360, Universitetsforlaget, Tromsö, Norway.

Khavkin, E. E., Misharin, S. E., Monastyreva, L. E., Polikarpochkina, R. T., and Sukhorzhevskaia, T. B., 1978*a*, Specific proteins maintained in maize callus cultures, *Z. Pflanzenphysiol.* **86**:273.

Khavkin, E. E., Misharin, S. E., Markov, Y. Y., and Peshkova, A. A., 1978*b*, Identification of embryonal antigens of maize: Globulins as primary reserve proteins of the embryo, *Planta* **143**:11.

King, T. P., Norman, P. S., and Connel, J. T., 1964, Isolation and characterization of allergens from ragweed pollen, *Biochemistry* **3**:458.

King, T. P., Norman, P. S., and Tao, N., 1974, Chemical modifications of the major allergen of ragweed pollen, antigen E, *Immunochem.* **11**:83.

Knox, R. B., 1971, Pollen-wall proteins: Localization, enzymic and antigenic activity during development in *Gladiolus* (Iridaceae), *J. Cell Sci.* **9**:209.

Knox, R. B., 1973, Pollen-wall proteins: cytochemical observations of pollen–stigma interactions in ragweed and *Cosmos* (Compositae), *J. Cell Sci.* **12**:421.

Knox, R. B., and Clarke, A. E., 1978, Localization of proteins and glycoproteins by binding to labelled antibodies and lectins, in: *Electron Microscopy and Cytochemistry of Plant Cells* (J. L. Hall, ed.), pp. 149–185, Elsevier North-Holland, Amsterdam.

Knox, R. B., and Heslop-Harrison, J., 1970, Pollen-wall proteins: Localization and enzymic activity, *J. Cell Sci.* **6**:1.

Knox, R. B., Willing, R. R., and Ashford, A. E., 1972, Role of pollen-wall proteins as recognition substances in interspecific incompatibility in poplars, *Nature* **237**:381.

Knox, R. B., Heslop-Harrison, J., and Heslop-Harrison, Y., 1975, Pollen-wall proteins, in: *The Biology of the Male Gamete* (J. G. Duckett and P. A. Racey, eds.), pp. 177–187, Academic Press, London and New York.

Knox, R. B., Clarke, A. E., Harrison, S., Smith, P., and Marchalonis, J. J., 1976, Cell recognition in plants: Determinants of the stigma surface and their pollen interactions, *Proc. Natl. Acad. Sci. USA* **73**:2788.

Kucera, V., and Polak, J., 1975, The serological specificity of S alleles of homozygous incompatible lines of the marrow-stem kale, *Brassica oleracea* var. *acephala* DC., *Biol. Plant* **17**:50.

Kumar, S., and Hecht, A., 1965, Inactivation of incompatibility in *Oenothera organensis* following ultraviolet irradiation, *Naturwissenschaften* **52**:398.

Landova, B., and Landa, Z., 1973, Immunochemicka detekee autoinkompatibilnich genotypu *Brassica oleracea* L., *Genet. Sel.* **9**:249.

Laties, G. G., 1975, Solute transport in relation to metabolism and membrane permeability in plant tissues, in: *Historical and Current Aspects of Plant Physiology: A Symposium*

*Honoring F. C. Steward* (J. P. Davies, ed.), p. 98, Cornell University, Ithaca, N.Y.

Lee, C. J., 1955, Fertilization in *Ginkgo biloba*, *Bot. Gaz.* **117**:79.

Lewis, D., 1952, Serological reactions of pollen incompatibility substances, *Proc. R. Soc. London Ser. B.* **140**:127.

Lewis, D., 1976, Incompatibility in flowering plants, in: *Receptors and Recognition* (P. Cuatrecasas and M. F. Greaves, eds.), Series A, Vol. 2, Ch. 4, p. 167, Chapman and Hall, London.

Lewis, D., and Crowe, L. K., 1958, Unilateral incompatibility in flowering plants, *Heredity* **12**:233.

Lewis, D., Burrage, S., and Walls, D., 1967, Immunological reactions of single pollen grains, electrophoresis and enzymology of pollen protein exudates, *J. Exp. Bot.* **18**:371.

Lindsay, D. W., Yeoman, M. M., and Brown, R., 1974, An analysis of the development of the graft union in *Lycopersicon esculentum*, *Ann. Bot.* **38**:639.

Linskens, H. F., 1960, Zur Frage der Abwehrkörper der Inkompatibilitätsreaktion von *Petunia*. III, *Z. Bot.* **48**:126.

Linskens, H. F., 1965, Biochemische aspecten van incompatibiliteitsverschijnselen bij de bevruchting der bloemplanten, Dodonaea, *Biol. Jaarb.* **33**:35.

Linskens, H. F., 1976, Specific interactions in higher plants, in: *Specificity in Plant Diseases* (R. K. S. Wood and A. Graniti, eds.), p. 311, Plenum Press, New York.

Linskens, H. F., and Esser, K., 1957, Über eine spezifische Anfärbung der Pollenschläuche im Griffel und die Zahl der Kallosepfropfen nach Selbstdung und Fremddung, *Naturwissenschaften* **44**:1.

Lundquist, A., 1975, Complex self-incompatibility systems in angiosperms, *Proc. R. Soc. London Ser. B.* **188**:235.

McKenzie, I. F. C., Clarke, A. E., and Parish, C. R., 1977, Ia antigenic specificities are oligosaccharide in nature: Hapten inhibition studies, *J. Exp. Med.* **145**:1039.

McNeil, M., Darvill, A. G., and Albersheim, P., 1979, The structural polymers of the primary cell wall of dicots, in: *Progress in the Chemistry of Organic Natural Products*, p. 39, Springer-Verlag, Berlin.

Makinen, Y. L. A., and Lewis, D., 1962, Immunological analysis of incompatibility proteins and of cross-reacting material in a self-compatible mutant of *Oenothera organensis*, *Genet. Res.* **3**:352.

Marchalonis, J. J., 1969, An enzymic method for the trace iodination of immunoglobulins and other proteins, *Biochem. J.* **113**:299.

Marchalonis, J. J., 1977, *Immunity in Evolution*, Harvard University Press, Cambridge, Mass.

Mattsson, O., Knox, R. B., Heslop-Harrison, J., and Heslop-Harrison, Y., 1974, Protein pellicle of stigmatic papillae as a probable recognition site in incompatibility reactions, *Nature* **247**:298.

Michurin, I. V., 1950, *Selected Works*, English ed., Moscow.

Misharin, S. I., Antipina, A. I., Reimers, F. E., and Khavkhin, E. E., 1974, Phase, tissue and organ specific proteins of corn germ plants (in Russian), Eng. trans. in *Doklady Biol. Sci.* **219**:516.

Nagata, T., and Takebe, I., 1970, Cell wall regeneration and cell division in isolated tobacco mesophyll protoplasts, *Planta* **92**:301.

Nasrallah, M. E., 1965, Physiological and immunogenetic studies on self incompatibility in *Brassica oleracea* var. *capitata*, Ph.D. thesis, Cornell University, Ithaca, N.Y.

Nasrallah, M. E., and Wallace, D. H., 1967*a*, Immunochemical detection of antigens in self-incompatibility genotypes of cabbage, *Nature* **213**:700.

Nasrallah, M. E., and Wallace, D. H., 1967*b*, Immunogenetics of self-incompatibility in *Brassica oleracea* L., *Heredity* **22**:519.

Nasrallah, M. E., Barber, J. T., and Wallace, D. H., 1970, Self-incompatibility proteins in plants: Detection, genetics, and possible mode of action, *Heredity* **25**:23.

Nasrallah, M. E., Wallace, D. H., and Savo, R. M., 1972, Genotype protein, phenotype relationships in self-incompatibility of *Brassica*, *Genet. Res.* **20**:151.

Nirk, H., 1959, Interspecific hybridization between *Lycopersicon esculentum* and *L. peruvianum*, *Nature* **184**:1819.

Nishio, T., and Hinata, K., 1977, Analysis of S-specific proteins in stigma of *Brassica oleracea* L. by isoelectric focussing, *Heredity* **38**:391.

Nishio, T., and Hinata, K., 1978, Stigma proteins in self-incompatible *Brassica campestris* L. and self-compatible relatives, with special reference to S-allele specificity, *Jpn. J. Genet.* **53**:27.

Nowak, P. T., Kobiler, D., Roel, L. E., and Barondes, S. H., 1977, Developmentally regulated lectin from embryonic chick pectoral muscle, *J. Biol. Chem.*, **252**:6026.

Pandey, K. K., 1976, Genetic transformation and graft hybridization in flowering plants, *Theor. Appl. Genet.* **47**:299.

Pettitt, J. M., 1977, Detection in primitive gymnosperms of proteins and glycoproteins of possible significance in reproduction, *Nature* **266**:530.

Preece, T. F., 1976, Some observations on leaf surfaces during the early stages of infection by fungi, in: *Biochemical Aspects of Plant-Parasite Relations* (J. Friend and D. R. Threlfass, eds.), Vol. I, pp. 1–10, Academic Press, London and New York.

Raff, J. W., Clarke, A. E., Harrison, S., and Knox, R. B., 1977, Identification of plants by their antigenic determinants, *Proc. Aust. Biochem. Soc.* **10**:24.

Raff, J. W., Hutchinson, J., McKenzie, I. F. C., Knox, R. B., and Clarke, A. E., 1978, Relationship between cellular determinants of plant organs and their derived callus cells, *Proc. Aust. Biochem. Soc.* **11**:34.

Raff, J. W., Hutchinson, J., Knox, R. B., and Clarke, A. E., 1979, Cell recognition; antigenic determinants of plant organs and their cultured callus cells, *Differentiation* **12**:179.

Robert, B., Robert, L., and Robert, A., 1973, Immunochimie des glycoprotéines, in: Methodologie de la Structure et du Metabolisme des Glycoconjugues, *Colloques Internationaux du CNRS* **2**:221.

Roggen, H. P., 1972, Scanning electron microscopical observations on compatible and incompatible pollen–stigma interactions in *Brassica*, *Euphytica* **21**:1.

Sedgley, M., 1974*a*, Assessment of serological techniques for S-allele identification in *Brassica oleracea*, *Euphytica* **23**:543.

Sedgley, M., 1974*b*, The concentration of S-protein in stigmas of *Brassica oleracea* plants homozygous and heterozygous for a given S-allele, *Heredity* **33**:412.

Shchori, Y., 1969, Self incompatibility studies in sunflower, *Res. Rep. Hebrew Univ. Jerusalem: Sci. Agric.* **1**:549 (abstr.).

Southworth, D., 1975, Lectins stimulate pollen germination, *Nature* **258**:600.

Stanley, R. G., and Linskens, H. F., 1974, *Pollen: Biology, Biochemistry, Management*, 307 pp., Springer-Verlag, Berlin and New York.

Sterba, S., 1975, Prispevek ke studiu antigennich vlastnosti extraktu topoloveho listu, *Pr. Vyzk. Ustavu Lesn. Hospod. Myslivosti* **46**:45.

Stone, B. A., and Clarke, A. E., 1980, *Biochemistry and Chemistry of 1,3β-D-Glucans*, Macmillan, London.

Strobel, G., 1974, Phytotoxins produced by plant parasites, *Ann. Rev. Plant Physiol.* **25**:541.

Tilney-Bassett, R. A. E., 1963, The structure of periclinal chimeras, *Heredity* **18**:265.

Tommerup, I. C., and Ingram, O. S., 1971, The life cycle of *Plasmiodophera brassicae* Woron. in *Brassica* tissue cultures and in intact roots, *New Phytol.* **70**:327.

Tran Thanh Van, K., 1977, Regulation of morphogenesis, in: *Plant Tissue Culture and Its Biotechnological Applications* (W. Barz, E. Reinhard, and M. H. Zenk, eds.), p. 367, Springer-Verlag, Berlin and New York.

Unestam, T., and Söderhall, K., 1977, Soluble fragments from fungal cell walls elicit defence reactions in crayfish, *Nature* **265**:45.

van den Ende, H., 1976, *Sexual Interactions in Plants*, Academic Press, London and New York.

van der Pluijm, J. E., and Linskens, H. F., 1966, Feinstruktur der Pollenschläuche im Griffel von *Petunia*, *Zuechter* **36**:220.

Vithanage, H. I. M. V., and Knox, R. B., 1977, Development and cytochemistry of the stigma surface and response to self and foreign pollination in sunflower, *Helianthus annuus*, *Phytomorphology* **27**(2):168.

Watkins, W. M., 1966, Blood group substances, *Science* **152**:172.

Watkins, W. M., 1972, Blood group specific substances, in: *Glycoproteins: Their Composition, Structure and Function*, 2nd ed. (A. Gotlschalk, ed.), Elsevier, Amsterdam and London.

Watson, L., and Knox, R. B., 1976, Pollen wall antigens and allergens: Taxonomically-ordered variation among grasses, *Ann. Bot.* **40**:399.

Williamson, F. A., Fowke, L. C., Constabel, F. C., and Gamborg, O. L., 1976, *Protoplasma* **89**:305.

Winkler, H., 1907, Über Pfropfbastarde und pflanzliche Chimären, *Ber. Dtsch. Bot. Ges.* **25**:568.

Yeoman, M. M., and Brown, R., 1976, Implications of the formation of the graft union for organisation in the intact plant, *Ann. Bot.* **40**:1265.

*Chapter 2*

# *Discrimination of Self and Non-self in Invertebrates*

**Michael J. Chorney and Thomas C. Cheng**

*Institute for Pathobiology*
*Center for Health Sciences*
*Lehigh University*
*Bethlehem, Pennsylvania 18015*

## I. INTRODUCTION

Conceptually, the basic mechanism common to both vertebrate and invertebrate immune systems is the recognition of and reaction against invading non-self materials and neoplastic cells. The information available on vertebrate immune systems has firmly established that both cell-mediated and humoral immune mechanisms occur. Furthermore, the cooperative effects of three classes of circulating leukocytes, namely B lymphocytes, T lymphocytes, and the highly phagocytic macrophages, are operative. The remarkable fact that has become evident from studies on vertebrate immune phenomena is that reactions against foreignness, involving the three mentioned cell types, exhibit a great deal of molecular specificity owing to the presence of antigen-specific receptors on the surfaces of both B and T lymphocytes.

Although it has been established that IgM and IgD immunoglobulins are the antigen receptors on B cells (Marchalonis, 1975; Nossal, 1977), the controversy regarding the nature of the antigen receptor on T cells, which has been reported to involve immunoglobulin heavy-chain variable regions (Binz and Wigzell, 1976), immunoglobulin $\kappa$ light chains and Fd heavy-chain sections (Marchalonis *et al.*, 1978), and/or products of the major histocompatibility locus (reviewed by Katz, 1977), still has not been resolved. Nevertheless, these receptors do confer a staggering amount of diversity and ultimate antigen-binding specificity to these classes of cells. In addition, the macrophages, which are generally considered essential nonspecific components in antibody processing and production, possess receptors specific for the immunoglobulin Fc portion (Dorrington, 1976) and for the C3b component of complement (Griffin *et al.*, 1975), both of which are important in facilitating the phagocytosis of foreign particles.

The reason for mentioning vertebrate immunologic cells and some of their known surface receptors is to reemphasize that reactions against antigen, both particulate and soluble, resulting in antibody formation and/or opsonization and ultimate phagocytosis, are mediated by an array of diverse membrane receptor molecules that elicit a high degree of binding specificity when presented with the proper complementary molecular configuration. Conversely, although the title of this contribution implies that antigen is recognized in invertebrates, as the available information indicates, the question becomes not merely by what mechanism(s) is antigen recognized, but develops into far broader questions, namely: (1) Do invertebrates show any degree of specificity in reaction to antigen? (2) What is the molecular basis for immunorecognition? and (3) Does a phylogenetic lineage of immunoreactive complexity exist, with increased specificity of antigen-binding receptors leading eventually to the vertebrate adaptive immune response? Although these questions appear rudimentary, satisfactory answers would provide an understanding of both the invertebrate and vertebrate immune systems.

At present, we are impeded in fully answering these questions because of three difficulties:

1. The task of synthesizing information pertaining to various immune phenomena as they occur in members of diverse phyla is extremely difficult. This is because of the extreme diversity among the invertebrates, and the few scattered reports regarding immune recognition in different phyla have prevented the formulation of any accurate scheme of phylogenetically emerging immune complexity leading to the vertebrates.
2. Comparative immunologists sometimes adapt vertebrate immunological terms to invertebrate systems, and some appear to be searching only for cellular phenomena and humoral immune molecules homologous to those of vertebrates. This approach has its drawbacks, for it can sometimes limit creativity and objectivity. In fact, distinguishable precursor immune systems and molecules homologous to those of the vertebrates may only have evolved in the more immediate ancestors of the vertebrate line, i.e., the urochordates or tunicates. Hence, such approaches to the study of invertebrate immune systems would be of limited and perhaps dubious value in protostomate schizocoelous phyla such as the Mollusca, Annelida, and Arthropoda.
3. The most important difficulty is due to the dearth of biochemical information on invertebrate immune systems.

Nevertheless, with the above three limitations in mind, we will attempt to answer our proposed queries by first addressing antigen clearance and presenting a critical review of the group of molecules known as agglutinins, or lectins. We will then discuss in a speculative manner the possible evolutionary advancements that led through the invertebrates and culminated in the complex vertebrate immune system.

## II. NON-SELF RECOGNITION

Although many invertebrate species have been shown to possess diverse populations of circulating leukocytes similar in morphology to certain vertebrate cells, the molecular basis of non-self recognition has remained virtually unexplored; reports of the existence of either membrane-bound or humoral antigen-specific receptors have been conjectural. To provide insights into invertebrate non-self recognition, investigators have utilized several basic experimental approaches. These include

1. Injection of particulate and soluble antigens into the circulatory system and the monitoring of their distribution as a function of time.
2. The study of the necessity of serum components for *in vitro* phagocytosis, and their possible opsonizing effect.
3. The search for possible precursor immune molecules, such as agglutinins and precipitins, and their bearing on immune recognition.
4. The examination of auto-, allo-, and xenografts and their relationship with host immune cells.
5. The morphological characterization of circulating leukocytes involved in phagocytosis, encapsulation, and graft rejection.

The initial studies by Stauber (1950), Tripp (1958, 1960), and Feng (1965, 1966) on the *in vivo* recognition and disposal of foreign materials in the mollusk *Crassostrea virginica* stimulated many similar investigations with other species of invertebrates, including the gastropods *Bullia laevissima* and *B. digitalis* (Brown and Brown, 1965), *Littorina scabra* (Cheng *et al.*, 1969), *Helix pomatia* (Bayne and Kime, 1970), and *Aplysia californica* (Pauley *et al.*, 1971); the bivalve *Tridacna maxima* (Reade and Reade, 1972); the echinoderm *Asterias vulgaris* (Reinisch and Bang, 1971); the tunicate *Molgula manhattensis* (Anderson, 1971); and a variety of arthropods, including the crustacean *Parachaeraps bicarinatus* (McKay and Jenkin, 1970*a*) and the cockroach *Periplaneta americana* (Ryan and Nicholas, 1972). In brief, all of the results clearly have shown that the non-self materials are rapidly recognized and sequestered by circulating and possibly fixed phagocytic cells (Reade, 1968); however, the molecular mechanism(s) for this non-self recognition has yet to be determined. Indeed, the idea of "non-self" recognition, stemming from the above experiments and being almost universally accepted, has even been challenged by those who feel that immune cells of primitive systems such as those of invertebrates are capable only of self-recognition. Burnet (1976) intriguingly proposes a system whereby invertebrate immune cells are activated against foreign material through the abrogation of the flow of self information from receptors on adjacent cells. However, it is apparent that the controversy will not be resolved until the molecular basis of recognition is established.

The elucidative soluble antigen clearance experiments by Hilgard *et al.* (1967), Crichton and Lafferty (1975), and Sloan *et al.* (1975) deserve special attention, for they have shown that the cells involved in recognition and endocytosis have a relatively refined discriminatory capacity and that elimination of different foreign proteins is effected by independent receptor systems. Crichton and Lafferty (1975) showed that clearance in the chiton *Liolophura gaimardi* of radiolabeled hemocyanins is a function of phylogenetic relatedness, with immunochemically cross-reacting hemocyanins of closely related species being eliminated more slowly than hemocyanins from phylogenetically distant species. They proposed that differences in clearance are attributable to structural differences in the proteins contributing to differences in size and/or charge. Hilgard *et al.* (1967) showed that in the echinoderm *Strongylocentrotus purpuratus* uptake of labeled bovine serum albumin (BSA) was uninhibited by simultaneously injected radiolabeled bovine gamma globulin, but was inhibited by injected unlabeled BSA. These competition experiments have revealed that the sea urchin possesses separate receptor molecules for antigenic discrimination, which ultimately led to the hypothesis that phagocyte membrane receptors are responsible for this recognition specificity (Hilgard *et al.*, 1974). Likewise, Sloan *et al.* (1975) performed uptake experiments with a crustacean and achieved similar results, although they did not speculate on the nature of the antigen receptors.

The significance of the experiments reviewed above is obvious, for although invertebrates lack the classic adaptive immune response centering on both cell-bound immunoglobulin receptors and secreted immunoglobulins, they appear to possess the ability to recognize slight differences in antigenic-determinant structures, perhaps by receptors on the phagocyte (fixed in these instances) surface. Although these recognition phenomena cannot be considered immunologic, the basic mode of molecular discrimination of non-self could possibly have been conserved and improved up the evolutionary ladder, thereby eventually providing the elementary basis for a true immune response possessing memory and specificity in those phyla directly progenitive for the vertebrates.

## III. SERUM FACTORS

Studies on *in vitro* phagocytosis have been performed with hemocytes from many invertebrates in order to assess the role of serum factors in phagocytosis.

Again, there is a great deal of diversity in reported serum requirements for *in vitro* phagocytosis; however, in several instances investigators have found that the uptake of bacteria, yeast, or red blood cells was enhanced by the presence of serum components termed opsonins (Tripp and Kent, 1967; Stuart, 1968; Prowse and Tait, 1969; McKay and Jenkin, 1970*b*; Tyson and Jenkin, 1973; Tyson *et al.*, 1974; Renwrantz and Mohr, 1978; and others). From the studies of McKay and Jenkin (1970*b*), Anderson and Good (1976), Arimoto and Tripp (1977), and Renwrantz and Mohr (1978), the presence of naturally occurring agglutinin molecules is believed to facilitate the phagocytosis of foreign cells. The possibility of lectins serving as invertebrate humoral-recognition molecules, stimulated by such opsonization experiments as those cited, has been considered by previous authors, including Burnet (1968), Acton and Weinheimer (1974), Cooper (1976*a*), and Jenkin (1976). Nevertheless, the critical review presented below may be useful.

Lectin, or agglutinin, molecules capable of binding specific sugar moieties appear to be ubiquitous throughout all plant and animal phyla (Gold and Balding, 1975). Hemagglutinating activity has been found in viruses, bacteria, algae, fungi, and flowering plants, and recent investigations into members of the Chordata have revealed the occurrence of lectins in chicken liver (Kawasaki and Ashwell, 1977), embryonic-chick pectoral muscle (Nowak *et al.*, 1977), and chick-embryo thigh muscle (Den and Malinzak, 1977). Bowles and Hanke (1977) have even reported agglutinating activity associated with the human red cell membrane protein, glycophorin.

In invertebrates, agglutinins have been demonstrated in an extensive list of species belonging to a variety of phyla. Aside from being found circulating in the hemolymph of the more advanced invertebrates, agglutinins have been isolated and characterized from tissue extracts of the sponges *Axinella polypoides* (see Bretting and Kabat, 1976) and *Aaptos papillata* (see Bretting *et al.*, 1976), and from the albumin gland of the gastropod *Helix pomatia* (see Hammarstrom and Kabat, 1969). The possible role(s) of invertebrate agglutinins have stimulated much discussion. These molecules have been hypothesized to serve as sugar carriers or calcium-transport molecules, to aid in the formation of multienzyme-glycoprotein complexes (Sharon and Lis, 1972), and to function as antimicrobial protection molecules, known as protectins (Prokop *et al.*, 1968). Of greatest interest, however, is their implicated role as non-self recognition factors.

It is noted that many of the opsonization studies mentioned are based on the investigator's ability to adsorb agglutinins with specific erythrocytes, thereby eliminating the increased uptake of foreign cells. Furthermore, several studies have shown that agglutinin adsorption by one cell type does not alter supposedly agglutinin-mediated opsonization of another cell type possessing differing terminal sugar residues. These experiments, although interesting, do not completely negate the possibility that a nonlectinlike opsonin-recognition molecule, of which diverse populations may exist in the hemolymph, was concomitantly adsorbed with the agglutinin. Also, immunocytochemical detection of opsonizing surface-attached agglutinins through utilization of ferritin-, fluorescein-, or peroxidase-labeled antibodies, and a characterization of agglutinin-specific receptor sites have yet to be performed.

In contrast, by isolating the agglutinins of the lobster *Homarus americanus*, Hall and Rowlands (1974*a*,*b*) were able to work with purified molecules, and they observed no *in vitro* phagocytosis of mammalian erythrocytes without the presence of agglutinins, thus suggesting the opsonic activity of the purified lectins. In addition, Anderson and Good (1976) have shown that the agglutinin obtained from the albumin gland of the snail *Otala lactea* is able to opsonize formalized sheep erythrocytes in an *in vitro* phagocytosis experiment. However, the role of the albumin gland agglutinin and its possible interaction with circulating hemolymph phagocytes requires clarification, for the hemolymph was shown not to possess agglutinating activity by Boyd *et al.* (1966). Similarly, Renwrantz and Mohr (1978) have demonstrated opsonic activity in the serum of *Helix pomatia* and they were able to increase the *in vivo* clearance rate of $A_1$ human erythrocytes by pretreating the cells with albumin-gland extracts of *H. pomatia* and *Cepaea nemoralis*. Intriguingly, the possibility was discussed of the strong anti-A agglutinin found in the albumin gland of *H. pomatia* acting as a serum opsonin; however, additional studies are needed to determine the validity of this hypothesis.

Care should be taken when assessing opsonic activity and attributing it to specific molecules. Rabinovitch and De Stefano (1970) found that a wider variety of modified sheep erythrocytes are endocytosed *in vivo* than *in vitro* by *Galleria mellonella* hemocytes, and that antiserum-treated sheep red blood cells are not phagocytosed appreciably *in vitro* by insect hemocytes. Interestingly, Rabinovitch and De Stefano (1974) showed that antiserum-, PHA-, and Con A-treated sheep cells resulted in increased phagocytosis by the soil amoeba *Acanthamoeba*, possibly by altering the surface charge of the red cells or by masking antiphagocytic red cell surface molecules. However, attachment and ingestion of antiserum-coated erythrocytes, two initial phases of endocytosis, obviously could not have been facilitated by complementary molecular ligand-receptor interaction, i.e., an Fc receptor; hence, nonspecific opsonization was involved. In addition, Rabinovitch and De Stefano (1971) showed that by treating sheep erythrocytes with aldehyde, tannic acid, polylysine, and other substances, uptake by *Galleria* hemocytes was likewise increased. Van Oss and Gillman (1975) and Stockem (1977) discussed particle charge and its relationship to nonspecific opsonization and internalization. We are of the opinion that in searching for invertebrate non-self recognition molecules based on opsonizing capacity attention must be directed not only to the charge characteristics of the test phagocytosis-inducing particles but also to all of hemolymph molecules present and to the extraneous culture-medium components being employed or accidentally introduced through adsorption.

Again, in attributing a common role to the agglutinins, namely as opsonins, difficulty is generally encountered owing to disparity among the various organisms investigated. Scott (1971), while finding hemagglutinating activity in the serum of the cockroach *Periplaneta americana*, was unable to demonstrate opsonic activity attributable to it. Conversely, Stuart (1968) was unable to find agglutinins in the serum of the lesser octopus, but was able to demonstrate that the serum of this cephalopod possesses opsonic activity, thereby indicating that opsonization in members of various phyla may be mediated by different molecules.

Attempts at immunizing invertebrates with foreign cells followed by the determination of agglutinin titers postimmunization have met with varied results. In general, agglutinin titers either remain unaltered (Wright and Cooper, 1975) or are slightly decreased (Pauley *et al.*, 1971), possibly owing to adsorption following immunization. However, Pauley (1973) reported a slight short-term increase in titer in the blue crab, *Callinectes sapidus*, postimmunization, perhaps attributable to the stress of injection. In general, attempts at increasing agglutinin levels in invertebrates through immunization have met with limited success, and the possible correlation between agglutinin levels and disease states has not been explored.

Recent studies have demonstrated agglutinating activity associated with circulating hemocytes in the lobster *Homarus americanus* (see Cornick and Stewart, 1973, 1978) and the insect *Leucophaea moderae* (see Amirante, 1976). Cornick and Stewart (1973) found an amoebocyte lysate to be 100 times greater in agglutinating activity than cell-free hemolymph and later hypothesized that the activity was associated with fixed phagocytes and/or with one of the four circulating types of phagocytic cells occuring in the hemolymph (Cornick and Stewart, 1978). Amirante (1976), using the fluorescent-antibody technique, immunocytochemically localized the agglutinins in circulating hemocytes. It still remains to be determined whether the agglutinins are synthesized intracellularly or are merely pinocytosed and concentrated within the cells. It would be of interest to determine the possible occurrence of intracellular hemagglutinins in the hemocytes of the many organisms possessing these molecules, and to investigate the intriguing question of whether these molecules are possibly membrane-embedded and secreted or are merely cytophilic and pinocytosed.

Gel-filtration chromatography experiments have shown that agglutinating activity is often associated with large molecular-weight components through weak noncovalent interactions in the hemolymph of various invertebrates (Acton *et al.*, 1969; Chorney, unpubl.) or high-molecular-weight hemocyanin complexes (Sullivan *et al.*, 1976). We suggest that the agglutinins may perhaps be involved in attachment of these components and respiratory pigments onto cell surfaces, thereby facilitating their transport across the membrane. Such agglutinins could also be involved in molecular linkage of various protein subunital structures. If these molecules are associated with the circulating cells, it is also possible that they play a role in cellular adhesion during leukocytic encapsulation.

According to Sharon (1975), of the 100 monosaccharides isolated from nature, 12 have been shown to be integral parts of glycoproteins. Accordingly, the combining specificities of invertebrate lectins have been shown to reside best in one of several monosaccharides capable of inhibiting the agglutination of cells or the precipitation of blood-group substances, although the possibility has been discussed that some lectins are capable of "possessing extended binding sites," which allow interaction with not only terminal monosaccharides but also adjacent sugar moieties (Sharon and Lis, 1972). The generation of diversity in lectin combining site specificity in relation to non-self discrimination is still an open question. Evolutionarily, the likelihood of any system involved in immunorecognition being molded to seemingly static binding complementarity would not impose a significant adaptive edge to any cellular or humoral non-self recognition system constantly being bombarded by an extremely large array of antigenic configurations. How sugar-binding molecules such as lectins could have been involved in the clearance phenomena of the related proteins mentioned above is difficult to surmise. We propose that only cell-bound or possibly still-unknown humoral factors capable of discerning tertiary structural alteration, as determined ultimately by the amino-acid primary sequence of the antigen, and not oligosaccharide side chains, could have effected these clearance phenomena.

In addition, an aspect of agglutinins not discussed at any length is their seeming lack of what we will term biological contextual information. For instance, few studies have been undertaken to investigate the binding kinetics among subunits and possible conformational changes upon initial sugar binding resulting in possible positive or negative cooperativity among remaining subunital binding, and how this may relate to cell-surface binding during putative opsonization, the inhibition of reactivity toward self molecules in general, and so on. Although the analogy is perhaps poor, it is noted that the Fc portion of immunoglobulin on binding with antigen undergoes a conformational change (Brown and Koshland, 1975), thereby increasing effector functioning, i.e., cytophilicity for the macrophage surface, complement fixation, and so on, among certain classes and subclasses of immunoglobulins. Lectins of invertebrate origin should be studied in a similar fashion in order to assess fully their biological function.

Two recent models proposed by Jenkin and Hardy (1975) and Parish (1977) attempt to explain non-self recognition through lectins by imparting binding-specificity variation to individual agglutinins. Parish's model emphasizes subunital structures acting as glycosyl transferases: After deposition of sugar residues on membrane receptors, the subunits combine into a complex of heterogeneous subunits, with one subunit conferring cytophilic properties to the aggregate for the amoebocyte surface by binding with a terminal carbohydrate residue. However, many of the lectins investigated possess homogeneous subunital binding specificity, although various agglutinins of dissimilar specificities do occur simultaneously in some organisms. Again, more work needs to be done in order to firmly establish the function of agglutinins in invertebrate immune systems.

Recently, Renwrantz and Cheng (1977*a*,*b*) and Warr *et al.* (1977) have started to map the topography of invertebrate immune cells by establishing the presence of carbohydrate receptors for various lectins of diverse origin. Renwrantz and Cheng (1977*a*), by studying the agglutinability of fixed cells, were able to demonstrate sugar receptors on the surface of fixed *Helix pomatia* hemocytes and were able to confirm their findings by studying lectin-mediated attachment of erythrocytes onto the surface (Renwrantz and Cheng, 1977*b*). Interestingly, it was found that *Helix* albumin gland agglutinin gave an extremely poor response, possibly because of low-density distribution of *N*-acetylgalactosamine, thus negating strong clumping of the hemocytes. Warr *et al.* (1977), working with lymphocytelike cells of the tunicate *Pyura stolonifera*, were able to demonstrate sugar receptors for the heterospecific lectins Con A, WGA, and soybean lectin; however, mitosis in the lymphocyte culture imparted by lectin binding was not demonstrated and hence differs from the situation with mammalian lymphocytes. A form of mixed lymphocyte reaction, in which allogeneic cells were allowed to interact, also does not provoke the lymphocytes to undergo mitosis and take up [$^{125}$I]deoxyuridine. Toupin *et al.* (1977) reported the lack of tritiated-thymidine uptake by the coelomocytes of the earthworm *Lumbricus terrestris* when cultured in a newly devised medium; however, the cells were not challenged with any known vertebrate mitogenic molecules. In contrast, Roch *et al.* (1975) observed uptake of tritiated thymidine by cultured coelomocytes of *Lumbricus* when challenged with Con A, and Toupin and Lamoureux (1976) observed mitosis in *Lumbricus* coelomocytes induced by PHA and were able to show coelomocyte-subpopulation cooperation in effecting this response. How this phenomenon may be associated, if at all, with leukocytosis following second-set xenografts in *Lumbricus* (see Cooper, 1976*b*) still requires elucidation. In addition, whether cell increases following xenografting and injury in *Lumbricus* are a result of recruitment or actual proliferation (Cooper, 1976*b*) requires clarification.

## IV. GRAFT STUDIES AND INVERTEBRATE HISTOCOMPATIBILITY ANTIGENS

The attractiveness of lectins in invertebrate immunology arises from their binding specificities; however, specificity alone is insufficient to relegate to lectins the role of immune factors. Although we are of the opinion that the present knowledge concerning the role of humoral factors in non-self recognition is still insufficient to explain responses to non-self by invertebrates, the experiments with tissue grafts by Hildemann, Cooper, and their co-workers strongly implicate lymphocytelike cells of *Lumbricus terrestris* (see Hostetter and Cooper, 1973) and of the echinoderm *Dermasterias imbricata* (see Karp and Hildemann, 1976) in mediating the rejection response to allografts and in generating short-term memory against second-set allografts. It is noted, however, that Parry (1978) has challenged the existence of specificity and memory in earthworms in response to grafted tissue.

Recently, Coffaro and Hinegardner (1977) observed allograft rejection in another echinoderm, *Lytechinus pictus*, and found a memory system to be operative, as demonstrated by increased rejection of second-set allografts. Surprisingly, Hildemann *et al.* (1977) also demonstrated a memory component in histoimmunorecognition in the coral *Montipora verrucosa* in response to second-set allografts, and found it to be unmediated by leukocyte infiltration. The tissue-incompatibility experiments mentioned, as well as others, demonstrate the general ability of invertebrates to recognize "non-self" allogeneic cells through histocompatibility differences generated by polymorphism of histocompatibility antigens, with increasing polymorphism existing in higher forms of invertebrates (Du Pasquier, 1974).

Bodmer (1972) and Burnet (1973) have discussed histocompatibility antigen polymorphism in relationship to mammals, primarily in human beings and the HL-A system. Relevant to this discussion, the underlying view is that histocompatibility antigens probably developed from cell–cell recognition factors involved in morphogenesis and structural homeostasis, and may still be operative in nonimmune-cell interaction, communication, and differentiation in the vertebrates (Katz, 1977). Because of the implicated role of histocompatibility antigens in various immune phenomena, a simplified system of evolutionary precursive histocompatibility antigens—pressured to evolve through molecular requirements for cellular adhesion in evolving metazoans of increasing complexity—may reside in higher invertebrate immune cells and function in "primordial cell-mediated" immune responses, in addition to antigen recognition. The evolutionary steps leading from weak reactions to the strongly accelerated reactions mediated by T cells in response to histocompatibility-antigen differences in the higher vertebrates have been the subject of much speculation. Burnet (1971, 1973) has postulated that the emergence of viviparity within the vertebrates and/or homospecific parasitism among cyclostomes and related species might have created the impetus to further refine self/non-self discrimination, thereby impeding invasive allogeneic cells through alterations in surface receptors involved in recognition. If a primitive cell-based immune response, lacking specificity and possessing short-term memory, is characteristic of the higher-invertebrate immune response, and T lymphocytes possessing a diverse contingent of surface histocompatibility antigens represent evolutionary products of invertebrate cells refined and altered through some unknown selective force, then the possible existence of surface recognition factors precursive to the histocompatibility antigens of vertebrates on invertebrate cells is a provocative speculation. These speculations, along with the hypotheses of Gally and Edelman (1972) and Peterson *et al.* (1975) that the histocompatibility-complex genes may have been precursors of those of the immunoglobulins, may shed some light on the evolutionary modification and refinement of self/non-self discrimination. Recent investigations have been undertaken in order to look for sequence homology between invertebrate agglutinins and mammalian antibodies, all of which have yielded negative results (Kaplan *et al.*, 1977). If cellular immune reactions possibly represent the main progression in immuno-recognition, with immunoglobulins appearing later in evolutionary time in the vertebrates as extensions of modified and amplified histocompatibility genes, then eventual comparisons of sequences of surface antigens on immune cells could possibly prove more fruitful in understanding the evolution of non-self recognition mediated by specific receptors. Marchalonis (1977), in discussing coelomocyte-mediated graft rejection in annelids, has stated that "the isolation, characterization, and comparison with vertebrate antibodies of the coelomocyte surface recognition unit are critical to establish homology with the immune response of vertebrates."

As presented, we propose that increasing complexity of immune systems in the invertebrates paralleled the emergence of increasing histocompatibility-antigen polymorphism, which in turn paralleled the possible development of highly specific antigen-binding cell-surface receptors residing on increasingly differentiated and active lymphoid cells. Other authors have expressed or implied ideas that have provoked our own thinking on this problem. Du Pasquier (1974), while discussing histocompatibility-antigen polymorphism and its relationship to allograft incompatibility, stated that the link between vertebrates and invertebrates resides in evolving histocompatibility structures involved in cell–cell recognition, as demonstrated through allograft experimentation. He presents the argument that in forms below the phylum Annelida, single haplotype differences in histocompatibility antigens do not cause aggressive reactions resulting in tissue incompatibility. He stated that the annelids therefore represent an important point in evolution, since a one-haplotype difference can lead to allograft recognition and tissue destruction. Cohen (1976), discussing the major histocompatibility complex of urodeles, stated that vestiges of vertebrate histocompatibility antigens could possibly be found in higher invertebrate forms. Cunningham (1976) postulated an even more vivid and exciting hypothesis, namely that $\beta_2$ microglobulin, found in all vertebrates and possessing sequence homology to immunoglobulin, could possibly be the molecular link between invertebrates and vertebrates. The possibility of finding an invertebrate $\beta_2$ "could have important implications for our understanding of the evolution of the immune system."

Hildemann (1974) first drew an evolutionary scheme of emerging immune systems based upon simple cellular recognition in lower invertebrates (coelenterates and related organisms), leading to immunorecognition–immunoincompatibility in higher invertebrates and finally ending in the vertebrate humoral and cell-mediated immune systems, paralleling the formulation and increasing sophistication of the lymphocyte-type cell. He based this evolutionary emergence upon the phenomenon of increasing antigraft reactivity found in higher invertebrates (linked to Du Pasquier's discussion of increasing polymorphism of histocompatibility antigens and the dose effect), and later expounded upon this idea by including a discussion of invertebrate histocompatibility antigens and their importance in mediating recognition phenomena (Hildemann, 1977). We agree with this pattern (although we are wary of using the term "cell-mediated immunity" to describe invertebrate responses, a term that implies T-cell functioning and T-cell subpopulations of helper and suppressor cells) and parallel this emergence not only with increasing complexity (polymorphism) of histocompatibility antigens, but also with increasing antigen-receptor specificity, which perhaps is intimately linked to the histocompatibility antigens themselves. These may be one and the same.

In lower invertebrates, maintenance of integrity involves the recognition of self surface molecules. With increasing structural complexity, the need arose for varying surface molecules involved not only in daily cell–cell communication and cohesion, but also in embryonic and morphogenetic design, and it could have created the necessary elements for a primitive antigen-recognition system amplified by increased vascularization and the concomitant occurrence of circulating leukocytes. Klein (1977) states that the large amount of progeny produced in the invertebrates and their short life spans could possibly have precluded the need for vertebratelike immune surveillance mechanisms to combat neoplastic cells with some degree of specificity and memory. According to Klein, the system of compatibility antigens, evolved in the invertebrates and designed for the maintenance of individuality, were later transformed and developed into the immunosurveillance-system receptors in the vertebrates. This then paralleled the coevolution of antigen recognition factors and improved cytotoxicity mechanisms. Our ideas on the underlying importance of histocompatibility antigens in maintaining self integrity and triggering invertebrate quasi-immune phenomena (allograft rejection) are very similar, yet at the emergence of circulating leukocytes a repertoire of polymorphic histocompatibility antigens had already become established on the cell surface and were the most likely candidates for not only self but eventual antigen recognition as well. Although it is premature to accurately identify the molecular beginnings of the vertebrate adaptive immune response within any invertebrate phyla, the possibility of finding the evolutionary antecedent of a dual recognition system (Zinkernagel *et al.*, 1978) would be of considerable interest. It is at this point in evolution that histocompatibility antigens branched into two groups: those still important in cell–cell contact and self recognition and those surface antigens that were modified and which concomitantly served as recognition factors for non-self antigenic configurations.

We do not refute the possibility of lectins serving as immune recognition molecules, but are of the opinion that more concrete evidence concerning their putative immune role is needed; and we feel that investigations are warranted into other serum molecules besides the lectins and their function as opsonins. In addition, we do not dismiss the possibility that the emergence of the immunoglobulins could have proceeded by another route independent of the histocompatibility antigens. The finding of a precursive serum molecule in higher invertebrates sharing sequence homology with immunoglobulins would not be surprising.

We have attempted to discuss available data on invertebrate immune systems in hopes of answering the questions of how antigen is recognized, and have dwelled primarily on the highly specific sugar-binding lectins. There also exists in most invertebrate phyla the possibility that specificity of antigen receptors may be totally absent and that other mechanisms are being employed that, though lacking molecular "lock and key" specificity, are nonetheless highly efficient in combating invasive organisms through phagocytosis and encapsulation. Although antigen is recognized in the invertebrates and at times in a discriminatory manner, we hope that the questions we have raised in the first section of this review will serve to motivate future investigations on this process.

## ACKNOWLEDGMENTS

The original information included in this article has resulted from research supported in part by a grant (AI 12355-03) from the National Institute of Allergy and Infectious Diseases, NIH, and in part by a grant (PCM77-23785) from the National Science Foundation.

## V. REFERENCES

Acton, R. T., and Weinheimer, P. F., 1974, Hemagglutinins: primitive receptor molecules operative in invertebrate defense mechanisms, in: *Contemporary Topics in Immunobiology*, Vol. 4 (E. L. Cooper, ed.), pp. 271–282, Plenum Press, New York.

Acton, R. T., Bennett, J. C., Evans, E. E., and Schrohenloher, R. E., 1969, Physical and chemical characterization of an oyster hemagglutinin, *J. Biol. Chem.* **244**:4128.

Amirante, G. A., 1976, Production of heteroagglutinins in haemocytes of *Leucophaea maderae* L., *Experientia* **32**:526.

Anderson, R. S., 1971, Cellular responses to foreign bodies in the tunicate *Molgula manhattensis* (DeKay), *Biol. Bull.* **141**:91.

Anderson, R. S., and Good, R. A., 1976, Opsonic involvement in phagocytosis by mollusk hemocytes, *J. Invert. Path.* **27**:57.
Arimoto, R., and Tripp, M. R., 1977, Characterization of a bacterial agglutinin in the hemolymph of the hard clam, *Mercenaria mercenaria*, *J. Invert. Pathol.* **30**:406.
Bayne, C. J., and Kime, J. B., 1970, *In vivo* removal of bacteria from the hemolymph of the land snail *Helix pomatia* (Pulmonata: Stylomatophora), *Malacol. Rev.* **3**:103.
Binz, H., and Wigzell, H., 1977, Antigen-binding, idiotypic receptors from T lymphocytes: An analysis of their biochemistry, genetics, and use as immunogens to produce specific immune tolerance, in: *Cold Spring Harbor Symp. Quant. Biol.* **41**:275.
Bodmer, W. F., 1972, Evolutionary significance of the HL-A system, *Nature* **237**:139.
Bowles, D. J., and Hanke, D. E., 1977, Evidence for lectin activity associated with glycophorin, the major glycoprotein of human erythrocyte membranes, *FEBS Lett.* **82**:34.
Boyd, W. C., Brown, R., and Boyd, L. G., 1966, Agglutinins for human erythrocytes in mollusks, *J. Immunol.* **96**:301.
Bretting, H., and Kabat, E. A., 1976, Purification and characterization of the agglutinins from the sponge *Axinella polypoides* and a study of their combining sites, *Biochemistry* **15**:3228.
Bretting, H., Kabat, E. A., Liao, J., and Pereira, M. E. A., 1976, Purification and characterization of the agglutinins from the sponge *Aaptos papillata* and a study of their combining sites, *Biochemistry* **15**:5029.
Brown, A. C., and Brown, R. J., 1965, The fate of thorium dioxide injected into the pedal sinus of *Bullia* (Gastropoda: Prosobranchiata), *J. Exp. Biol.* **42**:509.
Brown, J. C., and Koshland, M. E., 1975, Activation of antibody Fc function by antigen-induced conformational changes, *Proc. Natl. Acad. Sci. USA* **72**:5111.
Burnet, F. M., 1968, Evolution of the immune process in vertebrates, *Nature* **218**:426.
Burnet, F. M., 1971, "Self-recognition" in colonial marine forms and flowering plants in relation to the evolution of immunity, *Nature* **232**:230.
Burnet, F. M., 1973, Multiple polymorphism in relation to histo-compatibility antigens, *Nature* **245**:359.
Burnet, F. M., 1976, The evolution of receptors and recognition in the immune system, in: *Receptors and Recognition*, Vol. 1 (P. Cuatrecasas and M. F. Greaves, eds.), pp. 35–58, Chapman and Hall, London.
Cheng, T. C., Thakur, A. S., and Rifkin, E., 1969, Phagocytosis as an internal defense mechanism in the Mollusca: With an experimental study of the role of leucocytes in the removal of ink particles in *Littorina scabra* Linn, in: *Proceedings of the Symposium on Mollusca*, Part 2, pp. 546–563, Bangalore Press, Bangalore, India.
Coffaro, K. A., and Hinegardner, R. T., 1977, Immune response in the sea urchin *Lytechinus pictus*, *Science* **197**:1389.
Cohen, N., 1976, Phylogeny of the major histocompatibility complex: Theoretical implications of studies with urodele amphibians, in: *Phylogeny of Thymus and Bone Marrow–Bursa Cells* (R. K. Wright and E. L. Cooper, eds.), pp. 169–182, North-Holland, Amsterdam.
Cooper, E. L., 1976*a*, *Comparative Immunology*, Prentice-Hall, Englewood Cliffs, N.J.
Cooper, E. L., 1976*b*, The earthworm coelomocyte: A mediator of cellular immunity, in: *Phylogeny of Thymus and Bone Marrow–Bursa Cells* (R. K. Wright and E. L. Cooper, eds.), pp. 9–18, North-Holland, Amsterdam.
Cornick, J. W., and Stewart, J. E., 1973, Partial characterization of a natural agglutinin in the hemolymph of the lobster, *Homarus americanus*, *J. Invert. Pathol.* **21**:255.
Cornick, J. W., and Stewart, J. E., 1978, Lobster (*Homarus americanus*) hemocytes: Classification, differential counts, and associated agglutinin activity, *J. Invert. Pathol.* **31**:194.
Crichton, R., and Lafferty, K. J., 1975, The discriminatory capacity of phagocytic cells in the chiton (*Liolophura gaimardi*), in: *Immunologic Phylogeny* (W. H. Hildemann and

A. A. Benedict, eds.), *Advances in Experimental Medicine and Biology*, Vol. 64, pp. 89–98, Plenum Press, New York.

Cunningham, B. A., 1976, Structure and significance of $\beta_2$-microglobulin, *Fed. Proc. Fed. Am. Soc. Exp. Biol.* **35**:1171.

Den, H., and Malinzak, D. A., 1977, Isolation and properties of β-D-galactoside-specific lectin from chick embryo thigh muscle, *J. Biol. Chem.* **252**:5444.

Dorrington, K. J., 1976, Properties of the Fc receptor on macrophages, *Immunol. Commun.* **5**:263.

Du Pasquier, L., 1974, The genetic control of histocompatibility reactions: Phylogenetic aspects, *Arch. Biol.* **85**:91.

Feng, S. Y., 1965, Pinocytosis of proteins by oyster leucocytes, *Biol. Bull.* **129**:95.

Feng, S. Y., 1966, Experimental bacterial infections in the oyster *Crassostrea virginica*, *J. Invert. Pathol.* **8**:505.

Gally, J. A., and Edelman, G. M., 1972, The genetic control of immunoglobulin synthesis, in: *Annual Review of Genetics*, Vol. 6 (H. L. Roman, ed.), pp. 1–46, Annual Reviews Inc., Palo Alto, Calif.

Gold, E. R., and Balding, P., 1975, *Receptor-Specific Proteins–Plant and Animal Lectins*, American Elsevier, Amsterdam.

Griffin, F. M., Jr., Bianco, C., and Silverstein, S. C., 1975, Characterization of the macrophage receptor for complement and demonstration of its functional independence from the receptor for the Fc portion of immunoglobulin, *J. Exp. Med.* **141**:1269.

Hall, J. L., and Rowlands, D. T., Jr., 1974*a*, Heterogeneity of lobster agglutinins. I. Purification and physicochemical characterization, *Biochemistry* **13**:821.

Hall, J. L., and Rowlands, D. T., Jr., 1974*b*, Heterogeneity of lobster agglutinins. II. Specificity of agglutinin–erythrocyte binding, *Biochemistry* **13**:828.

Hammarström, S., and Kabat, E. A., 1969, Purification and characterization of a blood-group A reactive hemagglutinin from the snail *Helix pomatia* and a study of its combining site, *Biochemistry* **8**:2696.

Hildemann, W. H., 1974, Some new concepts in immunological phylogeny, *Nature* **250**:116.

Hildemann, W. H., 1977, Specific immunorecognition by histocompatibility markers: The original polymorphic system of immunoreactivity characteristic of all multicellular animals, *Immunogenetics* **5**:193.

Hildemann, W. H., Raison, R. L., Cheung, G., Hull, C. J., Akaka, L., and Okamoto, J., 1977, Immunological specificity and memory in a scleractinian coral, *Nature* **270**:219.

Hilgard, H. R., Hinds, W. E., and Phillips, J. H., 1967, The specificity of uptake of foreign proteins by coelomocytes of the purple sea urchin, *Comp. Biochem. Physiol.* **23**:815.

Hilgard, H. R., Wander, R. H., and Hinds, W. E., 1974, Specific receptors in relation to the evolution of immunity, in: *Contemporary Topics in Immunobiology*, Vol. 4 (E. L. Cooper, ed.), pp. 151–158, Plenum Press, New York.

Hostetter, R. K., and Cooper, E. L., 1973, Cellular anamnesis in earthworms, *Cell. Immunol.* **9**:384.

Jenkin, C. R., 1976, Factors involved in the recognition of foreign material by phagocytic cells from invertebrates, in: *Comparative Immunology* (J. J. Marchalonis, ed.), pp. 80–97, Blackwell Scientific Publications, Halstead Press, New York.

Jenkin, C. R., and Hardy, D., 1975, Recognition factors of the crayfish and the generation of diversity, in: *Immunologic Phylogeny* (W. H. Hildemann and A. A. Benedict, eds.), *Advances in Experimental Medicine and Biology*, Vol. 64, pp. 55–65, Plenum Press, New York.

Kaplan, R., Li, S. S.-L., and Kehoe, J. M., 1977, Molecular characterization of limulin, a sialic acid binding lectin from the hemolymph of the horseshoe crab, *Limulus polyphemus*, *Biochemistry* **16**:4297.

Karp, R. D., and Hildemann, W. H., 1976, Specific allograft reactivity in the sea star *Dermasterias imbricata*, *Transplantation* **22**:434.

Katz, D. H., 1977, T-lymphocyte receptors and cell interactions in the immune system, in: *International Cell Biology* (B. R. Brinkley and K. R. Porter, eds.), pp. 112–118, Rockefeller University Press, New York.

Kawasaki, T., and Ashwell, G., 1977, Isolation and characterization of an avian hepatic binding protein specific for N-acetylglucosamine-terminated glycoproteins, *J. Biol. Chem.* **252**:6536.

Klein, J., 1977, Evolution and function of the major histocompatibility system: Facts and speculations, in: *The Major Histocompatibility System in Man and Animals* (D. Götze, ed.), pp. 339–378, Springer-Verlag, New York.

McKay, D., and Jenkin, C. R., 1970*a*, Immunity in the invertebrates: The fate and distribution of bacteria in normal and immunised crayfish (*Parachaeraps bicarinatus*), *Aust. J. Exp. Biol. Med. Sci.* **48**:599.

McKay, D., and Jenkin, C. R., 1970*b*, Immunity in the invertebrates: The role of serum factors in phagocytosis of erythrocytes by hemocytes of the freshwater crayfish (*Parachaeraps bicarinatus*), *Aust. J. Exp. Biol. Med. Sci.* **48**:139.

Marchalonis, J. J., 1975, Lymphocyte surface immunoglobulins, *Science* **190**:20.

Marchalonis, J. J., 1977, *Immunity in Evolution*, Harvard University Press, Cambridge, Mass.

Marchalonis, J. J., Bucana, C., Hoyer, L., Warr, G. W., and Hanna, M. G., Jr., 1978, Visualization of a guinea pig T lymphocyte surface component cross-reactive with immunoglobulin, *Science* **199**:433.

Nossal, G. J. V., 1977, B-lymphocyte receptors and lymphocyte activation, in: *International Cell Biology* (B. R. Brinkley and K. R. Porter, eds), pp. 103–111, Rockefeller University Press, New York.

Nowak, T. P., Kobiler, D., Roel, L. E., and Barondes, S. H., 1977, Developmentally regulated lectin from embryonic chick pectoral muscle, *J. Biol. Chem.* **252**:6026.

Parish, C. R., 1977, Simple model for self–non-self discrimination in invertebrates, *Nature* **267**:711.

Parry, M. J., 1978, Survival of body wall autographs, allografts, and xenografts in the earthworm *Eisenia foetida*, *J. Invert. Pathol.* **31**:383.

Pauley, G. B., 1973, An attempt to immunize the blue crab, *Callinectes sapidus*, with vertebrate red blood cells, *Experientia* **29**:210.

Pauley, G. B., Krassner, S. M., and Chapman, F. A., 1971, Bacterial clearance in the California sea hare, *Aplysia californica*, *J. Invert. Pathol.* **18**:227.

Peterson, P. A., Rask, L., Sege, K., Klareskog, L., Anundi, H., and Östberg, L., 1975, Evolutionary relationship between immunoglobulins and transplantation antigens, *Proc. Natl. Acad. Sci. USA* **72**:1612.

Prokop, O., Uhlenbruck, G., and Köhler, W., 1968, Protecktine, eine neue Klasse antikörperähnlicher Verbindungen, *Dtsch. Gesundh. Wes.* **23**:318.

Prowse, R. H., and Tait, N. N., 1969, *In vitro* phagocytosis by amoebocytes from the haemolymph of *Helix aspersa* (Müller), *Immunology* **17**:437.

Rabinovitch, M., and De Stefano, M. J., 1970, Interactions of red cells with phagocytes of the wax-moth (*Galleria mellonella*, L.) and mouse, *Exp. Cell Res.* **59**:272.

Rabinovitch, M., and De Stefano, M. J., 1971, Phagocytosis of erythrocytes by *Acanthamoeba* sp., *Exp. Cell Res.* **64**:275.

Rabinovitch, M., and De Stefano, M. J., 1974, Antibody and plant agglutinins stimulate phagocytosis of erythrocytes by *Acanthamoeba*, *Nature* **234**:414.

Reade, P., and Reade, E., 1972, Phagocytosis in invertebrates. II. The clearance of carbon particles by the clam, *Tridacna maxima*, *J. Reticuloendothel. Soc.* **12**:349.

Reade, P. C., 1968, Phagocytosis in invertebrates, *Aust. J. Exp. Biol. Med. Sci.* **46**:219.

Reinisch, C. L., and Bang, F. B., 1971, Cell recognition: Reactions of the sea star (*Asterias vulgaris*) to the injection of amebocytes of sea urchin (*Arbacia punctulata*), *Cell. Immunol.* **2**:496.

Renwrantz, L., and Cheng, T. C., 1977*a*, Identification of agglutinin receptors on hemocytes of *Helix pomatia*, *J. Invert. Pathol.* **29**:88.

Renwrantz, L., and Cheng, T. C., 1977*b*, Agglutinin-mediated attachment of erythrocytes to hemocytes of *Helix pomatia*, *J. Invert. Pathol.* **29**:97.

Renwrantz, L., and Mohr, W., 1978, Opsonizing effect of serum and albumin gland extracts on the elimination of human erythrocytes from the circulation of *Helix pomatia*, *J. Invert. Pathol.* **31**:164.

Roch, P., Valembois, P., and Du Pasquier, L., 1975, Response of earthworm leukocytes to concanavalin A and transplantation antigens, in: *Immunologic Phylogeny* (W. H. Hildemann and A. A. Benedict, eds.), *Advances in Experimental Medicine and Biology*, Vol. 64, pp. 45–53, Plenum Press, New York.

Ryan, M., and Nicholas, W. L., 1972, The reaction of the cockroach *Periplaneta americana* to the injection of foreign particulate material, *J. Invert. Pathol.* **19**:299.

Scott, M. T., 1971, Recognition of foreignness in invertebrates. II. *In vitro* studies of cockroach phagocytic hemocytes, *Immunology* **21**:817.

Sharon, N., 1975, *Complex Carbohydrates*, Addison-Wesley, Reading, Mass.

Sharon, N., and Lis, H., 1972, Lectins: Cell-agglutinating and sugar-specific proteins, *Science* **177**:949.

Sloan, B., Yocum, C., and Clem, L W., 1975, Recognition of self from non-self in crustaceans, *Nature* **258**:521.

Stauber, L. A., 1950, The fate of India ink injected intracardially into the oyster, *Ostrea virginica* Gmelin, *Biol. Bull.* **98**:227.

Stockem, W., 1977, Endocytosis, in: *Mammalian Cell Membranes*, Vol. 5 (G. A. Jamieson and D. M. Robinson, eds.), pp. 151–195, Butterworth and Co., London.

Stuart, A. E.., 1968, The reticulo-endothelial apparatus of the lesser octopus, *Eledone cirrosa*, *J. Pathol. Bact.* **96**:401.

Sullivan, B., Bonaventura, J., Bonaventura, C., and Godette, G., 1976, Hemocyanin of the horseshoe crab, *Limulus polyphemus*, *J. Biol. Chem.* **251**:7644.

Toupin, J., and Lamoureux, G., 1976, Coelomocytes of earthworms: Phytohemagglutinin (PHA) responsiveness, in: *Phylogeny of Thymus and Bone Marrow–Bursa Cells* (R. K. Wright and E. L. Cooper, eds.), pp. 19–25, North-Holland, Amsterdam.

Toupin, J., Marks, D. H., Cooper, E. L., and Lamoureux, G., 1977, Earthworm coelomocytes *in vitro*, *In Vitro* **13**:218.

Tripp, M. R., 1958, Disposal by the oyster of intracardially injected red blood cells of vertebrates, *Proc. Natl. Shellfish Assoc.* **48**:143.

Tripp, M. R., 1960, Mechanisms of removal of injected micro-organisms from the American oyster, *Crassostrea virginica* (Gmelin), *Biol. Bull.* **119**:210.

Tripp, M. R., and Kent, V. E., 1967, Studies on oyster cellular immunity, *In Vitro* **3**:129.

Tyson, C. J., and Jenkin, C. R., 1973, The importance of opsonic factors in the removal of bacteria from the circulation of the crayfish (*Parachaeraps bicarinatus*), *Aust. J. Exp. Biol. Med. Sci.* **51**:609.

Tyson, C. J., McKay, D., and Jenkin, C. R., 1974, Recognition of foreignness in freshwater crayfish, *Parachaeraps bicarinatus*, in: *Contemporary Topics in Immunobiology*, Vol. 4 (E. L. Cooper, ed.), pp. 159–166, Plenum Press, New York.

van Oss, C. J., and Gillman, C. F., 1975, Phagocytosis and immunity, in *The Immune System and Infectious Diseases: Proceedings* (F. Milgrom and E. Neter, eds.), Proceedings of the Fourth International Convocation on Immunology, Buffalo, N.Y., June 1974, pp. 505–511, Karger, Basel.

Warr, G. W., Decker, J. M., Mandel, T. E., DeLuca, D., Hudson, R., and Marchalonis, J. J., 1977, Lymphocyte-like cells of the tunicate, *Pyura stolonifera:* Binding of lectins, morphological and functional studies, *Aust. J. Exp. Biol. Med. Sci.* **55**:151.
Wright, R. K., and Cooper, E. L., 1975, Immunological maturation in the tunicate *Ciona intestinalis*, *Am. Zool.* **15**:21.
Zinkernagel, R. M., Callahan, G. N., Klein, J., and Dennert, G., 1978, Cytotoxic T cells learn specificity for self H-2 during differentiation in the thymus, *Nature* **271**:251.

*Chapter 3*

# *Phylogeny of the Emergence of T-B Collaboration in Humoral Immunity*

**L. N. Ruben and B. F. Edwards**

*Department of Biology*
*Reed College*
*Portland, Oregon 97202*

## I. INTRODUCTION: PRIMARY AND SECONDARY LYMPHOID SITES

In order to deal effectively with the phylogeny of cellular collaboration in humoral immunity, it is first necessary to review briefly what is known of lymphoid heterogeneity within the ectothermic vertebrates. All extant vertebrates possess circulating lymphocytes. With the possible exception of the Agnatha (hagfish and lamprey), the most primitive jawless "fishlike" creatures, all vertebrates possess the requisite morphologic diversity of lymphopoietic sites. Only the thymus and spleen appear to be present consistently throughout vertebrate groups less primitive than the Agnatha.

The thymus is found to be comparable in structural complexity to its mammalian counterpart in members of all recently evolved species of the various vertebrate classes. However, it is less differentiated in those representative examples of more primitive groups that have been explored in this regard.

Aggregations of generative lymphoid tissue appear to be entirely absent from the pharyngeal region in larvae of the most primitive vertebrate, the hagfish (Good *et al.*, 1966). Nevertheless, adult hagfish reject allografts (Hildemann and Thoenes, 1969) and, what is more important to the subject of this chapter, are able to synthesize antigen-specific antibodies (Thoenes and Hildemann, 1970).

The development of pharyngeal aggregations homologus to the thymus of higher organisms has also been questioned recently for members of the other Agnathan order, the lamprey, by Cohen (1977).

The cartilaginous fish (Chondrichthyes), however, possess thymuses with corticomedullary distinctions and Hassal's corpuscles. Some primitive bony fish (Osteichthyes), e.g., the bowfin, bear thymuses that are less well differentiated in this regard. Snapper and grouper thymuses also lack clear corticomedullary distinctions. Since organ cultures of their thymuses will produce antibody following *in vivo* immunization, it seems that antibody-forming cells are either generated by or come to reside in this organ in at least some fish. We shall see later that thymic antibody-producing cells are not seen in all fish species (Ortiz-Muniz and Sigel, 1971). Primitive bony fish are particularly crucial with respect to considerations of subsequent terrestrial vertebrate evolution. The cartilaginous fish are thought to represent a separate branch from the now extinct ancestral gnathostomes (jawed fish) of the class Placodermi, and are therefore unable to provide us with useful information on the phylogeny of more recently evolved classes, e.g., Amphibia or Reptilia. The garpike, a member of the same superorder as the bowfin (Holostei), may develop thymuses early in its life history, but does not appear to bear them as an adult (McKinney *et al.*, 1976). Adult catfish (McKinney *et al.*, 1976) also appear to lack a thymus gland. While plaice possess thymuses, they do not appear to function as peripheral lymphoid organs, since no recirculating lymphocytes, injected carbon particles, or soluble antigens (Bogner and Ellis, 1977) enter them. They also involute very early at the time of sexual maturity. On the other hand, many of the more advanced bony fish, Teleostei–e.g., rainbow trout–(Bogner and Ellis, 1977) possess thymuses with clear corticomedullary differentiation.

The distinctions noted for fish can also be made within the class Amphibia. That is, the taillesss frogs and toads (Anura), which are representatives of the most recently evolved order, have thymuses that are more differentiated in terms of mammallike structure than those developed by the more primitive, tailed Amphibia (Urodela), the salamanders and newts. Corticomedullary regions are poorly delineated in thymuses of the Urodela. Furthermore, Hassal's corpuscles may also be absent (cf. Cohen, 1977).

Most members of the class Reptilia have structurally complex thymuses (cf. Cohen, 1977). The only exception to be noted is the discovery that two (individual) adult tuataras (*Sphenodon punctatum*) from New Zealand showed no evidence of thymus tissue. It is conceivable that while thymuses may have formed embryonically, early and complete involution obscured its presence in the limited number of adults available for observation. The investigators privileged to work with this precious protected resource material for evolutionary studies (Marchalonis *et al.*, 1969) also found that the spleen alone served as the primary site of lymphoid development and function. It should be noted that the spleen of adult *Sphenodon* is structurally primitive, in that the marginal zones, which usually serve as principal antigen-trapping regions in evolutionarily advanced vertebrate spleens, were missing. Furthermore, no germinal centers were observed. Germinal centers within secondary lymphoid sites are thought to represent memory B-cell compartments within follicular aggregations of mammals. They are also absent from the more advanced lizard *Calotes versicolor* and the more primitive turtle *Pseudemys scripta* (cf. Cohen, 1977).

The class Amphibia provides investigators with the extraordinary opportunity to study present-day members of different orders that may illuminate several vitally important phylogenetic transitions made in the evolution of higher vertebrates. One of these transitions concerns the utilization of bone marrow as a hematopoietic site. While adult anuran amphibians utilize bone marrow as a vascular-stem cell source, the more primitive salamanders and newts do not. Only one family of salamanders (Plethodontidae) uses bone marrow, but only as a granulopoietic site. Fish also lack hematopoietic bone marrow. Furthermore, larval anuran amphibians, which are immunocompetent, do not utilize bone marrow. Thus, the immunologist who uses both comparative and developmental approaches has a possibility of understanding the cellular and functional immunologic consequences of this shift as it may have occurred during evolution. Fish and urodeles commonly use the spleen for both erythro- and leukopoiesis (cf. Cohen, 1977).

Another transition available for study within the Amphibia is the generation of a small-molecular-weight-serum immunoglobulin (Ig) with a heavy chain different from $\mu$. Again, as in the preceding instance, the additional class of Ig is found among the anuran amphibians and not among the more primitive urodeles, or in fish (Atwell and Marchalonis, 1975). A 7 S IgM has been reported, however, for sharks, which also have a pentameric (19 S) IgM in the serum. The 7 S monomer does not appear to be a precursor or breakdown product of the pentamer. A 7 S serum Ig with a *non-*$\mu$ heavy chain has been reported for the lungfish (Latimeria), which evolved from ancestors of amphibians (Marchalonis, 1969). IgM is the primitive Ig class (Marchalonis, 1977). Since both the $\mu$ and $\kappa$ chains of primitive vertebrates are very similar to those of mammals, evolution must have dealt conservatively with gene selection related to their structure (Litman, 1976). But more important, at least with respect to the topic under consideration here, this transition may be related to thymic function in evolution, since thymic influence is known to affect the shift in Ig class (IgM → IgG) in rodents (cf. Katz and Benacerraf, 1972).

A third transition relates to the observation that anuran amphibians utilize lymphoid aggregations that are associated with a lymphatic circulation as antigen-trapping and immunologic structures. While these accessory sites in anurans may not represent true lymph nodes, which are found only in mammals, they do perform some analogous functions. They are usually found within lymphatic-vessel walls at critical junctions (cf. Cohen, 1977). Urodele amphibians and fish lack lymph nodes, as do primitive anurans, e.g., *Xenopus laevis*, the South African clawed toad (Good *et al.*, 1966; Manning and Horton, 1969).

Other accessory lymphopoietic sites, e.g., the anterior or head kidney, are utilized by many fish (Bogner and Ellis, 1977), and the kidney and the liver are utilized by amphibians (Cowden and Dyer, 1971). Additionally, some nodelike structures, e.g., the jugular and procoracoid bodies of advanced anurans drain vascular rather than lymphoid channels (Baculi *et al.*, 1970). Neither the primitive *Sphenodon* nor the more advanced alligators, both of which are ancestral to birds rather than mammals, possess definitive lymph nodes (Good *et al.*, 1966; Marchalonis *et al.*, 1969).

Finally, gut-associated lymphoid tissue (GALT) is present to a minor degree in all ectothermic gnathastomes, but it is particularly apparent in anuran amphibians. Goldstine *et al.* (1975) have examined four urodele and four anuran species. Their studies demonstrate the presence of well-organized, nodular GALT along anuran alimentary tracts. Urodeles, however, did not possess a comparable nodular distribution.

Thus, organized lymphopoietic sites can be described for all but one of the ectothermic vertebrate classes. The exception is the class Agnatha, the most primitive of the extant vertebrates. The Agnatha are capable of generating both cell-mediated and humoral immune responses, using circulating small lymphocytes. These cells provide a diffuse but functionally disparate immunologic system. No plasma cells or medium and large lymphocytes have been found in hagfish or lamprey specimens (Good *et al.*, 1966).

Plasma cells and the larger lymphocytes are found in cartilaginous fish, although mammalianlike "true" plasma cells may be restricted to the most advanced of the group (cf. Cohen, 1977). Large pyroninophilic lymphoid cells serve a similar function in the more primitive groups. The full range of functional cells of vascular tissue has been described for the remaining groups of ectotherms. The number of plasma cells found in fish and in urodele amphibians remains relatively small, however.

The distribution of cells and lymphoid organs within the ectothermic vertebrate classes is summarized in Table I. The reader who wishes to explore information on this subject in much greater depth is advised to see Cohen (1977).

Although humoral immune responses can be expressed by even the most primitive extant vertebrates, experimental evidence clearly showing that lymphocytes generated within varied developmental sites *function* differentially in humoral immunity is restricted to a relatively small number of species.

## II. EVIDENCE OF LYMPHOID HETEROGENEITY: DIFFERENTIAL MITOGENESIS

Mouse thymus (T)- and bone-marrow (B)-derived lymphocytes are stimulated to undergo lymphoblastosis by different plant-derived lectins (Greaves and Janossy, 1972). Phytohemagglutinin (PHA) and concanavalin A (Con A) specifically stimulate T cells, while membrane lipopolysaccharide (LPS) from *Escherichia coli* and purified protein derivative (PPD) from *Mycobacterium tuberculosis* can be used as mitogens specific for B cells.

**Table I. Distribution of Lymphoid Tissue in Ectothermic Vertebrates**

| Class | Thymus | Spleen | Other sites | Plasma cells |
|---|---|---|---|---|
| Agnatha | Diffuse? | Diffuse? | ? | – |
| Chondrichythes | | | | |
| Sharks | Discrete cortex and medulla; Hassal's corpuscles | Discrete red and white pulp | Some use renal, cranial, or gonadial tissue | + |
| Osteichthyes | | | | |
| Paddlefish, sturgeon | Lobular organization; Hassal's corpuscles | As above | Renal, alimentary canal | + |
| Bowfin, gar | Less well differentiated cortico-medullary distinction; absent in gar (?) | As above | ? | + |
| Recent bony fish | Well differentiated; Hassal's corpuscles | As above | Renal, pharyngeal | + |
| Amphibia | | | | |
| Salamanders, newts | Indistinct corticomedullary differentiation | White pulp not well defined; largely erythropoietic | Renal, hepatic | + |
| Primitive frogs, e.g., *Xenopus laevis* | Discrete cortex and medulla; Hassal's corpuscles | Discrete red and white pulp | Bone marrow, hepatic (larval), renal; GALT | + |
| Advanced frogs, e.g., Ranidae | As above | As above | Bone marrow, jugular bodies, variable accessory "nodes," renal (larval); GALT | + |
| Reptilia | | | | |
| Turtles | As above | As above but lack splenic nodules | Renal, alimentary canal, cloaca, bladder, lung, "nodes," bone marrow (snapping turtle); GALT (snapping turtle) | + |
| Tuatara | Not found | Center of lymphoid activity but structurally primitive | – | + |
| Lizards, snakes | As above | White pulp with diminished red pulp compartment | "Nodes," cloaca, bone marrow (snakes) | + |
| Alligator | Well differentiated | Discrete red and white pulp | Lymphoid "plexus," cloaca | + |

While a dose-dependent PHA response has been reported for an agnathan, the lamprey (cf. Cohen, 1977), no differential mitogenesis suggestive of the lymphoid heterogeneity that is characteristic of the dichotomous mouse model has yet been demonstrated. Results from experiments testing the effects of Con A and PHA on nurse shark (*Ginglymostoma cirratum*) peripheral-blood leukocytes (PBL) have suggested a degree of heterogeneity within this population (Lopez *et al.*, 1974). The reactivity of PHA-sensitive cells is suppressed by a subpopulation of PBL separable by Ficoll–Isopaque gradients.

The subpopulation that suppresses the PHA reactivity is responsive to Con A stimulation. As Cohen (1977) has pointed out, this finding suggests an analogy with the mouse system, in that Stobo and Paul (1973) have shown that mouse T-cell subsets respond differentially to PHA and Con A. It may be that lymphoid heterogeneity, with respect to mitogen sensitivity, evolved at least as early as the cartilaginous fish. There is no way of knowing whether this was an ancestral feature of this group of whether it subsequently appeared in other species by convergent evolution. We also do not know the basis for the suppression exerted by the Con A-sensitive PBL on those that are PHA-sensitive. The fact that very high concentrations of T-cell stimulators, e.g., Con A, are required in order to affect shark PBL is in accord with other data suggesting that T-cell functions are generally weak in this group (McKinney *et al.*, 1976).

Mitogens have also been used to stimulate lymphoblastosis in bony fish. Bogner (Bogner and Ellis, 1977), using rainbow trout (*Salmo gairdneri*), has shown that PBL respond to *in vivo* administration of PHA, Con A, and LPS. Furthermore, pyroninophilic blast cells were found in the immunologic organs, e.g., anterior kidney and spleen, following LPS injection. Etlinger and his colleagues (1976) have recently demonstrated lymphocyte subsets in this same species with *in vitro* application of mitogens. Thymocytes were reactive only to Con A, whereas anterior nephros cells responded well to LPS but poorly to Con A. PBL and splenic lymphocytes were found to be mixed populations, in that some members could respond to each of the three mitogens tested—Con A, LPS, and PPD. The authors provided additional evidence that LPS stimulates polyclonal-antibody formation and plasma-cell increase among PBL. The anatomical distribution of lymphocytes in rainbow trout subsets is similar to that found in the mouse. However, not all bony fish fit this distribution pattern. Both thymus and head nephros cells of the freshwater bluegill (*Lepomis macrochirus*) respond to PHA, Con A, and LPS *in vitro*. Nevertheless, it appears that at least two subsets of lymphocytes exist in this species as well. Rabbit anti-bluegill-brain serum plus complement will initiate lysis of some 50% of the lymphocytes of both organs. The survivors of this treatment have reactivity to only LPS (Cuchens and Clem, 1977). This suggests that in spite of their variant anatomical distribution, bluegill lymphoid-cell heterogeneity can be exposed. Moreover, it demonstrates that one of these subsets shares antigenicity with brain and is PHA- and Con A-sensitive, while the other does not share membrane antigens with brain and is LPS-sensitive. Thus, these two subsets of bluegill lymphocytes share at least these characteristics with mouse T and B cells. Cuchens and Clem (1977) have also shown that the subset that is PHA- and Con A-reactive, and shares antigenicity with brain, can also form spontaneous rosettes with rabbit erythrocytes. The LPS-sensitive population does not form comparable spontaneous rosettes. Bluegill MLR responses were found to be temperature-dependent, occurring at 32°C but not at 22°C. Furthermore, PHA and Con A sensitivities were exhibited only at substantially higher temperatures than those that represented the lower temperature limits of LPS reactivity. This is a particularly interesting finding in that it suggests that the lymphocyte subset that more closely matches mouse T cells in its characteristics may be responsible in ectotherms for the suppression of immunity that results from lowering environmental temperatures. Earlier, Avtalion and his colleagues (1976), working with carrier-specific enhancement of an antihapten response in carp, had noted that carrier-specific priming was the temperature-sensitive phase of the fish immune response. It seems likely that the temperature-sensitive population revealed by differential mitogenesis and carrier-specific-enhancement studies is the same. That is, the PHA- and Con A-sensitive carrier-specific helper cell of these fish is a subset of lymphocytes functionally equivalent to the mouse T cell. This analogy says nothing about the developmental origin of this subset, since it may or may not be the case that they are modified by or derived from the thymus in one or another species. We will consider this issue further in a subsequent section of this chapter.

Urodele amphibians, e.g., *Notophthalmus viridescens*, the common American newt, and *Ambystoma mexicanum*, the axolotl, have also been tested for differential effects of the T- and B-cell-specific mitogens of mice (Collins *et al.*, 1976). Spleen cells of both species respond to LPS *in vitro* with kinetics and a response intensity comparable to that found in mice. On the other hand, in higher animals response level was lower and the kinetics slower than one might expect when PHA or Con A stimulation was tested. This is true even when urodele mitogen responses are matched against comparable anuran-amphibian response standards. Although splenocytes of both of these urodeles and of the American grass frog, *Rana pipiens*, respond equally well to LPS, urodele cells in mixed leukocyte-culture reactions (MLR) or subject to Con A or PHA stimulation respond at levels substantially below those found with anuran splenocytes. Collins and Cohen (1976) studied the distribution of mitogen-reactive cells in spleen, peripheral blood, and thymus of axolotl. They found that unlike the situation in higher vertebrates and in advanced fish, thymocytes from this urodele did not respond to PHA, Con A, or LPS in a variety of culture conditions. Nonresponsive thymocytes did not exert any inhibitory influence when mixed with mitogen-responsive spleen cells.

Associated with this failure to respond to mitogens is the fact that thymocytes of axolotl, unlike those of frog or other vertebrates, will not serve as either stimulators or responder cells in MLR (Collins and Cohen, 1976). Axolotl splenocytes and PBL will respond to all three mitogens and perform MLR, though at relatively low indexes of activity. As in other urodeles, LPS produces much higher proliferative responses than does PHA or Con A. Moreover, passage of splenocytes through a nylon wool column substantially reduces LPS reactivity in the effluent population. As we noted in our earlier consideration of differential mitogenesis in fish, primative organisms clearly emulate mouse-T-cell activities less well than B-cell activities. But, with respect to the issue being considered here, lymphoid heterogeneity appears to be present.

Lymphoid heterogeneity has also been suggested for the common American newt as a consequence of injection *in vivo* of LPS 4 days prior to antigen (RBC) challenge. A cell population is generated that is hydrocortisone (HC)-insensitive and capable of participating in hormone-suppressed antierythrocyte responses (Ruben and Gwinnell, 1977). It is therefore distinguishable from the low-dose-sensitive helper-cell population that proved to be HC sensitive.

Differential mitogenesis has also been demonstrated in *Xenopus laevis*, the South African clawed toad. The combination of thymic ablation in early larval life with mitogen studies has confirmed that PHA and Con A reactivity in this species is related to thymus-derived lymphocytes. Reactivity to LPS or PPD was unaffected by early thymectomy, while PHA and Con A sensitivity was reduced to a low residual level (Tochinai and Katagiri, 1975; DuPasquier and Horton, 1976; Donnelly *et al.*, 1976; Manning *et al.*, 1976; Manning and Collie, 1977).

Temperature dependence and time relationships, particularly of activities initiated by T-cell stimulants, e.g., Con A, have also been studied with amphibians. Wright and Cooper (1977), using spleen cells of *Rana pipiens*, have analyzed the steps involved in mitogen stimulation. The initial steps of Con A binding and mitogen-induced cell agglutination take place at 15°C. In addition, they observe that lymphocyte activation but not mitotic division is evident at 15°C. All steps are obtainable at 22°C. They suggest, therefore, that environmental temperature depression prevents mouse T-cell equivalents in the frog from undergoing lymphoblastosis. Immunosuppression could result from inhibition of a relatively early temperature-sensitive event. They estimate that Con A-stimulated frog splenocytes divide at 2–4 days postexposure. This timing would be in agreement with the results of Avtalion and his colleagues (1976), who studied temperature-sensitive steps of immunized carp and frogs (*Rana ridibunda*), as well as other recent studies on temperature effects on different aspects of humoral immunity in amphibians (Ruben *et al.*, 1977*b*).

While poorer reactivity to T- than to B-cell mitogens has been reported for the more primitive vertebrate forms, the more recent groups, e.g., the anuran Amphibia, appear to reverse this condition. This lower response level to LPS can be enhanced substantially, however, by combination with suboptimal doses of Con A or PHA (Reddy and Wright, 1975), or by altering the nature of the media (Goldstine *et al.*, 1975). For instance, heat inactivation of the fetal-calf serum (FCS) with the addition of 2-mercaptoethanol (2-ME) significantly raised LPS response levels. Enhancement by heat-inactivated FCS suggests the presence of inhibitory factors in the FCS that mask LPS stimulatory capacities. The enhancement resulting from addition of low levels of Con A or PHA is suggestive of synergism between LPS-sensitive and T-cell-mitogen-sensitive cells.

Within the reptiles, differential mitogenesis has been studied using alligator PBL *in vitro* (Cuchens *et al.*, 1976). These cells were reactive to Con A and PHA but only seasonally reactive to LPS: LPS response was significantly lower during the winter months than at other times of the year. Evidence that two subsets of

**Table II. Evidence of Lymphoid Heterogeneity in Poikilotherms: Differential Mitogenesis**

| | PHA | Con A | | LPS | Organism studied |
|---|---|---|---|---|---|
| Cartilaginous fish | | | | | |
| PBL | (+) when Con-A cells absent | + | | | Nurse shark[a] |
| Bony fish | | | | | |
| PBL | | + | | + | Rainbow trout[b] |
| Spleen | | + | | + | Bluegill[c] |
| Thymus | | + | | – | Bluegill[c] |
| Anterior nephros | | – | | + | Bluegill[c] |
| Anterior nephros | + | + | | + | Bluegill[c] |
| Thymus | + | + | | + | Bluegill[c] |
| (Rabbit antibrain) | – | – | | + | Bluegill[c] |
| Tailed Amphibia | | | | | |
| PBL | + | + | < | + | Axolotl[d] |
| Spleen | + | + | < | + | Common American newt[e] |
| Tailless Amphibia | | | | | |
| Spleen | + | + | | + | South African clawed toad[f] |
| NTx spleen | – | – | | + | South African clawed toad[f] |
| Spleen | + | + | > | (+) synergistic enhancement | Grass frog[g] |
| PBL | + | + | > | (+) media-alteration enhancement | Grass frog[h] |
| Reptile | + | + | | (+) seasonal | Alligator[i] |

[a]Lopez *et al.*, 1974.
[b]Etlinger *et al.*, 1976.
[c]Cuchens *et al.*, 1976; Cuchens and Clem, 1977.
[d]Collins and Cohen, 1976.
[e]Collins *et al.*, 1976.
[f]Manning and Collie, 1975; Manning *et al.*, 1976.
[g]Reddy and Wright, 1975.
[h]Goldstine *et al.*, 1975.
[i]Cuchens *et al.*, 1976.

PBL were involved was derived from cell-separation studies using glass wool columns. Cells that passed the columns were found to be PHA- but not LPS-reactive, while those that stuck to the glass wool were strongly LPS-responsive. A summary of mitogenesis data is given in Table II.

## III. EVIDENCE OF LYMPHOID HETEROGENEITY FROM THYMUS ABLATION

Only a single report on early thymic ablation can be cited from experiments with fish. Removal of thymus glands from an immature, two-month-old Mozambique mouthbreeder (*Tilapia mozambique*), a teleost fish, will abrogate its capacity to generate an antierythrocyte response, as well as allograft rejection (Sailendri, 1973). This very interesting finding suggests that thymus-derived cells participate in fish humoral immune responses.

However, it will be necessary to show that T-independent stimuli are unaffected by early thymic ablation before one can conclude that only functional T cells have been removed. One could argue, for instance, that functional T *and* B cells may originate from the young thymus of this species. However, recent additional studies with members of this same species demonstrate that even ablation of adult thymuses will dramatically reduce response capacity against heterologous erythrocytes 14 to 16 weeks postthymectomy (Mohan, 1978).

Three recent reports, all from the same laboratory, have dealt with the effects of early thymic ablation in urodeles. In the first group of studies, cell-mediated immunity and humoral immunity were followed in *Triturus alpestris* and *Pleurodeles waltlii* Michah. The humoral responses were monitored by the technique of immunocytoadherence (Tournefier, 1976). Specific antigen-binding (rosette-forming) cell activity can be used to observe the kinetics of cellular aspects of humoral responses (Zaalberg, 1964). Serum-antibody characterization can be used, paralleling these antigen-binding-cell studies, to analyze the products of the cellular activity. In general, serum antibody titers continue to rise after immunization as the antigen-binding cell activity decreases in the various immunologic organs used as sources of sensitized cells. In the particular studies we are now considering, from one to four injections of sheep erythrocytes were used for immunization. The spleen cells that develop the induced antigen-binding cell activity are detectable by the fourth day after the final immunizing challenge. The activity reaches a peak two days thereafter. As one might expect, the unrelated individuals vary considerably with respect to the intensity of the response. Some do not respond at all. The important aspect of the data, with respect to the issue we are addressing here, is that early (9–10 weeks post-fertilization) thymectomy substantially reduced but did not abrogate the capacity of these urodeles to generate both spontaneous and immune antigen-binding cells. Where comparisons are possible from the original data presented, it would appear that spontaneous antigen binding in *Pleurodeles waltlii* was reduced by 53% as a consequence of early thymectomy. Moreover, we can compare the data provided for 25% horse red blood cell (HRBC) (i.p.)-immunized normal and thymectomized *T. alpestris* with respect to antigen-binding cell reduction as a consequence of early thymectomy. Of the three comparisons possible, one shows a reduction of 91%, while the other two, which can be made from the available data, show reductions of 96% and 97% respectively. Additionally, it should be noted that cell-mediated immunity, as reflected by allograft-rejection capacity, was permanently abrogated by early thymectomy. It would seem to be the case that these data indicate the presence of T cells that provide cytotoxic and helper-cell functions. As we have noted before, when considering thymic ablation in fish, it would also be interesting to know whether early thymectomy will also affect T-independent responses in urodeles. While the studies of serum antibodies in these species did not involve thymic ablation, another report of antierythrocyte responses in *Ambystoma mexicanum* (the axolotl) has dealt with this issue (Charlemagne and Tournefier, 1977*a*).

The six thymic lobes of the axolotl larva were extirpated five weeks after fertilization. HRBC served as the immunogen. Varied dosages from 25% to 0.0025% HRBC were injected intravenously and a high dose (0.2 ml of 25% HRBC) was given intraperitoneally in nonthymectomized controls. The thymectomized recipients of the immunizing challenge were 9 months old and received 0.2 ml of 25% HRBC i.p. Eighty days later they received a similar challenge. This timing corresponded to a point when a modest secondary response could be demonstrated in nonthymectomized controls. The maximum concentration of anti-HRBC antibody in the serum from a single challenge was achieved by 60 days and it declined thereafter. The authors found that under these experimental conditions the thymectomized animals gave statistically significant *higher* responses than the controls. Another group received only a single 0.2 ml of 0.25% HRBC challenge i.v., and once again the thymectomized axolotls produced higher serum antibody titers than the nonthymectomized controls! Thus, the authors suggest that in axolotl both the primary and secondary responses to heterologous erythrocytes are enhanced by early thymectomy. They therefore conclude the HRBC behaves in axolotl as if it were a T-independent immunogen for high doses given i.p. and low doses given i.v. However, one cannot know whether the *effective* dose, as far as the animal is concerned, may not be the same in both cases. In fact, given the evolutionary persistence in urodele adults of open ciliated nephrostomes, which function to clean the peritoneum directly, it could even be that the lowest i.v. dose tested represents a higher effective immunogenic dose than the highest one given i.p. If that is the case, then it may even be possible that the doses used in these experiments could have been high enough to obviate a minor T-dependent requirement in the axolotl antierythrocyte response. When sufficiently high doses are used in neonatally thymectomized mice, they are able to respond by producing adequate titers of normally T-dependent antierythrocyte antibody (Sinclair and Elliott, 1968). In the American common newt, *Notopthalmus viridescens*, hydrocortisone effectively eliminates antigen-binding responses initiated by 0.0025% HRBC given i.p. However, it can only reduce the antigen-binding-cell response to 25% HRBC i.p. by 41% (Ruben and Gwinnell, 1977). In rodents, T cells are more susceptible to low immunogen doses than are B cells (Trizio and Cudkowicz, 1978). Furthermore, helper T cells *responding* to immunogen *in vivo* especially sensitive to treatment with the hormone (Segal *et al*., 1972). By analogy with the rodent, it appears that the newt has a low-immunogen-dose-sensitive lymphocyte population, which is hydrocortisone-sensitive. It is not known whether this population is thymus-derived, however.

As a consequence of their experimental results with the axolotl, Charlemagne and Tournefier (1977*a*) have suggested, as others have for primitive fish (McKinney *et al*., 1976), that urodeles recognize *all* antigens as if they were T-independent. They provide additional argument for this by pointing out that the absence of a 7 S IgG-like immunoglobulin in fish and urodeles may be due to the absence of appropriate T cells. As we have noted earlier in this chapter, the shift from IgM to IgG has been determined to be under T-cell control in rodents (cf. Katz and Benacerraf, 1972). If fish and urodeles respond to all antigens as if they were T-independent, this too would fit with the observation that fish and urodeles generate only IgM serum antibodies (Marchalonis, 1974). It is worth noting that while the teleost *Tilapia mosambique* produces only IgM antibodies, early thymic ablation abrogates its capacity to generate an antierythrocyte response. Later on we shall present evidence that strongly suggests a helper role for thymus-derived cells in the goldfish *Carasius auratus*. Goldfish also have only serum IgM.

The third report on the effect of thymic ablation on urodele humoral responses deals with immunization of *Pleurodeles waltlii* Michah (Charlemagne and Tournefier, 1977*b*). Sixteen-month-old normal and thymectomized *P. waltii* were immunized with *Salmonella typhimurium* H (flagellar) and O (somatic) antigens. The H antigen is considered to be partially T-dependent and the O antigen is T-independent in rodents. The effectiveness of thymic ablation was tested by allografting. It was found that while early thymectomy completely abrogated allograft-rejection capacity, it had little effect on the generation of serum antibody to either antigen. Once again, their data suggest that thymic ablation does *not* remove the capacity to generate humoral immunity in urodeles. It is unfortunate in this regard that the single 0.2 ml challenge of $1.5 \times 10^9$ bacteria delivered i.p. was emulsified in Freund's complete adjuvant. The use of any general adjuvant of this kind is likely to reduce or eliminate any helper requirement, should one exist, by increasing macrophage involvement and antigen-delivery efficiency, and therefore B-cell-response capacity.

Taken as a group, these three recent reports provide strong evidence that there is present a cytotoxic T-cell subset that is involved in delayed-hypersensitivity types of responses, e.g., allograft rejection, although its activity is chronic only in urodeles. On the other hand, the presence of the regulatory thymus-derived cells of humoral immunity found in mice has been seriously questioned for primitive vertebrates. Urodeles do not respond well to soluble T-dependent antigens, such as bovine serum albumin, horseradish peroxidase, keyhole-limpet hemacyanin, or bovine gamma globulin (cf. Charlemagne and Tournefier, 1977*b*). This may imply a lack in the thymus-derived-cell population, and may be a reflection of a failure of antigen recognition by T cells rather than of ultimate response capacity. For instance, what would the consequences be of presenting these antigens in particulate form, as alum-precipitated or bentonite-coated antigens? Urodeles do have the capacity to respond well to particulate antigens, e.g., RBC or bacterial antigens.

While the situation in urodeles requires considerable clarification, early thymus ablation of *Xenopus laevis* seems to provide us with some unambiguous answers, particularly with respect to humoral immunity. Thymectomy five to seven days after fertilization, by either microcautery (Manning and Collie, 1975) or microsurgery (Tochinai and Katagiri, 1975; Tochinai, 1976), will eliminate the capacity to respond to heterologous erythrocytes or human gamma globulin *without* affecting responses to T-independent stimuli. Thymic ablation by microcautery at this time in development also suppresses but does not abrogate the toad's ability to reject primary allografts. Furthermore, it does not affect responses to second-set allografts. This picture appears to be nearly the reverse of the one we have just described with respect to the urodeles. If thymectomy is delayed for two weeks, allograft capacity is unaffected, while antierythrocyte responses remain blocked. It appears that developmental and functional heterogeneity within the T-cell pool can be exposed by microcautery thymus ablation (Horton *et al.*, 1976; Manning and Collie, 1977). This may be a most useful finding. It has been reported that microsurgical removal of thymus during the first week postfertilization completely abrogates allograft responses (Tochinai and Katagiri, 1975). The capacity for chronic allograft rejection following microcautery of the thymuses could be owing to some remnant of thymus surviving ablation. The prior seeding of cytotoxic T cells or the generation of a new cytotoxic T-cell population from an alternative (B cell?) developmental pathway could also account for the results, however. We have already noted that early thymectomy in this species reduces *in vitro* response capacity to Con A or PHA, T-cell mitogens, while B-cell mitogen activities remain unaffected (Manning and Collie, 1975). When one follows the residual T-mitogen capacities of animals thymectomized from 7 to 23 days, these remain at a constant level for many months into adulthood (Manning and Collie, 1977). This is strongly suggestive that development subsequent to larval thymectomy is *not* accompanied by enlargement of the available *T-cell* pool.

The thymus is the first organ to become lymphocytic in *Xenopus*. The development of the capacity to reject allografts coincides with the appearance of the first differentiated small lymphocytes within that organ (Horton, 1969; Horton and Manning, 1972; Ruben *et al.*, 1972). The humoral response to heterologous erythrocytes arises about one week later, when development is proceeding at 25°C. The onset of this immunocompetence coincides with the first appearance of differentiated small lymphocytes within spleen (Kidder *et al.*, 1973). It should be noted that these ontogenetic data that suggest a sequential appearance of cell-mediated and humoral response capacities correlate with the recent results from *Xenopus* thymic ablation studies we have just considered (Horton *et al.*, 1976). It may be that cytotoxic T cells differentiate and seed out peripherally earlier than T helper cells. An alternative possibility could involve simultaneous differentiation and seeding. Once peripheralized, however, the cytotoxic cells may become independent of thymic presence earlier than the helper cells.

Reconstitution of *Xenopus* humoral responses to heterologous erythrocytes after early thymectomy has been effected *in vivo* by the addition of histocompatible thymocytes (Tochinai *et al.*, 1976; Collie, 1976). Recently, this reconstitution has also been achieved *in vitro* using larval allogeneic thymocytes (Ruben *et al.*, 1977*a*). Since the thymuses themselves do not generate a demonstrable hemolytic response *in vitro*, the splenic hemolytic capacity is restored through a thymus–spleen interaction. This collaboration could have been mediated either by a factor derived from thymus–spleen allogeneic interaction or by the thymus's responding to antigen (RBC) and releasing a helper factor capable of activating B cells across allogeneic histocompatibility barriers. No functional or genetic restriction data about *any* regulatory lymphokine of ectotherms are available at present. In either case, the collaborative activity was antigen-specific, since the reconstituted spleens produced a hemolytic response against only the species of erythrocyte that had been used as the immunogen.

One might be tempted to argue that the embryonic thymus of this species serves as the source of both T- and B-type cells on grounds that early thymuses have a preponderance of membrane Ig-positive lymphocytes (DuPasquier *et al.*, 1972). Recent embryonic grafting experiments with *Xenopus*, however, suggest otherwise (Volpe *et al.*, 1977). Additionally, as we have already pointed out, early thymectomy does not affect those stimuli, e.g., LPS or polyvinylpyrolidone (PVP), that are T-independent polyclonal stimuli in rodents (Manning and Collie, 1975; Tochinai and Katagiri, 1975).

Recently, we have also demonstrated a similar thymus–spleen functional interaction that will restore hemolytic response capacity to young-adult splenic fragments that have lost that capacity as a consequence of sequential antigen competition (unpublished data). If spleens are removed from young-adult *Xenopus* four days following challenge with 0.2 ml of 25% sheep erythrocytes and these spleens are challenged with sonicated 25% HRBC *in vitro*, no anti-HRBC hemolytic response is generated 14 days later, when the fragments are assayed with intact HRBC and homologous complement. The addition of naive allogeneic thymocytes will restore response capacity to the previously *in vivo* primed spleen, however. The presence of thymus from the same previously primed spleen donor does not restore the response. Experiments are still in progress that may help us understand more about the nature of thymus-spleen collaboration in *Xenopus*, but there seems no doubt that one can readily show interactive events between the thymus and spleen that are suggestive of the kind of T–B collaboration so extensively studied in mice.

No early thymectomy experiments have been reported for reptiles. It has been found, however, that adult thymus ablation of the lizard *Calotes versicolor*, in combination with high doses of rabbit-anti-*Calotes* thymocyte serum, will abrogate antierythrocyte response capacity, as measured by plaque-forming cells. Recovery from antithymocyte suppression of the immune response requires the presence of the thymus (Muthukkaruppan *et al.*, 1976). Furthermore, since low doses of the antithymocyte serum enhance the response levels, it has been suggested that two subsets of T cells may be functioning in the lizard, one serving as helper, the other as suppressor.

Data with respect to thymic ablation have been summarized in Table III. It is noteworthy that the major point these data make is precisely how little has been learned from thymic ablation studies. Exploration of T-dependent *and*-independent phenomena has been performed solely with *Xenopus laevis*. It is obvious that there is much more to learn about the regulatory effects of thymus by utilizing ablation in a wide range of ectothermic organisms.

**Table III. Summary of Evidence of Lymphoid Heterogeneity from Thymic Ablation**

| Species | Antigen | T-dependent function | T-independent function |
|---|---|---|---|
| *T. mozambique* (teleost fish) | Sheep RBC | Abrogated (PFC) | NT[a] |
| *P. waltlii*, *T. alpestris* (urodele amphibia) | Sheep RBC | Severely inhibited (ABC) | NT |
| *P. waltlii* | Salmonella (H + O) | No significant change (serum antibody) | NT |
| *A. mexicanum* (urodele amphibian) | Horse RBC | No inhibition; enhanced (serum hemagglutinin) | NT |
| *X. laevis* (anuran amphibian) | Sheep RBC; human gammaglobulin | Abrogated (serum antibody) | unaffected (LPS, PVP) |
| *C. versicolor* (ATx + ATS) (lizard reptile) | Sheep RBC | Abrogated (PFC) | NT |

[a]NT, not tested.

Differential mitogenesis and thymus-ablation data strongly suggest that at least some fish, amphibians, and reptiles display lymphoid heterogeneity that parallels known lymphopoietic and immune functional diversity present in these species. In the final section we will consider whether this lymphoid heterogeneity in ectotherms provides the basis for T-B collaboration of the kind described for birds and mammals. Some of the evidence we have presented also suggests that the T-cell population itself may be heterogenous and that suppressor- and helper-cell populations may coexist, at least in some species.

## IV. EVIDENCE OF CELL–CELL COLLABORATION IN ECTOTHERMS

Carrier-specific enhancement of an antihapten response is indicative of T-B cell collaboration in birds (Warner *et al.*, 1962; Cooper *et al.*, 1966) and in mammals (Miller and Mitchell, 1968; Claman and Chaperon, 1969; Rajewski *et al.*, 1969). In rodents, carrier-specific helper cells are thymus-derived, while the antibody-secreting plasma cells are B- or bone-marrow-derived cells (Mitchell and Miller, 1968; Nossal *et al.*, 1968). Helper T cells recognize and respond to antigens but do not produce circulating antibody (Davies *et al.*, 1967; Falkoff and Kettman, 1972). There are a variety of models that offer possible mechanisms for collaborative activity. These T cells release an antigen-specific helper factor that, with the likely intermediary activity of adherent cells or macrophages, aids B cells in recognizing and responding to antigen (Feldmann and Nossal, 1972). One way this interaction between members of the two major immunocyte subsets has been demonstrated *in vivo* has been through the use of haptens on immunogenic carriers (Mitchison *et al.*, 1970). Preimmunization or priming with the carrier alone has been found to enhance a primary response to the hapten-carrier conjugate presented as a single challenge. Since only carrier has been added, it is reasonable to suggest that carrier priming stimulates a population of cells (helper cells) that in some way aid the antihapten response. The other aspect of carrier enhancement of the antihapten response is that it is carrier-specific. If an immunogen other than the one used as the carrier for the hapten is used to prime the response, no helper function is generated. Thus, helper activity is provided by carrier-specific cells. Helper function can then be measured in terms of the degree of carrier-specific enhancement (Miller, 1972).

Carrier-specific enhancement of an antihapten response has been reported for two marine teleosts (Yocum *et al.*, 1975), the sea robin (*Prionotus evolans*) and for the winter flounder (Stolen and Mäkelä, 1976). Additionally, carrier-specific enhancement of an antihapten response was found to be especially sensitive to lower environmental temperatures in the carp, a freshwater teleost (Weiss and Avtalion, 1977). This finding fits well with the temperature-sensitivity studies of differential mitogenesis we considered earlier. Taken together, they suggest that an early aspect of the progressive immune response is particular susceptibility to suppression by low environmental temperatures. Thus it would appear that helper function is likely to be involved in low-environmental-temperature inhibition of ectotherm immune response. It is not known for certain that helper function demonstrated in the species of fish noted above is a consequence of T-cell activity. A combination of thymic ablation, subsequent reconstitution, and hapten-carrier immunization will have to be employed in order to ascertain the origin of these helper cells. Recently, the common goldfish, *Carassius auratus*, has been similarly used to demonstrate carrier-specific enhancement (Ruben *et al*., 1977*c*). In this instance, nylon wool columns, of the kind used to enrich mouse helper-T-cell populations in the effluent, were used to separate two distinct populations of antigen-binding cells (ABC) from organs of immunized fish. Adult fish were injected with a carrier (RBC) dose known to generate maximal helper activity. Cell suspensions from both thymus and anterior nephros were passed over nylon wool. The column effluent was enriched 600- to 900-fold for ABC. The antigen-binding cell activity was monitored prior to and after column passage. This finding suggested that a population with comparable dosage sensitivity and response kinetics was present in *both* organs. These cells also share physical characteristics that allow passage through the nylon wool columns. T helper cells of the mouse are almost uniquely able to pass this type of column (Julius *et al*., 1973). Since fish thymocytes share these characteristics with a population of cells in the major immunologic organ, anterior nephros, the conclusion that helper cells are thymus-derived in this fish is not unreasonable. It should be noted that goldfish thymus will generate substantial antigen-binding cell activity (five times background levels) only in response to those low dosages of carrier (0.0025% HRBC) that generate maximum helper activity. High immunogen dosages (e.g., 25% HRBC) did not elicit high numbers of antigen-binding thymocytes nor did they provide for substantial carrier-specific helper activity for antihapten responses. It has been shown that in rodents low dose-carrier priming stimulates T but not B cells (Trizio and Cudkowicz, 1978).

When the full hapten-immunization protocol was used—that is, when low-dose carrier priming was followed in two to four days with a high-dose challenge of a hapten- (in this case, 2,4,6-trinitrophenyl) derived carrier, it was found that *no* thymocytes had TNP-binding specificity. Lymphocytes of the anterior nephros, on the other hand, did show TNP-binding specificity. The majority of ABC from the anterior nephros were of the secretory variety. That is, they bound several layers of carrier erythrocytes. The capacity to bind more than one layer of erythrocytes on the surface of immunized cells suggests that antibody has been released that allows for the binding (agglutination) of the additional RBC layers (Greaves *et al*., 1979; Haskill *et al*., 1972). Unlike the low-dose-sensitive helper antigen-binding cells, the hapten-specific binding cells of the anterior nephros were *retained* on the nylon wool columns. The absence of

TNP-specific binding cells in thymuses of the goldfish fits well with findings that the antigen-binding cells that do form in thymus are of the nonsecretory variety. Moreover, when plaque-forming-cell (PFC) assays, rather than antigen-binding-cell assays, were performed, no PFC were found in the thymus of immunized animals, whereas 8000 to 14,000 PFC could be demonstrated in the anterior nephros (Warr *et al.*, 1977). The data clearly suggest that two functionally different populations of goldfish lymphocytes can be distinguished by their antigen-dose sensitivity, response kinetics, and nylon wool binding properties. While prior studies with fish were not designed to determine whether carrier-specific enhancement and antibody secretion were functions of separate populations of cells, these goldfish studies are strongly suggestive that T-B collaboration is a component of humoral immunity. The goldfish has evolved relatively recently. We have less knowledge of this issue in the more primitive fish and in the Agnatha.

The question as to whether primitive vertebrates, e.g., the urodeles, possess regulatory T cells for humoral immunity has already been raised several times in conjunction with our consideration of developmental differential mitogenesis and thymic ablation studies. It is now necessary for us to take a fresh look at the evidence for non-antibody-producing regulatory cells from hapten-carrier studies.

Carrier-specific enhancement of an anti-hapten response was initially demonstrated with *Notophthalmus viridescens* by using 2,4,6-trinitrophenyl (TNP) as the hapten and several species of heterologous erythrocytes as carriers (Ruben *et al.*, 1973). The RBC carriers were used both for injection and for immunocytoadherence assays. Chicken (C) or toad (T) RBC were used as carriers and horse (H) RBC served as the assay species. An erythrocyte species other than the carrier was chosen for assay only for convenience, since it would reduce the large number of antigen-binding cells against the carrier immunogen, which would have to be counted if the assay were made with the homologous carrier species. We shall see later how important this decision in favor of convenience turned out to be. Sheep erythrocytes (SRBC) had been tried initially. Large, variably sized populations of spontaneous anti-SRBC-binding cells made experimentation with this RBC species impossible. Thus, regardless of the carrier species used, antigen binding was always measured against HRBC or TNP-HRBC. TNP-binding cells then would be defined as the excess number preferentially binding TNP-HRBC to HRBC. All assays were performed with spleen-cell populations pooled from three to six adult newts. Information concerning individual variability is lost as a consequence of pooling. The significant advantage is that pooling *dampens* the effect of individual variability. Additionally, pooling satisfies the practical need for sufficient numbers of sensitized spleen cells to provide for a grid of about 1500 lymphocytes per hemocytometer, so that several tests may be made of a common splenocyte population. In this way one can assay for binding specificity against both HRBC and TNP-HRBC in the presence or absence of specific blocking factors, e.g., TNP–human serum albumin (HSA) or TNP-glycine. Maximum responses produce between 1 and 2% ABC (1–2 $\times$ $10^4$ ABC/$10^6$ lymphocytes). No single spleen-cell pool taken from *unimmunized* adult newts has ever shown the presence of TNP-specific binding. This has been repeated many times over the years by a variety of workers in our laboratory. We shall note later that spleen-cell populations of the toad *Xenopus laevis* frequently show high "natural" anti-TNP-SRBC binding. But even in this case, the demonstrable binding is not TNP-specific binding. It can be shown to be related to TNP-SRBC but not to TNP-HRBC or TNP on guinea pig (GP) or human (Hu) erythrocytes. Moreover, it is not suppressible following incubation of the cells with appropriate concentrations of TNP-glycine. The important point to note here is that one must always test for TNP-binding specificity by using TNP on some nonparticulate carrier that does not add to the observable antigen-binding cell activity. While we have used TNP-HSA and even TNP–chicken RBC (which can be easily distinguished from mammalian RBC on morphological grounds) as blocking agents of TNP-binding activity, $10^{-7}$ M TNP-glycine, which has the advantage of its small molecular size, has been used most consistently and successfully in this regard (Edwards and Ruben, 1976). While it may seem that such experimental detail is out of place in a review of this kind, it is important to keep in mind when evaluating reports purporting to demonstrate "natural" anti-TNP activity (e.g., Charlemagne and Tournefier, 1977*a*).

The initial data demonstrated clearly that TNP-specific-binding cells are generated in the spleen of adult newts of this species only as a consequence of carrier-specific priming. They are not developed when priming is attempted with non-cross-reacting immunogens or by a single challenge of hapten carrier. In fact, no TNP-binding cells were produced following *two* challenges of TNP, when the hapten was presented on two different species of erythrocyte carriers (Ruben and Edwards, 1976).

As was reported for the goldfish, different immunogen (RBC) dosages elicit different antigen-binding cell kinetics, as well as predictable and consistent proportions of nonsecretory to secretory antigen-binding cells. These proportions are not altered when the sensitized cells are preincubated in the presence of either homologous serum taken late in the response, when specific antibody titer is high, or serum taken earlier, during the period of highest antigen-binding cell activity in the spleen. One can, however, increase the percentage of secretory antigen-binding cells by increasing the temperature, while the incubation of sensitized spleen cells and immunogen (RBC) is taking place. Significantly, this increase in numbers of secretory ABC can occur only when high-dosage-sensitized spleen-cell populations are taken late in the response, that is, when peak binding cell activity occurs (Ruben, 1975). Antigen-binding cells generated during the first four days after challenge do not show this alteration. As was the case with the goldfish, very low immunogen doses stimulate populations of splenic ABC to form very quickly and they are largely (90%) nonsecretory ABC. High immunogen doses, on the other hand, stimulate greater numbers of ABC to form 8 to 10 days later. About 50% of them are secretory cells. Three different populations of ABC are suggested by these immunogen-dosage studies: (1) a low-dose-sensitive population that does not secrete antibody, (2) a high-dose-sensitive population that does not secrete antibody (it is recoverable as a binding population long after binding activity of the low-dose-sensitive population has disappeared from the spleen), and (3) a high-dose-sensitive population that secretes antibody to form multilayered RBC antigen-binding cells. Just how these three populations relate to functions following hapten-carrier immunization can be exposed in part by studies of dosage and helper activity. The data in Fig. 1 indicate that low-dose priming stimulates maximum helper activity. This result, which has also been reported for the goldfish (Ruben *et al.*, 1977*c*), anuran amphibians (Ruben, 1976), and rodents (Mitchison, 1971), suggests that the low-dose-sensitive nonsecretory ABC population is the helper-lymphocyte subset. As we

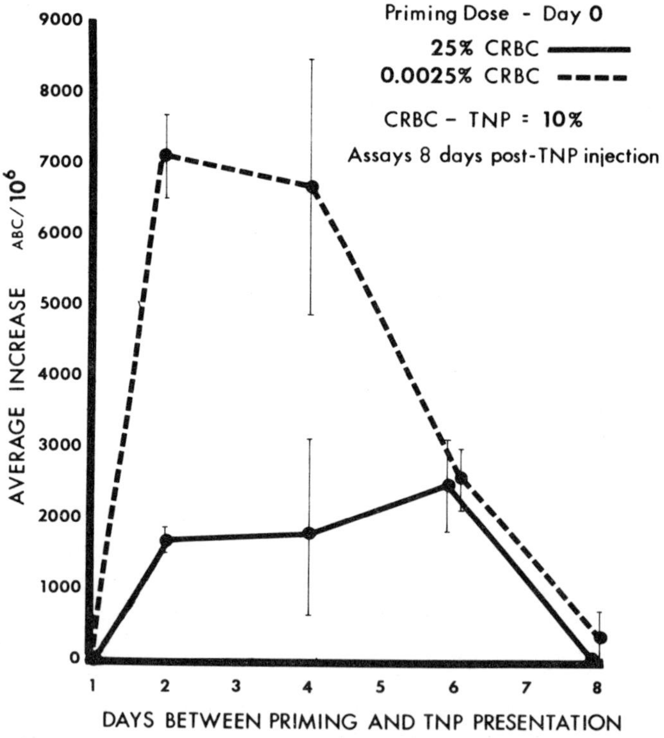


Figure 1. Enhancement of an anti-TNP response by carrier priming is both time-and dose-dependent. The response is monitored by immunocytoadherence of spleen cells of newts, *Notophthalamus viridescens*, which are immunized by intraperitoneal injection.

have indicated before, with the single exception of the toad *Xenopus laevis*, it is not yet possible to relate this helper-cell population to thymus derivation in ectotherms. Thymic-ablation studies have not progressed to the point of providing a distinction between helper T and antibody-forming "B" cells in the other species.

An association between secretory ABC with TNP-specific binding cells has also been made. It was found that the increase in antigen-binding cells achieved when the anti-TNP cells were generated following carrier priming was almost entirely (98%) in the secretory category of ABC. Thus the hapten-carrier data from studies with the newt suggested that one could visualize both helper and antibody-secreting ABC in terms of their dosage sensitivities, ABC kinetics, and ABC morphologies. The possibility remains, however, that these are not two different subsets but rather developmental stages, with functional differences, of a single lymphocyte subset: a subset that clearly differs from the cytotoxic cell population. We have already provided the evidence for this separation during our consideration of the three areas of investigation that precede this section.

The serendipity involved in the decision on grounds of convenience to assay antigen-binding cell activity with a species of erythrocyte different from the carrier immunogen became apparent after a series of experiments with newts in which this element of the protocol was varied (Ruben and Selker, 1975).

If adult newts are immunized in accordance with the schedule of low-dose (0.0025% RBC) carrier priming, followed in two to four days by a high-dose (25% RBC) challenge of TNP-RBC, and the assays for antigen-binding cell activity are performed eight days thereafter with the species of erythrocyte homologous with the immunogen carrier, *no TNP-specific binding is apparent.* The number of cells binding the carrier is the same as the number binding the TNP carrier. Furthermore, if $10^{-7}$ M TNP-glycine is used as a preincubation blocking agent prior to testing binding activity, the data show an equivalent reduction in the number of spleen cells binding carrier and the TNP conjugate of the carrier. TNP-glycine must therefore affect receptors on carrier-binding cells to the same extent as it does receptors on TNP-carrier-sensitized binding cells. We concluded that newt-spleen cells generated as a result of this immunization protocol bear receptors for *both* the hapten and the erythrocyte carrier. This suggestion was consistent with the results of earlier experiments in which newt spleen cells were sensitized to TNP on one species of RBC (e.g., TNP-HRBC) and preincubated with TNP on a heterlogous species of erythrocyte carrier (e.g., TNP-CRBC). Subsequent assays showed severely reduced binding to the immunogen-carrier species (HRBC). Similarly, preincubation with unconjugated carrier erythrocytes reduced spleen-cell binding to TNP on a heterologous carrier species. These data suggested that at least some newt-spleen cells have the capacity to bind both carrier and hapten (TNP-). We later tested this directly by using antigen-coated polyacrylamide beads (Ruben and Edwards,

1978). Beads conjugated with bovine-serum albumen (BSA) failed to bind newt spleen cells that had been immunized with HRBC and TNP-HRBC. However, if BSA-conjugated beads were additionally conjugated with TNP, some of the sensitized spleen cells bound on the surface of the beads. A second incubation in the presence of HRBC was then employed and some of the TNP-bound spleen cells now also bound erythrocytes. Preincubating TNP-HRBC-sensitized spleen cells with TNP-glycine and testing spleen cells immunized against HRBC alone confirmed that spleen-cell binding to TNP-BSA beads was TNP-related. Thus, one can visualize dual specificity on the part of some newt immunocytes. This finding raised interesting questions with respect to the evolution and development of phenotypic restriction of vertebrate lymphocytes. These questions are outside the scope of this paper, but relevant to the present discussion is a thought model that arose from these findings. It became possible to explain the results that had been reported up to that point for the newt without invoking cooperative cellular interactions. Priming by carrier should initiate clonal amplification of all immunocytes capable of recognizing any horse-erythrocyte membrane determinant. The challenge with TNP-conjugated HRBC that follows two days later can be thought of as acting by secondary amplification of those cells with receptor specificity for both the hapten *and* a carrier determinant, as well as those specific for only HRBC determinants. The preferential amplification of this subset of the dual specific immunocytes might occur because the presence of receptors for two different determinants confers greater antigen-binding affinity on these previously sensitized cells. Alternatively, preferential clonal expansion may result simply because cells with receptors for two epitopes are more apt to bind with one or the other determinant. This model suggests that one could explain all the early newt results in terms of selective proliferation of a single subset of immunocytes. Preferential binding to TNP-conjugated heterologous RBC, which has been shown to be TNP-specific by blocking with TNP, was enhanced by carrier-specific priming, but that enhancement might not have required T-B cooperation in this urodele system. Polyfunctionality for lymphocytes of primitive vertebrates, and particularly at their immunocompetent larval stages, is a very attractive concept, because so many of them have such small numbers of immunocytes available for response. In general, the numbers are so small that it would be difficult to conceive of their possessing even a single stem cell available for each potential antigenic determinant. Yet it is known that larval anurans can respond specifically to antigens at a time when the spleen has many fewer than $10^6$ lymphocytes. Furthermore, it seems clear, for at least one species of anuran, that when immunocompetence first arises in the larva, the organism can respond to a wide range of epitopes (Pross and Rowlands, 1975). Nothing is known of the development of immunologic specificity in urodeles, however. Obviously, the lack of phenotypic restriction for urodele adult lymphocytes could allow for organismic response diversity adequate to the task of protecting them against potential antigens in the environment. It is also conceivable that their aquatic environment has fewer potential epitopes than are found in terrestrial environments. This model of polyfunctionality for immunocytes of primitive vertebrates and its attendant suggestion that carrier-specific enhancement of a hapten response might be explicable on grounds other than cellular cooperation has been cited by McKinney *et al.* (1976) for fish and Charlemagne and Tournefier (1977*a*) for urodeles. It is supportive of their view that primitive vertebrates respond to mouse T-dependent antigens as if they were T-independent. The evidence for these views has already been discussed.

While it is still our opinion that all of the earlier data on hapten-carrier immunization in urodeles *could* be explained by selective proliferation of a single subset of lymphocytes, it is also very clear that recent experiments have provided results that *require* introduction of a concept, such as "second signal" or "carrier effect," in order to explain their causality (Ruben and Edwards, 1976). In other words, without recourse to analogy to mouse immunology—indeed, even if no such concept existed to explain carrier-specific priming of the antihapten response in mice—we should have had to develop one in order to account for the following results with the newt *Notophthalamus viridescens.* If, instead of priming with carrier, TNP-carrier RBC is used, and the major challenge that follows two days later is the unconjugated carrier, the ABC generated in the urodele spleen are different from those we considered earlier, when the immunization protocol was the reverse. The ABC generated from the protocol that uses the TNP carrier as the low-dose primer and the carrier as the second high-dose challenge are of two specificities, as before. However, in this instance, instead of their being 50% specific for HRBC determinants and 50% specific for TNP and a horse-membrane determinant, we now find about 50% to be specific for HRBC and 50% to be uniquely specific for the hapten TNP. This *restriction* to TNP specificity for these newt cells is suggested here only with respect to determinant specificities that were tested in our experiments. We have no way of knowing if receptors for different epitopes may be present. Priming with TNP carrier may stimulate short-term amplification of cells with (A) carrier specificity, (B) TNP-carrier (dual) specificities, or (C) TNP (but not carrier) specificity. The second challenge with high-dose unconjugated carrier could then reamplify those cells with carrier specificity or with dual specificity, but *not* those with only hapten specificity. Thus, the selective proliferation model does *not* provide an explanation of how this immunization protocol can generate such a large population of ABC that are uniquely TNP-specific. Moreover, TNP-glycine will block *only* binding to the TNP-carrier conjugate and does not affect those cells that bind unconjugated carrier following this reversed immunization protocol. In order to account for the evidence cited earlier that TNP-specific binding requires the same species of erythrocyte to be used in *both* the priming and secondary challenge, some sort of carrier-specific effect must be postulated. This carrier-specific effect would seem to represent a "second signal" generated by carrier-responsive cells, which provides for a proliferative stimulus on TNP-specific restricted cells. The kinetics of low-dose immunogen responses in newts are such that *no* TNP-specific restricted cells could be present in the spleen 10 days after priming without some type of reamplification. Thus, the large number actually found must have been generated as a consequence of the *second* challenge, which was with unconjugated erythrocytes! It is necessary to assume that the priming low-dose injection of TNP carrier activates the hapten-specific restricted cells so that they may respond to the second signal. This assumption is necessary in order to account for the lack of hapten-specific-restricted ABC generated by the reverse immunization protocol. Unconjugated-erythrocyte priming would not be expected to provide for this activation. Dual specific cells would be expected to arise in substantial numbers only when some selective advantage for their amplification is provided.

These newts produce only low serum-antibody titers after the immunization protocols described above. It is therefore not possible at this time to report on the question of whether dual specific cells generate two antibodies with unique specificities or a single antibody with both TNP and carrier specificity. When multiple injections of TNP carrier are made, adequate titers of hemagglutinin are obtained. Ireland (unpublished results) has tested the serum antibody generated after four weekly high-dose TNP-HRBC injections. By 35 days after the initial priming, 8 ± 2 wells of twofold serial-dilution microhemagglutinin assay, anti-HRBC and anti-TNP-HRBC-agglutinin activity had been produced. Background hemagglutinin levels to HRBC or SRBC were negligible ($<1$). When the antiserum was adsorbed three times with 0.1 ml pellets of packed HRBC, all activity against HRBC was removed, but 6 ± 2 wells of activity remained against TNP-HRBC. If the antiserum was similarly adsorbed with TNP-HRBC, activity was removed against both HRBC and TNP-HRBC. Adsorption with SRBC did not affect antibody titers against HRBC or TNP-HRBC. One can suggest, then, that after multiple stimulation with TNP-HRBC, two different antibody specificities can be demonstrated. That is, antibody activity against TNP, which is not cross-reactive with the carrier, has been indicated. It will be necessary to provide evidence from TNP-glycine blocking experiments before we can say with certainty that the antibody activity remaining against TNP-HRBC following HRBC adsorption is actually TNP-specific. The activity might be directed against a determinant created on the HRBC membrane as a consequence of TNP conjugation (Ruben and Edwards, 1976). This activity would not be completely suppressible with TNP-glycine, for instance.

Carrier-specific enhancement of a hapten response has also been demonstrated for the toad *Xenopus laevis* and the grass frog, *Rana pipiens* (Ruben and Edwards, 1977). Neither of these two species appears to generate cells of dual specificities within adult spleens. Moreover, blocking tests of their binding specificities within adult spleens. Moreover, blocking tests of their binding specificities demonstrate that they have much more precise antigen-determinant recognition than does the newt (Edwards and Ruben, 1976).

The question of the relationship between antigen-binding and antibody-forming cells has been satisfactorily dealt with in rodents (Greaves *et al.*, 1970; Haskill *et al.*, 1972). We have also been able to perform a series of tests with anuran ABC in order to determine whether a similar relationship can be demonstrated for these systems (Edwards *et al.*, 1975). The results indicate that the generation of secretory ABC depends on protein synthesis. Incubation of sensitized frog-spleen cells in emetine-HCl, a powerful inhibitor of protein synthesis, does not affect the overall number of cells binding the species of erythrocytes used originally as immunogen. However, no secretory or multilayered ABC appear. Paraformaldehyde, which effectively "freezes" the cell surface, also fails to reduce the number of ABC, and again no secretory cells are observed. Recently, we have incubated sensitized lymphocytes of the jugular bodies of *R. pipiens*, in the presence of the erythrocyte species originally used as the immunogen, overnight at 4°C in Cunningham-Szenberg chambers (Ruben and Edwards, unpublished results). The multilayered sensitized lymphocytes clearly (Fig. 2A) produced a halo of agglutination around themselves. Further, if fresh homologous serum (complement) is added to the chambers, typical lytic plaques will be generated (Fig. 2B). It should be noted that 4°C does not inhibit antigen-antibody complexing, complement activity, or antibody synthesis and secretion when amphibians are used as experimental material (Ruben *et al.*, 1977*b*).

Once again, we want to stress that blocking experiments must accompany tests of antihapten activity levels in order to be certain that preferential hemagglutination of hapten-conjugated erythrocytes is in fact related to TNP specificity and not to new membrane determinants created by the conjugation procedure. *Xenopus* provides the best example we have found for demonstrating this point. In assays for the TNP-SRBC binding activity of unimmunized splenic lymphocytes, high ($1\text{-}2 \times 10^4$ ABC/$10^6$) "natural" background levels of ABC are often found. This background of TNP-binding cells is not evident when TNP-human (HuRBC) or guinea-pig (GP-RBC) erythrocytes are used in the assays. Up until very recently, background TNP activity could not be found when TNP-HRBC was tested, but recently some *Xenopus* populations have been providing modest ($2 \times 10^3$ ABC/$10^6$ splenocytes) TNP-HRBC ABC background numbers (excess binding when compared with HRBC spontaneous ABC). These spontaneous TNP ABC can be found in spleen-cell populations, but not when thymocytes are tested. Incubation of the spleen cells in TNP-glycine does *not* alter the numbers of these spontaneous ABC. Since this "natural" activity is not TNP-suppressible and is almost uniquely related to TNP-SRBC, we suggest that the activity is really directed by memory cells against a new membrane determinant

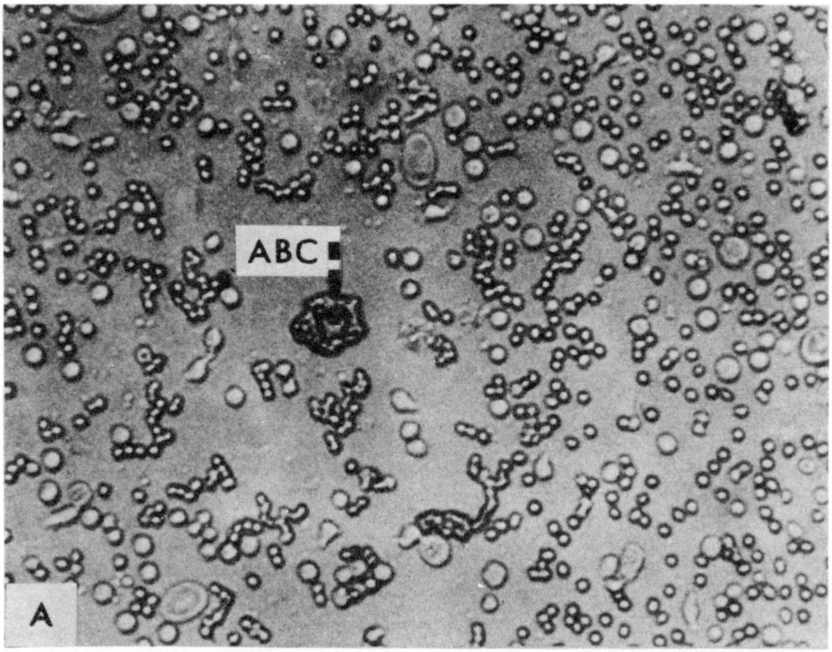
ABC
A

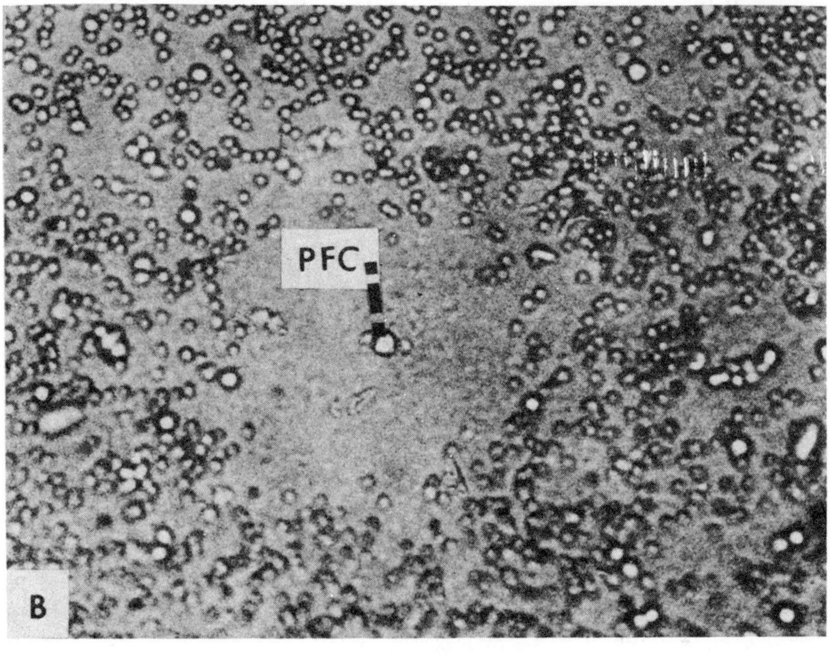
PFC
B

that is cross-reactive with some determinant these *Xenopus* had previously been exposed to. The serum picture with respect to "natural" anti-TNP activity seems even more confusing. Immunization with a single high-dose (20% RBC) injection of TNP-HuRBC generates no preferential cellular activity (ABC) against either TNP-HuRBC or TNP-HRBC. However, serum activity is generated that will agglutinate both TNP-HuRBC and TNP-HRBC, but not HRBC. It would appear that (A) there is a discrepancy between the cellular picture and serum activity and (B) the serum activity may in fact be against altered erythrocyte determinants and not TNP (Edwards and Ruben, unpublished results). This situation obviously requires clarification and there is little benefit to further speculation at this time. The reason we have called attention to these unexpected findings is to urge caution in evaluating work using haptenated RBC carriers.

One can also note more predictable discrepancies between cellular and serum data in these systems. For instance, while cellular binding activity in the spleen falls off to background levels 12 to 18 days post-high-dose immunization, serum-antibody levels continue to rise and persist for several weeks in anurans. This suggests that ABC may leave the spleen and continue to secrete serum antibody in some other site(s) (Edwards and Ruben, unpublished results).

It is particularly interesting that in all three of the amphibian species tested and in the goldfish, the enhancing effect by prior challenge with carrier is so short-lived. If the priming carrier challenge and the hapten-carrier challenge are separated by 7 to 10 days, no hapten-specific binding activity will be generated in the spleen. Cytotoxic-cell memory can be long-lived, even in the newt (Cohen, 1970), and adult thymic ablation studies with *Xenopus* suggest persistence of *potential* helper cells through at least 240 days (Horton *et al.*, 1977). It may be that antigen-responding helper cells and antigen-sensitive potential helper cells have very different viability periods available to them.

The two anurans *R. pipens* and *X. laevis* demonstrate dose sensitivities and ABC kinetics, as well as the morphological (nonsecretory or secretory) binding distinctions we have already seen to apply to the goldfish and newt. The advantage the anurans offer over the newts is that adult thymuses are large enough so that their cells can be pooled and monitored with respect to anti-erythrocyte responses.

As was the case with the goldfish, anuran thymocytes tend to bind as nonsecretory ABC regardless of the dose of erythrocyte immunogen used. This suggests that the thymuses of these species do not generate antibody-producing

←

Figure 2. (A) Multiple-layered (secretory) antigen-binding frog jugular body cells (ABC) will develop in Cunningham–Szenberg chambers at 4°C in the absence of complement. Additionally, a zone of secretion (hemagglutination) can be seen surrounding the ABC. (B) In the presence of homologous complement, typical plaque-forming cells can be visualized from the same cells. All other conditions remain the same.

cells. Some reports, however, suggest an antibody-producing role for the larval amphibian thymus (Moticka *et al.*, 1973). Ruben (1975) uses analogies among the amphibians to suggest that low-dose immunogen sensitivity, ABC kinetics, and nonsecretory ABC morphology—all characteristics that parallel induction of helper function—provide a firm basis for linking helper cells with T cells in these species. While this may turn out to be true, the reader should by now be aware that in our view this relationship of T-B collaboration can be strongly suggested only for early thymectomized *Xenopus laevis* (Manning and Collie, 1975; Ruben *et al.*, 1977*a*), and perhaps for the column-separable immunocytes of goldfish (Ruben *et al.*, 1977*c*). While we are convinced that collaborative interactions are demonstrable within the hapten-carrier immunization framework, we have as yet no evidence to offer *proving* that T cells play a role in any fish or other amphibian system.

## V. CONCLUSION: SOME SPECULATIONS WITH RESPECT TO THE EVOLUTION OF IMMUNITY

We noted in our introduction that data are available for only a few laboratory favorites. Whether information provided for these species will apply to more primitive extant vertebrates remains to be seen. Nevertheless, current information strongly suggests that collaborative cellular interactions in humoral immunity may have been a fundamental feature of vertebrate evolution. Certainly, these interactions did not await the evolution of a bursa of Fabricius or bone marrow as a hematopoietic source. Functional B cells are found in all extant vertebrates, since all have demonstrated the ability to generate antigen-specific antibody. What is not clear is whether the collaborative interactions that can be demonstrated in primitive vertebrates, e.g., the newt, involve T-B cooperation.

There is considerable evidence to suggest that all functions normally ascribed to T cells in the mouse are poorly performed in primitive vertebrates. Allograft rejection tends to be chronic rather than acute, MLR and GVHR are either poorly developed or absent, soluble macromolecules are nonimmunogenic, and responses to Con A and PHA stimulation tend to be less intense than mitogenic responses to LPS, for instance. If helper function is related to T-cell activity in these forms, it would have to be clearly in advance of the evolutionary trend exhibited by these other characteristics.

It is interesting that a heightened efficiency of T-cell functional activities can be observed within each of the ectothermic vertebrate classes. Moreover, this heightened activity is accompanied by increased structural differentiation of the thymus gland itself within each class.

Cohen (1977) has suggested that acute allograft rejection and MLR and GVHR capacity evolved several times, by convergent evolution, in each of the vertebrate classes. The evidence we have reviewed here argues for a similar view of convergent evolution with respect to all possible T-cell functions. If this is the situation, then it follows that an alternative may be offered to the more traditional view that in evolution T-cell activities preceded B-cell function (Cooper, 1977; Tam *et al.*, 1976). When vertebrates first evolved, *all* lymphocytes may have been similar to mouse B cells with respect to their capacity to synthesize immunoglobulin as a mediator of antigen recognition and response. The major alteration in immunity accompanying the evolution of vertebrates may then have been the development of immunoglobulin, IgM in particular. Certain functions currently ascribed to T-cell subsets of mice may have been managed with some success by this lymphocyte pool. Thus, weak graft-rejection capacity and cellular collaborative regulation of humoral immunity may be served in this way in some of the extant primitive vertebrates. As an alternative, self/non-self distinctions leading to rejection could conceivably be dealt with by a mechanism of molecular complementarity of the type exhibited by the still more primitive invertebrate groups.

In ancestral fish, buds of pharyngeal entoderm may have provided rudimentary thymuses and new tissue microenvironments for immigrant lymphoid-stem cells. Primitive thymuses lacked corticomedullary distinctions and may have produced little or no thymopoietin(s). While thymic lymphocytes may have been an early aspect of vertebrate evolution, they may not have been differentiated along functional "T-cell-like" pathways until further evolutionary progress was made in each of the vertebrate classes. The thymocytes of ancestral forms, then, may really have been mouselike "B cells." Extant primitive vertebrates might conceivably represent gradations of this evolutionary and developmental progression. This hypothesis may help us to understand why such a very high percentage of thymocytes of primitive vertebrates have surface immunoglobulin demonstrable by immunofluorescence (Ellis and Parkhouse, 1975; Charlemagne and Tournefier, 1975). There would seem to be a useful ontogenetic model available as well, since in the larvae of somewhat more advanced forms, e.g., *Xenopus laevis*, a vast majority of thymus cells have visualizable surface Ig, whereas adult thymocytes do not (DuPasquier *et al.*, 1972). Mouselike T cells seem likely to have evolved and to have developed from stem cells, which subsequently become modified by an appropriate thymus microenvironment. The more evolutionarily advanced or recent the organism, the more complete the subset conversion and the greater the cells' ability to perform those functions normally provided by T cells of the mouse. Thus it would be reasonable to expect to find that thymocytes and thymus-derived cells have visualizable and/or isolatable immunoglobulin on their surfaces (Warr, this volume). The thymus microenvironment could affect membrane Ig differentially, qualitatively and quantitatively, within each of the vertebrate classes. Thus, recently evolved fish, such as *Carassius auratus*, may have so much surface immunoglobulin on adult thymocytes that it can be visualized by immunofluorescence (Warr *et al.*, 1976; Ruben *et al.*, 1977), whereas the toad *Xenopus laevis* would not (Du-Pasquier *et al.*, 1972). Moreover, thymocyte-surface immunoglobulin may, in some instances, be typical of serum IgM, as in the bluegill (Clem *et al.*, 1977), or different from it, as in the goldfish (Warr and Marchalonis, 1977). What this hypothesis offers is the simplest possible genetic mechanism for providing comparable antigen-recognition specificity for T and B lymphocytes of advanced vertebrates. The immunoglobulin genes would determine it for *both* cell types.

The evolution of thymus within each vertebrate class may be viewed in terms of the evolution of cellular collaborative regulatory refinement, the fine tuning of humoral immune responses originally carried out by a homogenous lymphocyte pool that shared at least some characteristics with mouse B-like lymphocytes.

ACKNOWLEDGMENTS

The authors are grateful for support of work done in this laboratory through a grant (AI-12846) from the National Institutes of Health, Bethesda, Maryland, and for the technical assistance of Judith S. Ruben.

## VI. REFERENCES

Atwell, J. L., and Marchalonis, J. J., 1975, Phylogenetic emergence of immunoglobulin classes distinct from IgM, *J. Immunogenet.* **1**:367.

Avtalion, R. R., Weiss, E., and Moalem, T., 1976, Regulatory effects of temperature upon immunity in ectothermic vertebrates, in: *Comparative Immunology* (J. J. Marchalonis, ed.), pp. 227–238, Blackwell, Oxford.

Baculi, B. S., Cooper, E. L., and Brown, B. A., 1970, Lymphomyeloid organs of amphibia. V. Comparative histology in diverse anuran species, *J. Morphol.* **131**:315.

Bogner, K. H., and Ellis, A. E., 1977, Properties and functions of lymphocytes and lymphoid tissue in teleost fish, *Beitr. zur Histopath. Fische* **4**:59.

Charlemagne, J., and Tournefier, A., 1975, Cell surface immunoglobulins of thymus and spleen lymphocytes in the urodele amphibian, *Pleurodeles waltlii Salamanderidae*, *Adv. Exp. Biol. Med.* **64**:251.

Charlemagne, J., and Tournefier, A., 1977*a*, Anti-horse red blood cells anti-body synthesis in the Mexican axolotl (*Ambystoma mexicanum*): Effect of thymectomy, in: *Developmental Immunobiology* (J. B. Solomon and J. D. Horton, eds.), pp. 267–275, Elsevier North-Holland, Amsterdam.

Charlemagne, J., and Tournefier, A., 1977*b*, Humoral response to *Salmonella typhimurium* antigens in normal and thymectomized urodele amphibian *Pleurodeles waltlii*, Michah, *Eur. J. Immunol.* **7**:500.

Claman, H. N., and Chaperon, E. A., 1969, Immunological complementation between thymus and marrow cells: a model for a two cell theory of immunocompetence, *Transp. Rev.* **1**:92.
Clem, L. W., McLean, W. E., Shankey, V. T., and Cuchens, M. A., 1977, Phylogeny of lymphocyte heterogeneity. I. Membrane immunoglobulins of teleost lymphocyes, *J. Dev. Comp. Immunol.* **1**:105.
Cohen, N., 1970, Immunological memory involving weak histocompatability barriers in urodele amphibians, *Transplantation* **10**:382.
Cohen, N., 1977, Phylogenetic emergence of lymphoid cells and tissues, in: *The Lymphocyte* (J. J. Marchalonis, ed.), pp. 149–202, Marcel Dekker Inc., New York.
Collie, M. H., 1976, Ph.D. thesis, University of Hull, Hull, U. K.
Collins, N. H., and Cohen, N., 1976, Phylogeny of immunocompetent cells. II. *In vitro* behavior of lymphocytes from the spleen, blood, and thymus of the urodele, *Ambystoma mexicanum*, in: *Phylogeny of Thymus and Bone Marrow-Bursa Cells* (R. K. Wright and E. L. Cooper, eds.), pp. 143–151, Elsevier North-Holland, Amsterdam.
Collins, N. H., Manickavel, V., and Cohen, N., 1976, *In vitro* responses of urodele lymphoid cells: mitogenic and mixed lymphocyte culture reactivities, *Adv. Exp. Med. Biol.* **64**:305.
Cooper, E. L., 1977, Evolution of cell mediated immunity, in: *Developmental Immunobiology* (J. B. Solomon and J. D. Horton, eds.), pp. 99–105, Elsevier North-Holland, Amsterdam.
Cooper, M. D., Peterson, R. D., South, M. A., and Good, R. A., 1966, The functions of the thymus system and bursa system in the chicken, *J. Exp. Med.* **123**:75.
Cowden, R. R., and Dyer, R. F., 1971, Lymphopoietic tissue and plasma cells in amphibia, *Am. Zool.* **11**:183.
Cuchens, M. A., and Clem, L. W., 1977, Phylogeny of lymphocyte heterogeneity II. Differential effects of temperature on fish T-like and B-like cells, *Cell. Immunol.* **34**:219.
Cuchens, M. A., McLean, E., and Clem, L. W., 1976, Lymphocyte heterogeneity in fish and reptiles, in: *Phylogeny of Thymus and Bone-Marrow-Bursa Cells* (R. K. Wright and E. L. Cooper, eds.), pp. 205–213, Elsevier North-Holland, Amsterdam.
Davies, A. J. S., Leuchars, S. E., Wallis, V., Marchant, R., and Elliott, E. V., 1967, The failure of thymus derived cells to produce antibody, *Transplant* **5**:222.
Donnelly, N., Manning, M. J., and Cohen, N., 1976, Thymus dependency of lymphocyte subpopulation in *Xenopus laevis*, in: *Phylogeny of Thymus and Bone Marrow-Bursa Cells* (R. K. Wright and E. L. Cooper, eds.), pp. 133–141, Elsevier North-Holland, Amsterdam.
DuPasquier, L., and Horton, J. D., 1976, The effect of thymectomy on the mixed leukocyte reaction and phytohemagglutinin responsiveness in the clawed toad, *Xenopus laevis*, *Immunogenetics* **3**:105.
DuPasquier, L., Weiss, N., and Loor, F., 1972, Direct evidence for immunoglobulins on the surface of thymus lymphocytes of amphibian larvae, *Eur. J. Immunol.* **2**:366.
Edwards, B. F., and Ruben, L. N., 1976, The precision of combining site discrimination within the amphibia as tested by selective blocking of antigen-binding splenocytes, in: *Phylogeny of Thymus and Bone Marrow-Bursa Cells* (R. K. Wright and E. L. Cooper, eds.), pp. 153–159, Elsevier North-Holland, Amsterdam.
Edwards, B. F., Ruben, L. N., Marchalonis, J. J., and Hylton, C., 1975, Surface characteristics of spleen cell erythrocyte rosette formation in the grass frog, *Rana pipiens*, *Adv. Exp. Med. Biol.* **64**:387.
Ellis, A. E., and Parkhouse, P. M. E., 1975, Surface immunoglobulins on the lymphocytes of the skate, *Raja naevus*, *Eur. J. Immunol.* **5**:726.
Etlinger, H. M., Hodgins, H. O., and Chiller, J. M., 1976, Evolution of the lymphoid system.

I. Evidence for lymphocyte heterogeneity in rainbow trout revealed by the organ distribution of mitogenic responses, *J. Immunol.* **116**:1547.

Falkoff, R., and Kettman, J., 1972, Differential stimulation of precursor cells and carrier-specific thymic derived cell activity in the *in vivo* response to heterologous erythrocytes in mice, *J. Immunol.* **108**:54.

Feldmann, M., and Nossal, G. J. V., 1972, Tolerance, engancement and regulation of interactions between T cells, B cells and macrophages, *Transpl. Rev.* **13**:3.

Goldstine, S. N., Collins, N. H., and Cohen, N., 1975, Mitogens as probes of lymphocyte heterogeneity in anuran amphibians, *Adv. Exp. Med. Biol.* **64**:343.

Goldstine, S. N., Manickavel, V., and Cohen, N., 1975, Phylogeny of gut-associated lymphoid tissue, *Am. Zool.* **15**:107.

Good, R. A., Finstad, J., Pollara, B., and Gabrielson, A. E., 1966, Morphologic studies on the evolution of the lymphoid tissues among the lower vertebrates, in: *Phylogeny of Immunity* (R. T. Smith, P. A. Miescher, and R. A. Good, eds.), pp. 149–168, University of Florida Press, Gainesville.

Greaves, M. F., and Janossy, G., 1972, Elicitation of selective T and B lymphocyte responses by cell surface binding ligands, *Transpl. Rev.* **11**:87.

Greaves, M. F., Möller, E., and Möller, A., 1970, Studies on antigen-binding cells. II. Relationships to antigen-sensitive cells, *Cell. Immunol.* **1**:386.

Haskill, J. S., Elliot, B. E., Kerbel, R., Axelrad, M. A., and Eidinger, D., 1972, Classification of thymus-derived and marrow-derived lymphocytes by demonstration of their antigen-binding characteristics, *J. Exp. Med.* **135**:1410.

Hildemann, W. H., and Thoenes, G. H., 1969, Immunological responses of Pacific hagfish. I. Skin transplantation immunity, *Transplant* **7**:506.

Horton, J. D., 1969, Ontogeny of the immune response to skin allografts in relation to lymphoid organ development in the amphibian *Xenopus laevis* (Daudin), *J. Embryol. Exp. Morphol.* **22**:265.

Horton, J. D., and Manning, M. J., 1972, Response to skin allograft in *Xenopus laevis* following thymectomy at early stages of lymphoid organ maturation, *Transplant* **14**:141.

Horton, J. D., and Manning, J. J., 1974, Effect of early thymectomy on the cellular changes occurring in the spleen of the clawed toad following administration of soluble antigen, *Immunol.* **26**:797.

Horton, J. D., Rimmer, J. J., and Horton, T. L., 1976, The effect of thymectomy at different stages of larval development of the immune response of the clawed toad to sheep erythrocytes, *J. Exp. Zool.* **196**:243.

Horton, J. D., Rimmer, J. J., and Horton, T. L., 1977, Critical role of the thymus in establishing humoral immunity in amphibians: Studies on *Xenopus* thymectomized in larval and adult life, *J. Dev. Comp. Immunol.* **1**:119.

Julius, M. H., Simpson, E., and Herzenberg, L. A., 1973, A rapid method for isolation of functional thymus-derived murine lymphocytes, *Eur. J. Immunol.* **3**:645.

Katz, D. N., and Benacerraf, B., 1972, The regulatory influence of activated T cells on B cell responses to antigen, *Adv. Immunol.* **15**:1.

Kidder, G. M., Ruben, L. N., and Stevens, J. M., 1973, Cytodynamics and ontogeny of the immune response of *Xenopus laevis* against sheep erythrocytes, *J. Embryol. Ex. Morphol.* **29**:73.

Litman, G. W., 1976, Physical properties of immunoglobulins of lower species: A comparison with immunoglobulins of mammals, in: *Comparative Immunology* (J. J. Marchalonis, ed.), pp. 239–275, Blackwell, Oxford.

Lopez, D. M., Sigel, M. M., and Lee, J. C., 1974, Phylogenetic studies on T cells. I. Lymphocytes of the shark with differential response to phytohemagglutinin and concanavalin A, *Cell. Immunol.* **10**:287.

McKinney, E. C., Ortiz, A., Lee, J. C., Sigel, M. M., Lopez, D. M., Epstein, R. W., and McLeod, T. F., 1976, Lymphocytes of fish: Multipotential or specialized? in: *Phylogeny of Thymus and Bone Marrow-Bursa Cells* (R. K. Wright and E. L. Cooper, eds.), pp. 73–82, Elsevier North-Holland, Amsterdam.

Manning, M. J., and Collie, M. H., 1975, Thymic function in amphibians, *Adv. Exp. Med. Biol.* **64**:353.

Manning, M. J., and Collie, M. H., 1977, The ontogeny of thymic dependence in the amphibian, *Xenopus laevis*, in: *Developmental Immunobiology* (J. B. Solomon and J. D. Horton, eds.), pp. 291–298, Elsevier North-Holland, Amsterdam.

Manning, M. J., and Horton, J. D., 1969, Histogenesis of lymphoid organs in larvae of the South African Clawed toad, *Xenopus laevis* (Daudin), *J. Embryol. Exp. Morphol.* **22**:265.

Manning, M. J., Donnelly, N., and Cohen, N., 1976, Thymus-dependent-independent components of the amphibian immune system, in: *Phylogeny of Thymus and Bone-Marrow-Bursa Cells* (R. K. Wright and E. L. Cooper, eds.), pp. 123–132, Elsevier North-Holland, Amsterdam.

Marchalonis, J. J., 1969, Isolation and characterization of immunoglobulinlike proteins of the Australian lungfish (*Neoceratodus forsteri*), *Aust. J. Exp. Biol. Med. Sci.* **47**:405.

Marchalonis, J. J., 1974, Phylogenetic origins of antibodies and immune recognition, in: *Progress in Immunology*, Vol. 2 (L. Brent and J. Holborow, eds.), pp. 249–259, North-Holland, Amsterdam.

Marchalonis, J. J., 1977, *Immunity in Evolution*, Edward Arnold, London.

Marchalonis, J. J., Ealey, E. H. M., and Diener, E., 1969, Immune response of the tuatara, *Sphenodon punctatum*, *Aust. J. Exp. Biol. Med. Sci.* **47**:367.

Miller, J. F. A. P., 1972, Lymphocyte interactions in antibody responses, *Int. Rev. Cytol.* **33**:77.

Miller, J. F. A. P., and Mitchell, G. F., 1968, Cell to cell interaction in the immune response. I. Hemolysin forming cells in neonatally thymectomized mice reconstituted with thymus or thoracic duct lymphocytes, *J. Exp. Med.* **128**:810.

Mitchell, G. F., and Miller, J. F. A. P., 1968, Cell to cell interaction in the immune response II. The Source of hemolysin forming cells in irradiated mice given bone marrow and thymus or thoracic duct lymphocytes, *J. Exp. Med.* **128**:821.

Mitchison, N. A., 1971, The relative ability of T and B lymphocytes to see protein antigen, in: *Cell Interactions and Receptor Antibodies in Immune Responses* (O. Mäkelä, A. Cross, and T. U. Kosunen, eds.), pp. 149–160, Academic Press, New York.

Mitchison, N. A., Taylor, R., and Rajewski, K., 1970, Cooperation of antigenic determinants in the induction of antibodies, in: *Developmental Aspects of Antibody Formation and Structure* (J. Sterzl, ed.), pp. 547–561, Czechoslovakian Academy of Science, Prague.

Mohan, R., 1978, Ph.D. thesis, Madurai University, Madurai, India.

Moticka, E. J., Brown, B. A., and Cooper, E. L., 1973, Immunoglobulin synthesis in bullfrog larvae, *J. Immunol.* **110**:855.

Muthukkaruppan, V. R., Pitchappan, R. M., and Ramila, G., 1976, Thymic dependence and regulation of the immune response to sheep erythrocytes in the lizard, in: *Phylogeny of Thymus and Bone Marrow-Bursa Cells* (R. K. Wright and E. L. Cooper, eds.), pp. 185–193, Elsevier North-Holland, Amsterdam.

Nossal, G. J. V., Cunningham, A., Mitchell, G. F., and Miller, J. F. A. P., 1968, Cell to cell interaction in the immune response. III. Chromosomal marker analysis of single antibody forming cells in reconstituted irradiated or thymectomized mice, *J. Exp. Med.* **128**:839.

Ortiz-Muniz, G., and Sigel, M. M., 1971, Antibody synthesis in lymphoid organs of two marine teleosts, *J. Retic. Endoth. Soc.* **9**:42.

Pross, S. H., and Rowlands, D. T., 1975, Immunity in the developing amphibian, *Adv. Exp. Med. Biol.* **64**:373.

Rajewski, K., Schirrmacher, V., Nase, S., and Jerne, N. K., 1969, The requirement of more than one antigenic determinant for immunogenicity, *J. Exp. Med.* **129**:1131.

Reddy, A. L., and Wright, R. K., 1975, Synergistic and antagonistic effects of mitogens on proliferation of lymphocytes from spleens of *Rana pipiens*, *Adv. Exp. Med. Biol.* **64**: 335.

Ruben, L. N., 1975, Ontogeny, phylogeny and cellular cooperation, *Am. Zool.* **15**:93.

Ruben, L. N., 1976, The phylogeny of cell–cell cooperation in immunity, in: *Comparative Immunology* (J. J. Marchalonis, ed.), pp. 120–166, Blackwell, Oxford.

Ruben, L. N., and Edwards, B. F., 1976, The inference of lymphoid cell heterogeneity in the newt *Triturus viridescens* from hapten-carrier antigen binding studies, in: *Phylogeny of Thymus and Bone Marrow-Bursa Cells* (R. K. Wright and E. L. Cooper, eds.), pp. 161–168, Elsevier North-Holland Biomedical Press, Amsterdam.

Ruben, L. N., and Edwards, B. F., 1977, Phenotypic restriction of antigen-binding specificity on immunized amphibian spleen cells, *Cell. Immunol.* **33**:437.

Ruben, L. N., and Edwards, B. F., 1978, The visualization of bispecific immunized splenocytes of the newt, *Triturus viridescens*, *J. Dev. Comp. Immunol.* **2**:175.

Ruben, L. N., and Gwinnell, E., 1977, The effects of hydrocortisone and bacterial lipopolysaccharide on the anti-erythrocyte response in the spleens of adult *Triturus viridescens*, *J. Exp. Zool.* **200**:137.

Ruben, L. N., and Selker, E. U., 1975, Polyfunctional antigen-binding specificity in hapten-carrier responses of the newt, *Triturus viridescens*, *Adv. Exp. Med. Biol.* **64**:387.

Ruben, L. N., Stevens, J. M., and Kidder, G. M., 1972, Suppression of the allograft response by implants of mature lymphoid tissues in larval *Xenopus laevis*, *J. Morphol.* **138**:457.

Ruben, L. N., van der Hoven, A., and Dutton, R. W., 1973, Cellular cooperation in hapten-carrier responses in the newt (*Triturus viridescens*), *Cell. Immunol.* **6**:300.

Ruben, L. N., Clothier, R. H., Hodgson, R., and Balls, M., 1977*a*, The *in vitro* reconstitution of a thymus cell dependent humoral immune response in spleens of thymectomized *Xenopus laevis* with allogeneic thymocytes, in: *Developmental Immunobiology* (J. B. Horton, eds.), pp. 277–282, Elsevier North-Holland, Amsterdam.

Ruben, L. N., Edwards, B. F., and Rising, J., 1977*b*, Temperature variation and the function of complement and antibody in amphibia, *Experientia* **33**:1522.

Ruben, L. N., Warr, G. W., Decker, J. M., and Marchalonis, J. J., 1977*c*, Phylogenetic origins of immune recognition: Lymphoid heterogeneity and the hapten/carrier effect in the goldfish, *Carassius auratus*, *Cell. Immunol.* **31**:266.

Sailendri, K., 1973, Ph.D. thesis, Madurai University, Madurai, India.

Segal, S., Cohen, I. R., and Feldman, M., 1972, Thymus-derived lymphocytes: Humoral and cellular reactions distinguished by hydrocortisone, *Science* **175**:1126.

Sinclair, N. R., and Elliott, E. V., 1968, Neonatal thymectomy and decrease in antigen-sensitivity of the primary response and immunological "memory" systems, *Immunology* **15**:325.

Stobo, J. D., and Paul, W. E., 1973, Functional heterogeneity of murine lymphoid cells. III. Differential responsiveness of T cells to phytohemagglutinin and concanavalin A as a probe for T cell subsets, *J. Immunol.* **110**:362.

Stolen, J. S., and Mäkelä, O., 1976, Cell collaboration in a marine fish: The effect of carrier preimmunization on the anti-hapten response to NIP and NNP, in: *Phylogeny of Thymus and Bone Marrow-Bursa Cells* (R. K. Wright and E. L. Cooper, eds.), pp. 93–97, Elsevier North-Holland, Amsterdam.

Tam, M. R., Reddy, A. L., Karp, R. D., and Hildemann, W. H., 1976, Phylogeny of cellular immunity among vertebrates, in: *Comparative Immunology* (J. J. Marchalonis, ed.), pp. 98–119, Blackwell, Oxford.

Thoenes, G. H., and Hildemann, W. H., 1970, Immunological responses of Pacific hagfish. II. Serum antibody production to soluble antigen, in: *Developmental Aspects of Antibody Formation and Structure* (J. Sterzl, ed.), pp. 711–722, Czechoslavakian Academy of Science, Prague.

Tochinai, S., 1976, Demonstration of thymus-independent immune response in *Xenopus laevis:* Response to polyvinylpyrrolide, *Immunology* **31**:125.

Tochinai, S., and Katagiri, C., 1975, Complete abrogation of the immune response to skin allografts and rabbit erythrocytes in the early thymectomized *Xenopus*, *Dev. Growth Different.* **17**:383.

Tochinai, S., Nagata, S., and Katagiri, C., 1976, Restoration of immune responsiveness in early thymectomized *Xenopus* by implanation of histocompatible adult thymus, *Eur. J. Immunol.* **6**:711.

Tournefier, A., 1976, Ph.D. thesis, Université Pierre et Marie Curie, Paris.

Trizio, D., and Cudkowicz, G., 1978, The effect of selective T cell priming on anti-sheep and anti-hapten humoral responses. II. Separation by nylon-wool columns of the activated lymphocytes, *J. Immunol.* **120**:1028.

Volpe, E. P., Tompkins, R., and Reinschmidt, D., 1977, Experimental studies on the embryonic derivation of thymic lymphocytes, in: *Developmental Immunobiology* (J. B. Solomon and J. D. Horton, eds.), pp. 109–114, Elsevier North-Holland, Amsterdam.

Warner, N. L., Szenberg, A., and Burnet, F. M., 1962, The immunological role of different lymphoid organs in the chicken. I. Dissociation of immunological responsiveness, *Aust. J. Exp. Biol. Med. Sci.* **40**:373.

Warr, G. W., and Marchalonis, J. J., 1977, Lymphocyte surface immunoglobulin of the goldfish differs from its serum counter part, *J. Dev. Comp. Immunol.* **1**:15.

Warr, G. W., Deluca, D., and Marchalonis, J. J., 1976, Phylogenetic origins of immune recognition: Lymphocyte surface immunoglobulins in the goldfish, *Carassius auratus*, *Proc. Natl. Acad. Sci. USA* **73**:2476.

Warr, G. W., DeLuca, D., Decker, J. M., Marchalonis, J. J., and Ruben, L. N., 1977, Lymphoid heterogeneity in teleost fish: Studies on the genus *Carassius*, in: *Developmental Immunobiology* (J. B. Solomon and J. D. Horton, eds.), pp. 241–248, Elsevier North-Holland, Amsterdam.

Weiss, E., and Avtalion, R. R., 1977, Regulatory effects of temperature and antigen upon immunity in ectothermic vertebrates. II. Primary enhancement of the anti-hapten antibody response at high and low temperatures, *J. Dev. Comp. Immunol.* **1**:93.

Wright, R. K., and Cooper, E. L., 1977, Lymphocyte activation: Effects of temperature on polyclonal expansion of anuran amphibian (*Rana pipiens*) lymphocytes, in: *Developmental Immunobiology* (J. B. Solomon and J. D. Horton, eds.), pp. 249–258, Elsevier North-Holland, Amsterdam.

Yocum, D., Cuchens, M., and Clem, L. W., 1975, The hapten-carrier effect in teleost fish, *J. Immunol.* **114**:925.

Zaalberg, O. B., 1964, A simple method of detecting single antibody forming cells, *Nature* **202**:1231.

*Chapter 4*

# *Lymphoid-Cell Cooperation in Immune Responses of the Chicken*

**G. Jeanette Thorbecke, Michael A. Palladino, and Stephen P. Lerman**

*Department of Pathology*
*New York University School of Medicine*
*New York, New York 10016*

Our knowledge of cellular interactions in the immune response of chickens is in a primitive stage as compared with the degree of sophistication with which such interactions are being interpreted for mouse cells. Relatively little use has been made of the unique position that the bursa occupies in the ontogeny of B cells, as initially shown by the experiments on bursectomy by Glick *et al.* (1956), Mueller *et al.* (1960), and Warner *et al.* (1962). Although there is still some difference of opinion about this (Jankovic *et al.*, 1975), it seems likely that the chicken has no other source of virgin B cells (Kincade *et al.*, 1973) and that the bursa is, from approximately day 13 until day 19 of ontogeny, the only site of B-cell formation and Ig synthesis (Thorbecke *et al.*, 1968; Kincade and Cooper, 1971). The lymphoid follicles in the bursa arise from the influx of hematopoietic cells into the epithelial site near the cloaca (Moore and Owen, 1965, 1966). This influx starts during the 8th day and continues until at least the 15th day of incubation (Houssaint *et al.*, 1976). Once cells have differentiated in the bursa, they have different surface antigens from those of cells in the thymus (Albini and Wick, 1974; Galton and Ivanyi, 1977; Donnelly *et al.*, 1975; McArthur *et al.*, 1971; Forget *et al.*, 1970), are slightly larger (Sherman and Auerbach, 1966), and have a somewhat different chromatin distribution (Olson *et al.*, 1973).

Various experimental results indicate that T-B-cell interactions in the chicken are needed for the primary antibody response to some antigens and not to others. The first data suggesting this were obtained with intraperitoneal bursa-cell trans-

**Table I. Ability of i.p.-Injected 1-2 × $10^8$ Cells from Various Lymphoid Organs of 4-Week-Old Chickens to Transfer Antibody Responses to Different Antigens[a]**

| Cells transferred | Primary responses | | | | Secondary[b] responses | |
|---|---|---|---|---|---|---|
| | BA | SE | Ferritin | Bov. γ-glob. | BA | SE |
| Bursa | ++ | – | – | – | ++ | ± |
| Spleen | ++ | ++ | + | + | ++++ | +++ |
| Thymus | ± | – | – | – | ++ | + |
| Bone marrow | tr | – | N.D. | N.D. | N.D. | N.D. |

[a]Donors immunized by i.v. injection of *Brucellus abortus* or SE, 7–17 days prior to transfer.
[b]Results summarized from Gilmour *et al.* (1970) and W. P. McArthur and G. J. Thorbecke (unpublished observations). Recipient serums titrated for antibody 7 days after transfer.

fer and antigen challenge in X-irradiated immature recipients. Bursa cells from young (⩽4-weeks-old) donors transferred a higher response to *Brucellus abortus* (BA) than did an equal number of spleen cells, while spleen but not bursa cells transferred a response to sheep erythrocytes (SE). Neither thymus nor bone-marrow cells transferred much of a response to these antigens (Table I). When responses to other antigens were studied, it was found that protein antigens in general could induce a response in spleen but not bursa cells (W. P. McArthur, D. G. Gilmour, and G. J. Thorbecke, unpublished observations).

After a primary injection of BA into donor chickens the responsiveness of spleen cells increased much more than that of bursa cells, and thymus cells also became able to transfer antibody production. Similarly, both thymus and bursa cells from chickens primed to SE transferred antibody production to this antigen, but spleen cells were still much more effective. These findings were interpreted as showing that bursa could by itself transfer responses to BA, a thymus-independent antigen, whereas both thymus-derived and bursa-derived cells were needed for the response to SE and protein antigens. The results obtained with transfer of secondary responses illustrated the enormous degree of cross-contamination of thymus with B cells and of bursa with T cells, as well as the presence of primed B cells in all the lymphoid organs of primed chickens.

Simultaneous experiments in the mouse showed very similar results for the BA and SE antigens, in that the adoptive primary and secondary responses of spleen cells to BA were just as good in the presence as in the absence of T cells (Takahashi *et al.*, 1971*a*), while both primary and secondary responses to SE were markedly decreased after treatment with anti-Thy 1.2 + C. These experiments were summarized in Table II for comparison with Table III, presenting data for chicken experiments in which use was made of rabbit antisera to chicken T and B cells (described by McArthur *et al.*, 1971; Thorbecke *et al.*, 1971). Pretreatment of spleen cells with anti-T + C greatly reduced the ability of the chicken spleen cells to respond to SE both *in vitro* and upon transfer to

**Table II. Effect of Antisera to Mouse T Cells (Anti-THY 1.2), Plasma Cells Anti-PC 1), or Mouse IG + C on Ability of Primed Mouse Spleen Cells to Give Secondary Responses to Sheep Erythrocytes and *B. abortus* *in Vitro* and *in Vivo*[a]**

| Incubation medium[b] | % Cytotoxicity | | Antibody response[c,d] | | |
|---|---|---|---|---|---|
| | Spleen cells | Indirect PFC | $10^7$ cells per dish SE | i.v. transfer of 1–2 × $10^7$ cells/recipient SE | i.v. transfer of 1–2 × $10^7$ cells/recipient BA |
| Normal MS + C | <10 | 0 | 100% (2,000–16,500 IPFC/dish) | 100% (73–75 × $10^3$ IPFC/spleen) | 100% ($\log_2$ = 7.2 serum titer) |
| R. anti-mouse Ig + C | 50 | | 7–40% | 17–28% | 74% |
| Anti-PC-1 + C | <10 | 81 | | 100% | |
| Anti-thy 1.2 + C | 30 | N.D. | 2–12% | <1 | 98% |

[a] Data summarized from Takahashi *et al.* (1970, 1971) and Mond *et al.* (1972).
[b] BALB/c mice; recipients were X-irradiated one day prior to transfer (650 R).
[c] PFC/dish determined on day 4 of culture; PFC/spleen and anti-BA agglutinin titers on day 7 after transfer.
[d] SE, sheep erythrocytes; BA, *B. abortus.*

irradiated recipients, whereas the response to BA remained unaffected. The specificity of the antisera was illustrated by their ability to kill a large percentage of spleen cells without affecting PFC, similar to the effect of anti-Thy 1.2 + C on mouse spleen cells (Takahashi *et al.*, 1970*b*). Pretreatment of mouse spleen cells with anti-PC.1 + C, a serum specific for a plasma-cell antigen, did not affect the ability of spleen cells to transfer either response, but caused killing of PFC (Takahashi *et al.*, 1970*a,b*). This was somewhat different from the effect of anti-bursa serum + C on chicken spleen cells, which affected both PFC and to some extent the response to SE (Thorbecke *et al.*, 1971). The effect of pretreatment with anti-Ig + C was quite similar for the two species (Mond *et al.*, 1972; Takahashi *et al.*, 1971*b*; Thorbecke *et al.*, 1971; McArthur *et al.*, 1971).

The effect of thymectomy (TX) in the chicken was relatively difficult to study in view of the frequency with which thymic remnants remained (Graetzer *et al.*, 1963). Reports have appeared showing an inhibiting effect of TX on antibody production, but the investigators usually needed a combination of TX with irradiation or with duck antilymphocyte serum to obtain the effect (Ivanyi and Salerno, 1971; Rouse and Warner, 1972; Cooper *et al.*, 1966).

The formal proof that thymus and bursa cells needed to cooperate in the response to SE came later, also from transfer experiments. The positive interaction could not be shown readily with intraperitoneal transfer (Hala, 1973; Gilmour *et al.*, 1970), but was particularly clear when 1- to 2-week-old donors were used for both thymus and bursa cells and $10^7$ cells of each were transferred

**Table III. Effect of Rabbit Antiserums to Chicken Thymus, Bursa, or Ig + C on Ability of Chicken Spleen Cells to Give Immune Responses to Sheep Erythrocytes and *B. abortus***

| Incubation medium[a] | % Cytotoxicity[b] | | | Antibody response | | |
|---|---|---|---|---|---|---|
| | Spleen cells | PFC Direct | PFC Indirect | $10^7$ cells/dish[c] in vitro SE | i.v. transfer of $10^7$ cells/recipient[d] SE | i.v. transfer of $10^7$ cells/recipient[d] BA |
| Normal RS + C | <10 | 0 | 0 | 100% (550–3000 IPFC per dish) | 100% (2000–2600 IPFC per dish) | 100% ($\log_2$ = 3.8 serum titer) |
| R-anti-chick L chain + C | 33 | 77 | 44 | 2–20% | | |
| R-anti-chick-Ig + C | 40 | 69 | 32 | 3% | N.D. | 100% |
| R-anti-bursa #1 + C | 28 | 33 | 72 | 20–44% | 17% | 100% |
| R-anti-bursa #2 + C | 38 | 22 | 65 | 46% | | |
| R-anti-thymus #1 + C | 52 | 10 | 12 | 0–23% | 7% | 92% |
| R-anti-thymus #2 + C | 57 | 10 | 11 | 2% | | |

[a] Antiserum treatment of $10^7$ cells/ml for 1 hr at 37°C at 1:20 final dilution, with guinea pig C at 1:12. Data from McArthur *et al.* (1971) and Thorbecke *et al.* (1971).
[b] Results of several experiments; spleen cells taken 5–10 days after i.v. injection of SE. Indirect to direct PFC ratio ranged from 10 to 25.
[c] Ranges given for results of 3–4 experiments. PFC determined on day 4 of culture. Primed spleen cells taken for culture on days 7–10 after i.v. injection of 0.2 ml 20% SE.
[d] Spleen cells taken from 4-week-old chickens, challenged in recipients either with 0.1 ml 20% SE or with $4 \times 10^8$ killed *B. abortus* organisms. Results are expressed as $\log_2$ serum agglutinin titers (for BA) or as indirect PFC per spleen (for SE) on day 7 after transfer.

intravenously. The data indicated that addition of $2 \times 10^7$ irradiated spleen cells (McArthur *et al.*, 1973) or $1.5 \times 10^6$ bone-marrow cells to the thymus + bursa mixtures allowed better results, suggesting that a relative deficit of a macrophagelike (A-cell) component in neonatal irradiated recipients was limiting the height of the response (Table IV). Filtering of the irradiated spleen cells through cotton removed their activity on T-B-cell cooperation.

This approach also allowed the examination of bone marrow for the presence of B-cell precursors. It was found that bone marrow and thymus did cooperate in the response to SE, but only when bone marrow was taken from donors more than 1 week of age (Table IV). Since bursa cells taken from 1-week-old donors responded, it was concluded that bone marrow B cells might be

**Table IV. Synergism between Transferred Thymus and Bone Marrow or Bursa Cells in the Splenic PFC Response to Sheep Erythrocytes**

| Donor age (days) | Cells transferred[a] ($\times 10^{-6}$) | | | Mean of geom. means ± S.E. PFC/SPL in recipients[b] of | | | | | Number of expts.[c] |
|---|---|---|---|---|---|---|---|---|---|
| | Thy | BM | BU | Thy | BM | BU | BM + T | BU + T | |
| 6–7 | 9 | 45 | | 1 | 1 | | 2 | | 2 |
| 14–26 | 4.5–18 | 18–45 | | 12 ± 4 | 32 ± 19 | | 403 ± 159 | | 6 |
| 6–7 | 9–10 | | 7.5–9 | 1 | | 3 | | 32 | 2 |
| 12–16 | 9–10 | | 7.5–12 | 7 ± 2 | | 80 ± 45 | | 567 ± 274 | 6 |
| 12–18 | 9–10 | 1.5 | 7.5–12 | 38 ± 23 | | 36 ± 3 | | 3898 ± 2470 | 3 |

[a] Cells were injected i.v. together with 0.2 ml 20% SE on day 0. A second dose of SE was given on day 3 and recipient spleens were assayed for PFC on day 7.
[b] 3- to 7-day-old recipients were used that had been treated with cyclophosphamide at hatching and received gamma irradiation (660 R) on the day of cell transfer.
[c] Data summarized from McArthur *et al.* (1973).

bursa-derived. A similar conclusion has been reached by Eskola and Tiovanen (1976).

Studies by Sarvas *et al.* (1974) have shown that priming with small doses of carrier protein in complete Freund's adjuvant (CFA) could increase the subsequent humoral response to hapten presented on that carrier in the chicken, just as was described originally for the mouse by Rajewsky (1971). The possibility of obtaining helper cells from totally agammaglobulinemic (A$\gamma$) donors made the chicken an attractive species with which to study further the nature of the carrier effect, shown in the mouse by Mitchison (1971) to be the result of T-cell priming. Spleen cells taken from A$\gamma$ animals that had been sensitized with bovine serum albumin (BSA) and CFA allowed spleen cells from normal chickens preimmunized to trinitrophenylated hemocyanin (TNP-KLH) to respond to challenge with TNP-BSA in recipients, as determined both by height of splenic PFC response and by 2- to 3-log differences in serum titers to TNP in recipients (Table V). In view of the complete absence of B cells in the primed T-cell donors, any contribution of antibody to the carrier protein in this T-B cell cooperation was formally excluded by these results.

The induction of delayed hypersensitivity (DH) in the chicken follows rules similar to those observed in other species. Presentation of the antigen with CFA is virtually obligatory for obtaining a good DH response. Recently, however, Palladino *et al.* (1978) have been able to obtain a certain degree of sensitization for DH to the protein antigen human Ig (HGG) by presentation in incom-

**Table V. Cooperation in Irradiated Recipients between Transferred TNP-KLH-Immune B Cells and BSA- or HGG-Immune T Cells**

| Cells[a] transferred | Geometric mean PFC/spleen $\overset{\times}{\div}$ S.E.[b] | | | |
|---|---|---|---|---|
| | Expt. 1[c] | Expt. 2[c] | Expt. 3[d] | Expt. 4[d] |
| B cells (1–2 × $10^7$) | 7 $\overset{\times}{\div}$ 2.6 | 135 $\overset{\times}{\div}$ 6.3 | 316 $\overset{\times}{\div}$ 1.6 | 16 $\overset{\times}{\div}$ 2.5 |
| $T_H$ cells (2–3 × $10^7$) | 2 $\overset{\times}{\div}$ 1.7 | 14 $\overset{\times}{\div}$ 3.3 | | |
| B + $T_H$ cells | 565 $\overset{\times}{\div}$ 1.5 | 4441 $\overset{\times}{\div}$ 1.3 | 2512 $\overset{\times}{\div}$ 1.4 | 1995 $\overset{\times}{\div}$ 1.4 |
| B + $T_{Tol.}$ cells | | | 200 $\overset{\times}{\div}$ 1.8 | 20 $\overset{\times}{\div}$ 2.2 |

[a] In expts. 1 and 2, helper cells ($T_H$) were spleen cells from BSA + CFA-sensitized A$\gamma$ chickens, and the challenging antigen was $TNP_{13}$-BSA; in expts. 3 and 4 helper cells came from HGG + CFA-sensitized A$\gamma$ chickens and the challenging antigen was $TNP_8$-HGG. Chickens injected with HGG i.v., followed by HGG + CFA 1 week later, donated the tolerant cells ($T_{Tol.}$). All $T_H$-cell donors had been tested and were positive for delayed hypersensitivity to either BSA or HGG, while $T_{Tol.}$ donors were negative. Normal chickens immunized with $TNP_{8-11}$-KLH i.v. donated the immune B cells. Donors and recipients were strain 96 in expts. 1 and 2, and strain FP in expts. 3 and 4.

[b] PFC (indirect) per spleen were determined on day 5–7 after transfer.

[c] Data from Weinbaum *et al.* (1973).

[d] Data from Grebenau and Thorbecke (1978).

plete adjuvant containing peptidoglycan, an *Escherichia coli* constituent, or the water-soluble *N*-acetylmuramyl-L-ala-D-glu-α-$NH_2$ (Adam *et al.*, 1973). Both of these agents can also serve as substitutes for mycobacteria in the induction of DH in guinea pigs (Fleck *et al.*, 1974).

It was noted that the ability of chickens to give DH reactions to BSA in their wattles correlated with their ability to show BSA-specific T-helper activity in their spleen cells. More recent studies in this laboratory have shown that i.v. injection of HGG prior to sensitization to HGG in CFA prevented the protection of DH as well as of specific helper T cells to this antigen (Grebenau and Thorbecke, 1978). However, spleen cells taken 1 week after i.v. injection of HGG did not suppress help afforded by spleen cells from chickens with DH to HGG. In fact, such spleen cells sometimes provided TNP-primed B cells with a low degree of carrier help. Thus, tolerization by i.v. injection of HGG appeared to lead to a deletion of T cells responsible for DH and for carrier help in the absence of demonstrable suppressor cells (Grebenau *et al.*, 1979).

A T-cell-tolerizing i.v. injection of 5-50 mg ultracentrifuged HGG into normal chickens led to primary anti-HGG 19 S antibody production within 1 week. Further challenge with 0.2 mg HGG in CFA, which in control animals induced high titers of both 7 S and 19 S anti-HGG, caused a reduction rather than a rise in the antibody of the i.v.-injected chickens (Grebenau and Thorbecke, 1978). Thus, while antibody production could apparently be initiated in the relative absence of T help, the humoral response could not be maintained and 7 S antibody levels remained minimal. This is in agreement with findings in mice, which may give fair primary responses but never good secondary responses or high-titered 7 S antibody in the relative absence of T help (reviewed and discussed in Mond *et al.*, 1974, and Thorbecke and Lerman, 1976). Previous studies in this laboratory have emphasized germinal-center production, particularly in the mouse and rabbit, and its relationship to memory-B-cell formation (Thorbecke and Lerman, 1976). The complete dependency of germinal center and memory-B-cell formation on thymus help was clearly shown by studies on thymusless mice (Jacobson *et al.*, 1974). This particular form of T-B interaction has received relatively little attention, but may be of paramount importance for the generation of 7 S antibody formation and for the expression of B-cell memory.

Studies by Toivanen *et al.* (1974, 1977) indicated that T-B-cell interaction might also be of great importance for germinal-center formation in the chicken, since reconstitution of cyclophosphamide-treated chickens with bursa cells—with respect to bursa-follicle, germinal-center, and plasma-cell production 4 weeks later—could be accomplished only in syngeneic, not allogeneic, 4-day-old recipients. When thymus cells of the same donor strain were given along with the bursa cells, germinal-center production and secondary antibody production (Toivanen and Toivanen, 1977) could be shown even in allogeneic recipients, suggesting that syngeneic T and B cells needed to interact for the production of these splenic centers of B-cell proliferation. Recent experiments in our laboratory suggest that transferred bursa cells, upon stimulation with the T-independent antigen BA, can produce germinal centers in syngeneic recipients within 1 to 2 weeks after transfer, but only when a source of T helper cells is present (Chi *et al.*, unpublished observations). This production of germinal centers, as in mice, appears correlated with the ability to give secondary, 19 S + 7 S, antibody responses to BA.

One aspect of T-B-cell interaction *in vivo* appears somewhat different in the chicken than in the mouse. It is known in the mouse that free carrier either interferes with or does not affect the immune response to hapten or another carrier, whether cross-reacting or not (Mitchison, 1971; Weinbaum *et al.*, 1974). In the chicken we have done studies in which BSA-primed Aγ-donor spleen cells were transferred together with TNP-KLH-primed spleen cells and challenged by TNP or other albumins with and without added BSA (Table VI). It was shown that while TNP-HSA did not itself challenge a good memory response under these conditions, the combination of BSA and TNP-HSA did (Lerman, Weinbaum, and Thorbecke, unpublished observations). A curious aspect of these results was that BSA, added to a non-cross-reacting hapten conjugate such as TNP-ovalbumin or TNP-mouse albumin, did not raise the response. These preliminary findings suggest that the chicken might be a good species in which to search for a humoral factor mediating T-B-cell cooperation *in vivo*.

The ability of T cells from Aγ donors, sensitized to BSA, to recognize and respond to a variety of cross-reacting serum albumins was also investigated (Ler-

**Table VI. Cooperation in Recipients between Transferred TNP-KLH-Immune B Cells and BSA-Immune T Cells to Various TNP-Albumin Conjugates: Effect of Added BSA[a]**

| Cells[b] transferred | Challenge antigen(s) | Geometric mean PFC/spleen on day 7 $\times\!\!\div$ S.E. | | |
|---|---|---|---|---|
| | | Expt. 1 | Expt. 2 | Expt. 3 |
| B cells | TNP-BSA | 275 $\times\!\!\div$ 1.9 | 3 $\times\!\!\div$ 3.5 | 18 $\times\!\!\div$ 1.7 |
| B + T cells | TNP-BSA | 8,812 $\times\!\!\div$ 1.3 | 758 $\times\!\!\div$ 1.4 | 1,318 $\times\!\!\div$ 2.2 |
| B + T cells | TNP-HSA | 2,754 $\times\!\!\div$ 1.3 | 158 $\times\!\!\div$ 2.9 | |
| B + T cells | TNP-HSA + BSA | 10,232 $\times\!\!\div$ 1.4 | 1,820 $\times\!\!\div$ 1.4 | |
| B + T cells | TNP-OV | | 31 $\times\!\!\div$ 3.0 | 17 $\times\!\!\div$ 2.2 |
| B + T cells | TNP-OV + BSA | | 112 $\times\!\!\div$ 1.9 | 11 $\times\!\!\div$ 3.0 |
| B + T cells | TNP-MSA | | | 91 $\times\!\!\div$ 3.1 |
| B + T cells | TNP-MSA + BSA | | | 26 $\times\!\!\div$ 4.2 |

[a] Donors and recipients were from strain 96. Recipients irradiated (660 R) 1 day prior to transfer.

[b] B cells: 5–10 × $10^6$ TNP-KLH-immune spleen cells from normal chickens. T cells: 1.6–2 × $10^7$ BSA-immune spleen cells from agammaglobulinemic chickens.

man, Weinbaum, Gilmour, Butchko, Thorbecke, and Nisonoff, unpublished observations). Methods used in this study were similar to those used in a parallel study in mice (Weinbaum *et al.*, 1974). The results are presented in Table VII. Although slight differences were found, the results indicated a striking similarity in the degree with which chicken serum anti-BSA interacted with the various albumins tested, and the degree to which BSA-primed T cells responded with a helper effect on TNP-primed B cells upon challenge with TNP albumins. This result was comparable to that of the parallel study in mice and suggested a fine degree of specific recognition at the level of the T cell in the chicken, as in mammals. The discriminatory capacity of T-cell receptors and its similarity to that of serum antibody were discussed in detail elsewhere (Weinbaum *et al.*, 1974).

In the studies on T-B-cell interaction mentioned above, T cells from Aγ birds were usually the source of "helper" T cells. It should be noted that caution has to be exerted in this type of cooperation experiment to avoid the now well-documented suppressor effect that Aγ spleen cells may exert on B cells (Blaese *et al.*, 1974; Palladino *et al.*, 1976; Grebenau *et al.*, 1976). In assays of suf-

**Table VII. Cross-reactivity of Chicken Anti-Bovine Serum Albumin[a] with Various Heterologous Albumins: Comparison with Cross-reactivity at the T-Cell Level**

| | Chicken anti-BSA[b] | | |
|---|---|---|---|
| Albumin | Binding capacity for [$^{125}$I]albumin (μg/ml) | 30% inhibition of [$^{125}$I]-BSA binding (μg required) | Ability of TNP albumins[c] to challenge BSA-sensitized T cells % of PFC response to TNP-BSA |
| Bovine | 108 | <0.1 | 100 |
| Sheep | 24 | 1.0 | >100 |
| Goat | | 2.5 | 31 |
| Rabbit | 11 | 3.5 | |
| Horse | 0.6 | 20 | |
| Pig | 8 | >20 | 62 |
| Human | 3 | >20 | 21 |
| Dog | 3 | >20 | 69 |
| Guinea pig | 0.1 | >20 | |
| Rat | 0.07 | >20 | |
| Mouse | <0.05 | >20 | 6 |
| Duck | <0.05 | >20 | 0 |

[a] Anti-BSA prepared by injection of 1 mg BSA in CFA i.m., followed 6–8 weeks later by i.v. challenge with 10 mg in saline. Chickens were bled 1 week after challenge.
[b] Interaction between 0.1 ml antiserum and 50 μl (0.125 μg) [$^{125}$I]-BSA. Methods as described in Weinbaum *et al.* (1974).
[c] Expressed as % of the PFC response obtained in recipient spleens 6 days after challenge by TNP-BSA of transferred TNP-KLH-sensitized B cells and BSA-sensitized T cells. Range for 100% was 408 to 8853 PFC/spleen.

ficiently short duration, and particularly when A$\gamma$ donors less than 4 months of age are used, the demonstration of helper effects is not noticeably influenced by this phenomenon. The tendency of A$\gamma$ spleen cells to suppress antibody and Ig production, however, becomes quite evident when such cells are transferred together with B cells (bursa or spleen) into irradiated recipients and the study of antibody production is extended over more than 1 week after transfer. Furthermore, when A$\gamma$ donors have previously been injected with a source of syngeneic B cells, their spleen-cell suppressive activity for antibody and Ig production can be detected within a few days after transfer together with B cells into recipients (Grebenau *et al.*, 1976). Further studies on this peculiar "autoimmunization" to B cells, which A$\gamma$ T cells appear to be prone to, go beyond the scope of this review and have been described elsewhere (Lerman *et al.*, 1978).

Another form of cellular interaction that has been noted in the chicken occurs during graft-versus-host (GVH) reactions. It has been shown that most of the mitotic activity leading to splenomegaly in embryos undergoing GVH reactions is due to host cells, possibly yolk-sac-derived stem cells (Walker *et al.*, 1973) that are recruited into the proliferative reaction induced by the injection of allogeneic adult peripheral-blood cells (Burnet and Boyer, 1961; Nisbet and Simonsen, 1967; Biggs and Payne, 1959; Weber, 1970). Experiments in this laboratory on irradiated $F_1$ hybrid mice undergoing GVH reaction after i.v. injection of parental lymph node cells have demonstrated that approximately 50% of the proliferating activity in host spleens, as judged by [$^3$H]thymidine incorporation, is due to non-T cells recruited into the response, although the reaction is clearly initiated by donor T cells, even when given after exposure to mitomycin C *in vitro* (Romano *et al.*, 1976). Similar experiments have been carried out using 2-week-old heavily irradiated FP chicks as recipients and SC spleen cells from adult donors for the induction of GVH reactions.* Untreated SC spleen cells ($2 \times 10^7$) cause significantly increased [$^3$H]thymidine incorporation in spleens of recipients by day 4 after injection (Table VIII, line 6). Mitomycin-C-treated SC spleen cells (mito. spl.) or spleen cells treated with anti-T + C usually do not raise the splenic [$^3$H]thymidine incorporation over that in uninjected controls (Table VIII, lines 2 and 3). However, the combination of these two treated-spleen-cell preparations causes a significant proliferative activity in recipient spleens (Table VIII, line 1). This can be interpreted as showing recruitment of non-T spleen cells into proliferation under the influence of mito. spl. The mito. spl. is just as active when taken from A$\gamma$ donors (Table VIII, expt. 5), suggesting the T-cell nature of the cells causing the recruitment. Mito.-thymus cells (not in table) also cause recruitment of anti-T + C-treated spleen cells, which is in agreement with the observation that thymus induces GVH in the chicken (Nisbet *et al.*, 1969). The recruited cell is obviously resistant to treatment with anti-T + C and cannot be demonstrated in bursa-cell suspensions

*FP strain = $B_{15}B_{21}$, SC strain = $B_2B_2$ chickens.

**Table VIII. Recruitment into Proliferation of Non-T Spleen but Not of Bursa Cells under Influence of Mitomycin-C-Treated SC Spleen Cells in Irradiated FP Recipients[a]**

| Donor cells[b] 2 × $10^7$, i.v., day 0 | Splenic [$^3$H]thymidine incorporation on day 4 (cpm)[c] | | | | |
|---|---|---|---|---|---|
| | Expt. 1 | Expt. 2 | Expt. 3 | Expt. 4 | Expt. 5 |
| Mito. spl. + anti-T + C spl. | 24,807 | 15,544 | | 14,855 | 11,450 |
| Mito. spl. | 18,293 | 8,654 | 13,105 | 7,589 | 7,427 |
| Anti-T + C spl. | 14,605 | 9,189 | | 4,809 | 9,987 |
| Bursa | 12,662 | 12,477 | 13,462 | 7,512 | |
| Mito. spl. + Bursa | 19,497 | 13,135 | 16,555 | 9,226 | |
| Untreated spl. | 31,268 | 32,397 | 37,944 | 29,445 | 20,030 |

[a] Recipients were exposed to 440 R (day −2), 825 R (day −1), and 715 R (day 0) gamma irradiation ($^{137}$Cs source).
[b] Normal SC spleen cells in all experiments except in expt. 5, in which Aγ spleen cells were used; mitomycin-C treatment was for 45 min at 37°C at 50 μg and $10^7$ cells/ml. Recruited anti-T-treated spleen or bursa cells were from FP chickens in expts. 1 and 2, and from SC chickens in other experiments; incubation with anti-T (1 : 75) and gp C (1 : 18) for 45 min at 37°C.
[c] 50 μC: [$^3$H]thymidine (0.36 C:/mM) injected i.p. 2 h before assay. Methods as described in Romano *et al.* (1976).

(Table VIII, line 5). It has been shown in other studies, however, that bursa cells are capable of causing increased splenic proliferation when exposed to dextran sulfate or *E. coli* endotoxin in recipients (data not shown; Palladino and Thorbecke, manuscript in preparation). Thus, the recruitment phenomenon is very similar in chickens to that observed in rodents, i.e., that caused by T cells and exerted on non-T cells (Howard *et al.*, 1961; Piquet *et al.*, 1977; Romano *et al.*, 1976; Rolstad, 1976). Another interesting feature of the results reported here is that mito.-SC spl. cells recruit anti-T + C-treated FP spl. cells as well as SC spl. cells, suggesting that histocompatibility at the major *B* locus is not needed for this recruitment to occur. This result was not unexpected in view of the obvious recruitment into chorioallantoic-pock formation occurring in embryos under the influence of allogeneic cells during GVH (Weber, 1970; Walker *et al.*, 1973). Further experiments are needed to analyze in more detail the nature of the recruitable cell in these experiments, whether a mature B cell (not present in bursa), a monocyte, or a null cell. Preliminary findings suggest the presence of the recruited cell in anti-T + C-treated spleen from Aγ chickens, strongly supportive of an important role for non-T, non-B cells in this recruitment phenomenon (Palladino *et al.*, 1980).

Recent experiments in this laboratory have established that interaction between T cells and monocytes appears to be extremely important for the expression of tumor immunity to transplantable carcinogen-induced fibrosarcomas in the chicken (Palladino and Thorbecke, 1978*b*). Data illustrating this type of cellular interaction are summarized in Tables IX and X. These studies were carried out in SC chickens with the use of histocompatible transplantable tumor lines (Lerman *et al.*, 1976), to which immunity could be generated with the aid of bacterial adjuvants such as *C. parvum* and BCG (Palladino and Thorbecke, 1978*a*). This immunity was tumor-line specific in a manner totally similar to that described for carcinogen-induced tumors in mice (Old *et al.*, 1962). Winn tests (Winn, 1961) in wing webs of recipients could be used to demonstrate adoptive immunity in spleen and peripheral blood cells from tumor-immune donors, whether Aγ or normal (Table IX). The cells responsible for this immunity were shown to be mitomycin-C-resistant, gamma-irradiation-sensitive peripheral T cells (Table IX, Palladino and Thorbecke, 1978*a*,*b*).

Since tumor-immune donors showed DH reactions to irradiated tumor cells, the immune T cell involved could be of the type mediating DH reactions. It was noted, in addition, that recipients contributed an important component to the tumor-growth inhibition in Winn tests. Trypan-blue-treated, silica-treated, or heavily irradiated recipients were not capable of supporting the expression of tumor immunity (Table X). Trypan blue was thought to act through inhibition of macrophage function, as was suggested by Hibbs (1976), and silica was shown

**Table IX. Identification and Properties of T Cells Mediating Adoptive Tumor Immunity to SCFS in Wing Webs of Normal SC Recipients**

| Immune cell source[a] | Pretreatment of immune cells *in vitro*[b] | Tumor growth on days 7–10 | |
|---|---|---|---|
| | | Tumor size ± S.E. (cm) | % sites with tumor (*n*) |
| None | | 0.78 ± 0.05 | 100 (30) |
| N1 peripheral blood | None | 0.31 ± 0.07 | 100 (4) |
| Aγ peripheral blood | None | 0.27 ± 0.04 | 100 (5) |
| Thymus | None | 0.80 ± 0.05 | 100 (8) |
| Aγ spleen | None | 0.07 ± 0.04 | 17 (18) |
| N1 spleen | None | 0.14 ± 0.05 | 45 (20) |
| | Mitomycin C | 0.00 ± 0.00 | 0 (5) |
| | 500–2000 R | 0.81 ± 0.04 | 100 (24) |
| | NRS + C | N.D. | 12.5 (8) |
| | Anti-T + C | N.D. | 100 (8) |
| | Nylon wool nonadh. | 0.04 ± 0.01 | 10 (10) |
| | Nylon wool adh. | 0.91 ± 0.07 | 100 (8) |

[a] $2 \times 10^7$ cells from N1 (*not* bursectomized) or Aγ chickens immunized to SCFS with the aid of *C. parvum* or BCG injected together with $10^6$ SCFS in wing web; spleen cells from unimmunized donors, or from donors immunized with *C. parvum* or BCG alone, did not affect tumor growth under these conditions.

[b] Mitomycin-C treatment was by incubation at 37°C for 45 min with 100 μg/ml; gamma irradiation dose rate: 630 R/min ($^{137}$Cs); NRS or anti-T used at 1:75, gpC at 1:18, and cells at $10^7$/ml for 45 min at 37°C; nylon wool column incubation in RPMI 1640 + 2% chicken serum for 45 min at 37°C.

**Table X. Effect of Monocyte Inhibition and Reconstitution in Host on the Ability to Support Adoptive Tumor Immunity to SCFS**

| Pretreatment of recipients[a] | Method of reconstitution[b] | Immune-donor T cells[c] added to SCFS in wing web | Tumor growth on day 7–10: Tumor size ± S.E. (cm) | Tumor growth on day 7–10: % sites with tumors ($n$) |
|---|---|---|---|---|
| None | None | – | 0.68 ± 0.09 | 100 (43) |
| | None | + | 0.11 ± 0.05 | 38 (50) |
| Trypan blue | None | + | 0.48 ± 0.03 | 100 (10) |
| Silica | None | + | 0.68 ± 0.02 | 100 (8) |
| Silica + PVNO | None | + | 0.29 ± 0.05 | 86 (14) |
| 1260 R gamma irradiation | None | + | 0.54 ± 0.03 | 100 (18) |
| | i.v. Aγ BM ($2 \times 10^8$) | + | 0.01 ± 0.00 | 18 (6) |
| | i.v. Aγ spl ($2 \times 10^8$) | + | 0.02 ± 0.02 | 16 (7) |
| | Wing-web Aγ spl ($4–20 \times 10^6$) | + | 0.14 ± 0.06 | 83 (6) |
| | Wing-web monocytes ($10^6$) | + | 0.11 ± 0.06 | 30 (10) |
| | None | – | 0.59 ± 0.04 | 100 (8) |

[a] Trypan blue: 5 mg i.v. day –3 and 2 × 5 mg i.v. day –1; silica: 2 × 3 mg i.v. day –1 and 0; PVNO: 150 mg/kg subc. day –2; gamma irradiation ($^{137}Cs$) 2 × 630 R days –3 and –2.

[b] i.v. injection of bone marrow (BM) or spleen (spl) cells from unimmunized Aγ donors on day –2, or of spleen or monocytes from Aγ donors together with SCFS and immune T cells in wing web.

[c] Nylon wool nonadherent spleen cells from tumor-immune donors used in most experiments; $1–2 \times 10^7$ injected with $10^6$ SCFS in wing web.

to act on macrophages by the observation that pretreatment with poly-2-vinyl pyridine-*N*-oxide (PVNO) protected against its effect. In addition, gamma irradiation also acted via monocyte inactivation, since the defect caused by irradiation was readily reconstituted by i.v., injection of spleen or bone-marrow cells from nonimmune A$\gamma$ donors, or by wing-web injection of isolated peripheral-blood monocytes at the time of the Winn test (Table X; for more details on experiments, see Palladino and Thorbecke, 1978*b*). Additional studies, not in the tables, showed clearly that local DH reactions to unrelated antigens, such as HGG or *C. parvum*, also caused a significant retardation, or in some cases permanent inhibition, of growth of $10^5$ SCFS* cells (Palladino and Thorbecke, 1978*c*). Thus, an interaction between DH-sensitive T cells and monocytes, such as described for mice in the response to viable intracellular microorganisms (Collins and Mackaness, 1970) and parasites (Remington *et al.*, 1972), and for DH reactions in general (Lubaroff and Waksman, 1968), appears also to occur in the chicken, and, at least in this SCFS model, is of importance for tumor-growth inhibition. The mechanism is likely to involve activation of macrophages that become either cytotoxic or cytostatic for tumor cells, as has been suggested to occur in mice (Hibbs, 1976). In agreement with the conclusion that T cell–monocyte interaction may be an important component of the immune response in the chicken is the report by Pierce and Long (1965) showing that TX inhibits development of immunity to infection with the parasite *Eimeria tenella* more than does BX, even though antibodies fail to develop in the BX chickens.

## ACKNOWLEDGMENTS

This work was supported by Grants AI-3076 and AI-14829 from the USPHS. Michael A. Palladino is a Fellow under USPHS Training Grant 5TO1-GM00127. Stephen P. Lerman is a Special Fellow of the Leukemia Society of America.

## REFERENCES

Adam, A., Ciorbaru, R., Petit, J. F., Lederer, E., Chedid, L., Lamensans, A., Parant, F., Parant, M., Rosselet, J. P., and Berger, F. M., 1973, Preparation and biological properties of water soluble adjuvant fractions from delipidated cells of *Mycobacterium smegmatis* and *Nocardia opaca*, *Infect. Immunol.* **7**:855.

Albini, B., and Wick G., 1974, Delineation of B and T lymphoid cells in the chicken, *J. Immunol.* **112**:444.

Biggs, P. M., and Payne, L. N., 1959, Cytological identification of proliferating donor cells in chick embryos injected with adult chicken blood, *Nature* **184**:1594.

*SCFS = carcinogen-induced transplantable fibrosarcoma in SC chickens.

Blaese, R. M., Weiden, P. L., Koski, I., and Dooley, N., 1974, Infectious agammaglobulinemia: transmission of immunodeficiency with grafts of agammaglobulinemic cells, *J. Exp. Med.* **140**:1097.

Burnet, F. M., and Boyer, G. S., 1961, The chorio-allantoic lesion in the Simonsen phenomenon, *J. Pathol. Bacteriol.* **81**:141.

Collins, F. M., and Mackaness, G. B., 1970, The relationship of delayed hypersensitivity to acquired anti-tuberculosis immunity. I. Tuberculin sensitivity and resistance to reinfection in BCG-vaccinated mice, *Cell Immunol.* **1**:253.

Cooper, M. D., Peterson, R. D. A., South, M. A., and Good, R. A., 1966, The functions of the thymus system and the bursa system in the chicken, *J. Exp. Med.* **123**:75.

Donnelly, N., Brand, A., and Gilmour, D. G., 1975, Bursal and thymic alloantigen expression in lymphoid tissues of the chicken, in: *Immunologic Phylogeny* (W. H. Hildemann and A. A. Benedict, eds.), pp. 293–302, Plenum Press, New York.

Eskola, J., and Toivanen, A., 1976, Cell transplantation into immunodeficient chicken embryos: Reconstituting capacity of cells from the bursa of Fabricius, spleen, bone marrow, thymus, and liver of 18-day-old embryos, *Cell. Immunol.* **26**:68.

Fleck, J., Mock, M., Tytgat, F., Nauciel, C., and Minck, R., 1974, Adjuvant activity in delayed hypersensitivity of the peptidic part of bacterial peptidoglycans, *Nature* **250**:517.

Forget, A., Potworowski, E. F., Richer, G., and Borduas, A. G., 1970, Antigenic specificities of bursal and thymic lymphocytes in the chicken, *Immunology* **19**:465.

Galton, J., and Ivanyi, J., 1977, Detection of bursa and thymus-specific alloantigens in the chicken, *Eur. J. Immunol.* **7**:457.

Gilmour, D. G., Theis, G. A., and Thorbecke, G. J., 1970, Transfer of antibody production with cells from bursa of Fabricius, *J. Exp. Med.* **132**:134.

Glick, B., Chang, T. S., and Jaap, R. G., 1956, The bursa of Fabricius and antibody production, *Poultry Sci.* **35**:224.

Graetzer, M. A., Wolfe, H. R., Aspinall, R. L., and Meyer, R. K., 1963, Effect of thymectomy and bursectomy on precipitin and natural hemagglutinin production in the chicken, *J. Immunol.* **90**:878.

Grebenau, M. D., and Thorbecke, G. J., 1978, T cell tolerance in the chicken. I. Parameters affecting tolerance induction to human $\gamma$-globulin in agammaglobulinemic and normal chickens, *J. Immunol.* **120**:1046.

Grebenau, M. D., Lerman, S. P., Palladino, M. A., and Thorbecke, G. J., 1976, Suppression of adoptive antibody responses by addition of spleen cells from agammaglobulinaemic chickens "immunised" with histocompatible bursa cells, *Nature* **260**:5546.

Grebenau, M. D., Chi, D. S., and Thorbecke, G. J., 1979, T cell tolerance in the chicken. II. Lack of evidence for suppressor cells in tolerant agammaglobulinemic and normal chickens, *Eur. J. Immunol.* **9**:477.

Hala, K., 1973, Adoptive transfer of antibody formation by various cell types in chickens and an attempt to demonstrate synergism, *Folia Biol.* **19**:262.

Hibbs, J. B., 1976, Role of activated macrophages in nonspecific resistance to neoplasia, *J. Reticuloendothel. Soc.* **20**:223.

Houssaint, E., Belo, M., and le Douarin, N. M., 1976, Investigations on cell lineage and tissue interactions in the developing bursa of Fabricius through interspecfic chimeras, *Dev. Biol.* **53**:250.

Howard, J. G., Michie, D., and Simonsen, M., 1961, Splenomegaly as a host response in graft-versus-host disease, *Br. J. Exp. Pathol.* **42**:478.

Ivanyi, J., and Salerno, A., 1971, Impairment of humoral antibody response in neonatally thymectomized and irradiated chickens, *Eur. J. Immunol.* **1**:227.

Jacobson, E. B., Caporale, L. H., and Thorbecke, G. J., 1974, Effect of thymus cell injections on germinal center formation in lymphoid tissues of nude (thymusless) mice, *Cell. Immunol.* **13**:416.

Jankovic, B. D., Knezevic, Z., Isakovic, K., Mitrovic, K., Markovic, B. M., and Rajcevic, M., 1975, Bursa lymphocytes and IgM-containing cells in chicken embryos bursectomized at 52–64 hours of incubation, *Eur. J. Immunol.* **5**:656.

Kincade, P. W., and Cooper, M. D., 1971, Development and distribution of immunoglobulin-containing cells in the chicken, *J. Immunol.* **106**:371.

Kincade, P. W., Self, K. S., and Cooper, M. D., 1973, Survival and function of bursa-derived cells in bursectomized chickens, *Cell. Immunol.* **8**:93.

Lerman, S. P., Palladino, M. A., and Thorbecke, G. J., 1976, Chemical carcinogen-induced transplantable fibrosarcomas in histocompatible chickens. I. Incidence of tumor induction in normal and bursectomized chickens, *J. Natl. Cancer Inst.* **57**:295.

Lerman, S. P., Grebenau, M. D., Palladino, M. A., Galton, J., Chi, D. S., and Thorbecke, G. J., 1978, The agammaglobulinemic chicken as a model for T-cell mediated B-cell suppression, in: *Comparative and Developmental Aspects of Immune Disease* (M. E. Gershwin and E. L. Cooper, eds.), pp. 110–121, Pergamon Press, Elmsford, NY.

Lubaroff, D. M., and Waksman, B. H., 1968, Bone marrow as source of cells in reactions of cellular hypersensitivity,. II. Identification of allogeneic or hybrid cells by immunofluorescence in passively transferred tuberculin reactions, *J. Exp. Med.* **128**:1437.

McArthur, W. P., Chapman, J., and Thorbecke, G. J., 1971, Immunocompetent cells of the chicken. I. Specific surface antigenic markers on bursa and thymus cells, *J. Exp. Med.* **134**:1036.

McArthur, W. P., Gilmour, D. G., and Thorbecke, G. J., 1973, Immunocompetent cells in the chicken. II. Synergism between thymus cells and either bursa or bone marrow cells in the humoral immune response to sheep erythrocytes, *Cell. Immunol.* 8:103.

Mitchison, N. A., 1971, The carrier effect in the secondary response to hapten–protein conjugates, *Eur. J. Immunol.* **1**:18.

Mond, J. J., Takahashi, T., and Thorbecke, G. J., 1972, Surface antigens of immunocompetent cells. III. In vitro studies of the role of B and T cells in immunological memory, *J. Exp. Med.* **136**:663.

Mond, J. J., Caporale, L. H., and Thorbecke, G. J., 1974, Kinetics of B cell memory development during a thymus "independent" immune response, *Cell Immunol.* **10**:105.

Moore, M. A. S., and Owen, J. J. T., 1965, Chromosome marker studies on the development of the hematopoietic system in the chick embryo, *Nature* **208**:956.

Moore, M. A. S., and Owen, J. J. T., 1966, Experimental studies on the development of the bursa of Fabricius, *Dev. Biol.* **14**:40.

Mueller, A. P., Wolfe, H. R., and Meyer, R. K., 1960, Precipitin production in chickens. XXI. Antibody production in bursectomized chickens and in chickens injected with 19-nortestosterone on the fifth day of incubation, *J. Immunol.* **85**:172.

Nisbet, N. W., and Simonsen, M., 1967, Primary immune response in grafted cells: Dissociation between the proliferation of activity and the proliferation of cells, *J. Exp. Med.* **125**:967.

Nisbet, N. W., Simonsen, M., and Zaleski, M., 1969, The frequency of antibody sensitive cells in tissue transplantation: a commentary of clonal selection, *J. Exp. Med.* **129**:459.

Old, L. J., Boyse, E. A., Clark, D. A., and Carswell, E. A., 1962, Antigenic properties of chemically induced tumors, *Ann. N.Y. Acad. Sci.* **101**:80.

Olson, G. B., Wied, G. L., and Bartels, P. H., 1973, Differentiation of chicken thymic and bursal lymphocytes by cell image analysis, *Acta Cytol.* **17**:454.

Palladino, M. A., and Thorbecke, G. J., 1978*a*, Immunity to transplantable carcinogen-induced fibrosarcomas in B2/B2 chickens. I. Use of bacterial adjuvants in induction of immunity demonstrable in Winn tests, *Cell. Immunol.* **38**:336.

Palladino, M. A., and Thorbecke, G. J., 1978*b*, Immunity to transplantable carcinogen-induced fibrosarcomas in B2/B2 chickens. II. Macrophage dependency of adoptive T cell mediated tumor immunity, *Cell. Immunol.* **38**:350.

Palladino, M. A., and Thorbecke, G. J., 1978*c*, Immunity to transplantable, carcinogen-induced fibrosarcomas in B2/B2 chickens. III. Tumor growth inhibition by local delayed hypersensitivity reactions to unrelated antigens, *Eur. J. Immunol.* **8**:257.

Palladino, M. A., Lerman, S. P., and Thorbecke, G. J., 1976, Transfer of hypogammaglobulinemia in two inbred chicken strains by spleen cells from bursectomized donors, *J. Immunol.* **116**:1673.

Palladino, M. A., Grebenau, M. D., and Thorbecke, G. J., 1978, Requirements for induction of delayed hypersensitivity in the chicken, *Dev. Comp. Immunol.* **2**:121.

Palladino, M. A., Blyznak, N., and Thorbecke, G. J., 1980, Recruitment of null cells during graft versus host reactions in the chicken, *Cell. Immunol.*, in press.

Pierce, A. E., and Long, P. L., 1965, Studies on acquired immunity to coccidiosis in bursaless and thymectomized fowls, *Immunology* **9**:427.

Piquet, P.-F., Dewey, H. K., and Vassalli, P., 1977, Orgin and nature of the cells participating in the popliteal graft versus host reaction in mouse and rat, *Cell. Immunol.* **31**: 242.

Rajewsky, K., 1971, The carrier effect and cellular cooperation in the induction of antibodies, *Proc. R. Soc. London Ser. B.* **176**:385.

Remington, J. S., Krahenbuhl, J. L., and Mendenhall, J. W., 1972, A role for activated macrophages in resistance to infection with toxoplasma, *Infect. Immun.* **6**:829.

Rolstad, B., 1976, The host component of the graft-versus-host reaction, *Transplantation* **21**:117.

Romano, T. J., Ponzio, N. M., and Thorbecke, G. J., 1976, Graft vs. host reactions in $F_1$ mice induced by parental lymphoid cells: nature of recruited cells, *J. Immunol.* **116**: 1618.

Rouse, B. T., and Warner, N. L., 1972, Depression of humoral antibody formation in the chicken by thymectomy and antilymphocyte serum, *Nature New Biol.* **236**:79.

Sarvas, H., Makela, O., Toivanen, P., and Toivanen, A., 1974, Effect of carrier pre-immunization on the anti-hapten response in the chicken, *Scand. J. Immunol.* **3**:455.

Sherman, J., and Auerbach, R., 1966, Quantitative characterization of chick thymus and bursa development, *Blood* **27**:371.

Takahashi, T., Carswell, E. A., and Thorbecke, G. J., 1970*a*, Surface antigens of immunocompetent cells. I. Effect of Θ and PC.1 alloantisera on the ability of spleen cells to transfer immune responses, *J. Exp. Med.* **132**:1181.

Takahashi, T., Old, L. J., and Boyse, E. A., 1970*b*, Surface alloantigens of plasma cells, *J. Exp. Med.* **131**:1325.

Takahashi, T., Old, L. J., McIntire, K. R., and Boyse, E. A., 1971*a*, Immunoglobulin and other surface antigens of cells in the immune system, *J. Exp. Med.* **134**:815.

Takahashi, T., Mond, J. J., Carswell, E. A., and Thorbecke, G. J., 1971*b*, The importance of Θ and Ig bearing cells in the immune response to various antigens, *J. Immunol.* **107**: 1520.

Thorbecke, G. J., and Lerman, S. P., 1976, Germinal centers and their role in immune responses, in: *The Reticuloendothelial System in Health and Disease: Functions and Characteristics* (S. M. Reichard, M. R. Escobar, and H. Friedman, eds.), pp. 83–100, Plenum Press, New York.

Thorbecke, G. J., Warner, N. L., Hochwald, G. M., and Ohanian, S. H., 1968, Immune globulin production by the bursa of Fabricius of young chickens, *Immunolgy* **15**:123.

Thorbecke, G. J., Takahashi, T., and McArthur, W. P., 1971, Surface antigens of immunocompetent cells, in: *Morphological and Functional Aspects of Immunity* (K. Lindahl-Kiessling, G. Alm, and M. Hanna, eds.), pp. 467–478, Plenum Press, New York.

Toivanen, A., and Toivanen, P., 1977, Histocompatibility requirements for cellular cooperation in the chicken: generation of germinal centers, *J. Immunol.* **118**:431.

Toivanen, P., Toivanen, A., and Sorvari, T., 1974, Incomplete restoration of the bursa-dependent immune system after transplantation of allogenic stem cells into immunodeficient chicks, *Proc. Natl. Acad. Sci. USA* **71**:957.

Toivanen, A., Viljanen, M., and Tamminen, P., 1977, Histocompatibility requirements for cellular cooperation in the chicken, *Adv. Exp. Med. Biol.* **88**:257.

Walker, K. Z., Lafferty, K. J., and Schoefl, G. I., 1973, Pathogenesis of the graft-versus-host reaction in chicken embryos: requirement of yolk sac-derived stem cells for the development of proliferative lesions, *Aust. J. Exp. Biol. Med. Sci.* **51**:347.

Warner, N. L., Szenberg, A., and Burnet, F. M., 1962, The immunological role of different lymphoid organs in the chicken. I. Dissociation of immunological responsiveness, *Aust. J. Exp. Biol. Med. Sci.* **40**:373.

Weber, W. T., 1970, Analysis of host and donor cell proliferation in chorioallantoic pocks, *Transplantation* **10**:275.

Weinbaum, F. I., Gilmour, D. G., and Thorbecke, G. J., 1973, Immunocompetent cells of the chicken. III. Cooperation of carrier sensitized T cells from agammaglobulinemic donors with hapten immune B cells, *J. Immunol.* **110**:1434.

Weinbaum, F. I., Butchko, G. M., Lerman, S., Thorbecke, G. J., and Nisonoff, A., 1974, Comparison of cross-reactivities between albumins of various species at the level of antibody and helper T cells—studies in mice, *J. Immunol.* **113**:257.

Winn, H. L., 1961, Immune mechanisms in homotransplantation. II. Quantitative assay of the immunologic activity of lymphoid cells stimulated by tumor homografts, *J. Immunol.* **86**:228.

Chapter 5

# *Salamanders and the Evolution of the Major Histocompatibility Complex*

**Nicholas Cohen**

*Department of Microbiology*
*Division of Immunology*
*University of Rochester*
*School of Medicine and Dentistry*
*Rochester, New York 14642*

## I. INTRODUCTION

All species of eutherian mammals and birds that have been systematically investigated possess one homologous system of closely linked gene loci that is intimately involved with the immune responses of that species (Götze, 1977). This gene cluster is called the major histocompatibility complex, or MHC. Products of genes within this complex induce differentiation of T cells, as measured by blast-cell transformation, clonal expansion, and the development of cytotoxic effectors. MHC gene products also induce B-cell differentiation, resulting in antibody production. Recently, the MHC has been recognized to be intimately involved in the recognition of a multiplicity of non-self antigenic determinants, with the acquisition of the T-cell repertoire, and with the cooperative interactions between subsets of T cells, between T and B cells, between lymphocytes and macrophages, and between cytotoxic effectors and their specific targets (Möller, 1978). Finally, constituent loci of the MHC are involved, either structurally or in some regulatory fashion, in the biosynthesis and activation of at least some components of the complement system (Meo *et al.*, 1975; Lachman and Hobart, 1978).

In the hope of unifying the diverse nomenclature of components of the MHCs of different species and in the interest of relating homologous regions by their phylogenetic origins, Klein (1977) recently suggested that we should divide the MHC into three regions, designated simply as class I, class II, and class III. Those portions of the MHC that historically were defined serologically, such as the paired *D* and *K* regions of the mouse *H-2* MHC, are categorized in class I. Class II regions describe those portions of the MHC that were first detected by the ability of their products to incite proliferation in the mixed-lymphocyte reaction. These regions would then include the *I* and the *D* regions of the mouse and human MHCs, respectively. Class-III regions are those involved in complement.

Questions and theories concerning the evolutionary origins of the MHC have captured the interest, imagination, and prose of at least three classes of scientists. Class I investigators are immunobiologists who, because of their keen awareness of the cellular events leading to an immune response, are enticed to speculate extensively, and often with perspicacity, as to the raison d'être of the MHC. An implicit (or even explicit) derivative of their contributions is the conviction that the complete homologue of the MHC must have appeared very early in vertebrate evolution, because: (1) the MHC is present in all endothermic (warm-blooded) vertebrates; (2) the MHC is of critical importance in the self/non-self discriminatory systems of these endotherms; and (3) all ectothermic (cold-blooded) vertebrates are similar to birds and mammals with respect to fundamental expressions of immune competence (lymphocytes, allograft rejection, antibody production, memory, specificity) (Manning and Turner, 1976; Marchalonis, 1977; Cooper, 1976). Class II investigators are biochemists and geneticists who deal with more restricted (and often better-substantiated) theories of MHC phylogeny. For example, while it has been suggested for many years that the paired arrangement of class I regions of mammalian species' MHC is indicative of gene duplication (Shreffler *et al.*, 1971), it is only recently that class II investigators have supported this hypothesis with solid data disclosing extensive amino acid sequence homology between the products of the *D* and *K* regions of the mouse (Silver *et al.*, 1977; Strominger *et al.*, 1977; Barnstable *et al.*, 1978). Similarly, the hypothesis that the class I regions of vertebrates are evolutionarily related and have descended from some common ancestral gene is at least partially substantiated by the striking amino acid sequence homology of the relevant class I region molecules of mouse and man. Class III investigators are those comparative immunologists who struggle to fathom the cellular and humoral non-self recognition systems of extinct creatures of bygone eras by describing the immune and quasi-immune systems of a plethora of extant invertebrates and ectothermic vertebrates. These investigators are interested in whether a given species of so-called primitive vertebrate *has* an MHC, not in whether it *should* have one.

The theoretical and practical contributions of class I and II investigators are extensively promulgated in the recent literature, while those of the comparative immunologists who are interested in MHC evolution lag far behind. In an attempt to offset this imbalance, this chapter will focus almost exclusively on recent published and unpublished studies with amphibians that bear directly and theoretically on the evolution of the MHC.

## II. DOES THE MHC EXIST IN ANY ECTOTHERMIC VERTEBRATE?

Pioneering studies by Du Pasquier and his co-workers have supported the hypothesis that the ancestral homologue of the complete MHC emerged prior to the appearance of birds and mammals. They selected a set of classic functional properties of the MHC of mammals, found that they could be detected in the South African clawed frog, *Xenopus laevis*, and then demonstrated that these markers segregated together within a family produced by mating two outbred adults (Du Pasquier *et al.*, 1975; Kobel and Du Pasquier, 1977). These markers include: strong proliferative responses in the mixed-lymphocyte reaction (MLR), acute allograft rejection, cell-mediated lympholysis (L. Du Pasquier, personal communication), and serologically defined erythrocyte and lymphocyte alloantigens. Although in mammals these functions are associated with linked class I and II region genes, formal proof that in the frog they are also controlled by linked loci, rather than by a single gene locus, is not yet available. Similarly, definitive studies that associate inheritance of complement components with the other markers in this species, and that provide evidence for biochemical homologies, seem a long way off.

As exciting and as important as these findings with *Xenopus* are, they do not tell us when during vertebrate or even anuran phylogeny the MHC first appeared. Neither do they permit us to make the generalization that all other orders of extant amphibians (Urodela and Apoda) have a comparable MHC, or whether all extant species of frogs are similar to *Xenopus* with respect to this genetic system. Similarly, studies with *Xenopus* do not warrant making the deductive step that since reptiles have evolved more recently than frogs, all reptiles have an MHC. Studies with other ectothermic vertebrates, however, do speak to these issues. A recently published collation of information (Cohen and Collins, 1977) concerned with the presence or absence of some of the aforementioned functional markers of the MHC has led to the argument that part, or all, of the MHC may have evolved at least four separate times during vertebrate evolution. That is, MHC phylogenesis may reflect convergent gene evolution (Cohen, 1976, 1979). Thus, one finds acute allograft rejection, lethal graft-versus-host reactions (GVHR), and strong and reproducible MLR (functional markers of disparities associated with the MHC) in "advanced" anuran amphibians (e.g., ranid and pipid frogs), birds (i.e., advanced reptiles?), and mammals. Some or all of these markers are either absent or undetectable in "primitive" fishes (agnathans, chondrichthians, chondrosteans, holosteans), "primitive"

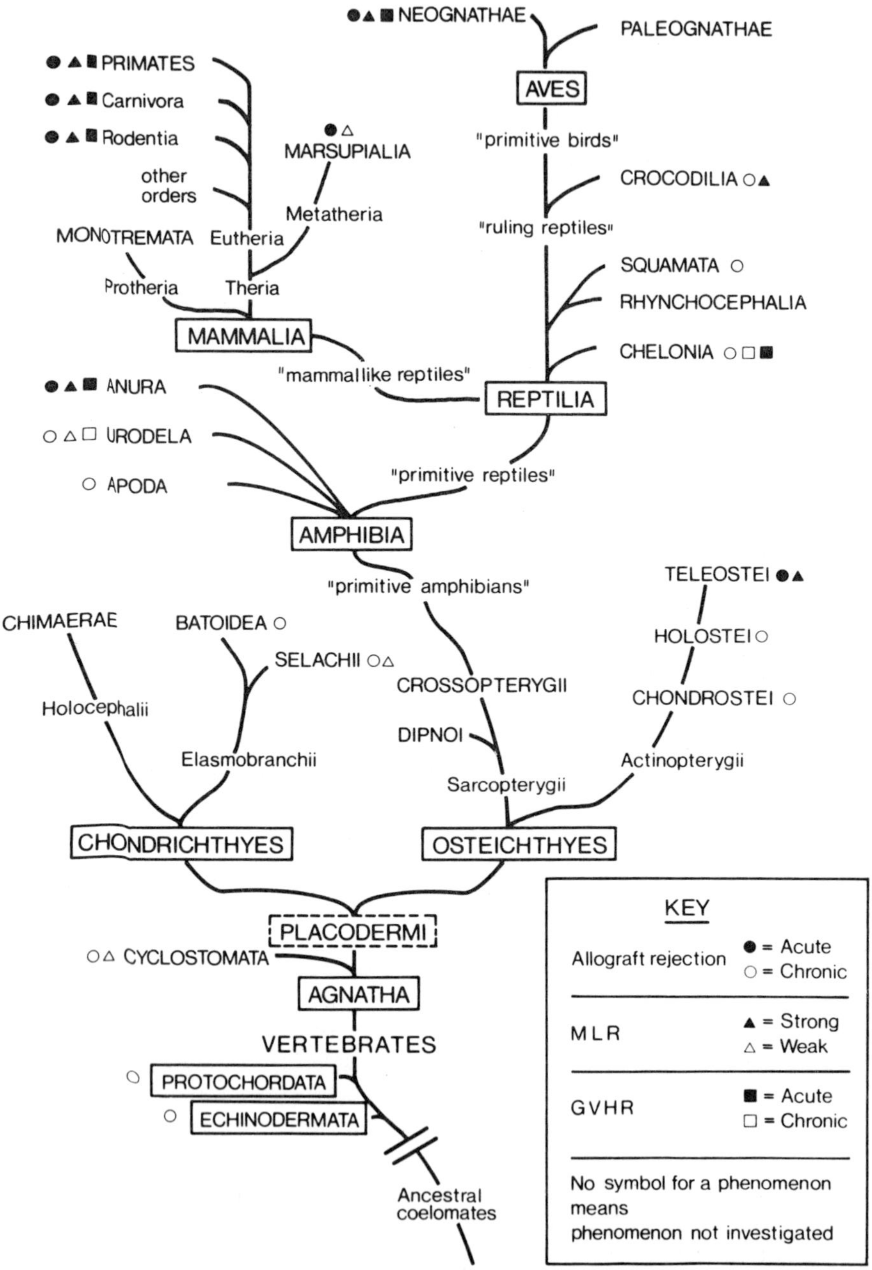


Figure 1. Evolutionary trends in the rapidity of allograft rejection, lethality of GVHR, and intensity of MLR. Modified from Cohen (1976); original is copyrighted by Elsevier North-Holland Publishing Co., Amsterdam.

amphibians (urodeles, apodans, and perhaps, some discoglossid frogs), and some (if not all) reptiles. The phylogenetic tree in Fig. 1 and Cohen and Collins's review (1977) illustrate our current knowledge about the phylogeny of these MHC markers.

## III. DO SALAMANDERS HAVE THE MHC?

Urodele amphibians are the most extensively studied group of vertebrates that fail to *routinely* display these three markers of MHC function. In a few recent publications (Cohen, 1976, 1979), I attempted to relate the absence of these markers to the presence or absence of the MHC regions that control such functions in mammals. The most straightforward explanation of the urodele situation is that, unlike frogs, salamanders lack the entire MHC. There are, however, certain alternatives that also fit existing data. For example, salamanders could have a genetic system that exhibits homology with class I but not with the class II regions. Salamanders could also have the homologue of the complete MHC if allelic polymorphism at one or more regions were minimal. Finally, some data are consistent with the hypothesis that salamanders have the MHC but lack the relevant subset of lymphocytes that recognize and react to class II region products. In this chapter I will discuss, in some detail, published and new unpublished data that bear on the immunogenetic basis of allograft rejection and mixed-lymphocyte reactivity of salamanders. Although these data bear on MHC evolution, I shall not speculate extensively in this area for I now know too much, and, therefore, too little, to do so with any conviction.

### A. The Immunogenetic Basis of Allograft Rejection

Alloreactivity directed against skin transplants has been studied for salamander species from 12 genera and about 6 different families (Cohen, 1971*a*). A rather consistent picture of this aspect of alloimmunity has emerged. All allografts resemble autografts (which survive indefinitely) for a 1- to 3-week period. Termination of this so-called latent period of healing-in and revascularization is registered grossly by vessel dilation and hemorrhaging. Histologically, an initial influx of lymphoid cells is seen. These events herald the onset of rejection, a phase that usually lasts for another 1 to 3 weeks. Macroscopically, the rejection phase is characterized by hemostasis, hemorrhaging, and pigment-cell destruction. Histologically, an increase in lymphocyte infiltration can be correlated with epidermal-, glandular-, and pigment-cell death (Cohen, 1968). Based on the survival end point of total pigment-cell death, median survival times (MSTs) of skin allografts for many species range between 26 and 55 days.

MSTs, however, fail to reveal fully the variability (i.e., number of *H* loci; polymorphism at each locus) of individual survival times that characterize chronic rejection reactions in salamanders. For example, individual survival end points of thousands of skin allografts on the newt *Notophthalmus v. viridescens* range from as early as 7 days (indicative of the immune-response potential of these animals) to as late as 200 days postgrafting. In addition, a significant number of allografts that enjoy indefinite survival (>400 days) have also been reported for this and for other species (Cohen, 1971*a*).

Reciprocal skin xenografts have been exchanged between salamanders from four genera. In six combinations, chronic rejection occurred (MSTs of 32–50 days); in two other combinations, rejection was subacute (MSTs of 19 and 24 days). It is noteworthy that, like allografts, some xenografts can also survive indefinitely (Cohen, 1969*a*,*b*). Of course, this is in marked contrast to the fate of orthotopically transplanted xenografts in anuran, avian, and mammalian species, in which rejection is more rapid and vigorous than is seen for allografts.

Other aspects of transplantation alloreactivity in outbreeding salamanders are also noteworthy. First, rejection is clearly an immune phenomenon, as witnessed in accelerated second-set rejection and allospecificity (Cohen, 1971*a*). Second, this rejection is thymus-dependent, as demonstrated by the failure of adults, thymectomized as young larvae, to reject allografts (Cohen, 1969*b*; Tournefier, 1973). Third, organ allografts often enjoy a more prolonged survival than skin grafts, even on hosts that have been hyperimmunized by several skin transplants (Cohen, 1971*a*; Cohen and Rich, 1970). Fourth, it is relatively easy to specifically and nonspecifically immunosuppress transplantation immunity. Finally, failure to reject rapidly is not a function of a deficient immune system, in that, under certain conditions, acute rejection has been recorded (Baldwin and Cohen, 1972; Cohen and Hildemann, 1968; Cohen, 1973). Indeed, chronicity appears to result in part from an active suppression elicited by the antigens of the transplant themselves (Cohen *et al.*, 1975; Manickavel and Cohen, 1975).

These observations with outbred salamanders are quite different from those recorded for outbred frogs, birds, or mammals in which skin allografts are destroyed acutely within the first 2 weeks after grafting. Comparable acute rejection also occurs when skin grafts are exchanged between two strains of mice that are congenic for all *H* loci save those that characterize their MHC (Démant, 1973). Indeed, *in vivo* alloimmunity in outbreeding salamanders is remarkably similar to *in vivo* alloimmunity in strains of mice that are bred for compatibility at their MHC but incompatibility at multiple minor *H* loci. It is primarily for this reason (reviewed more extensively by Cohen and Collins, 1977) that I proposed that salamanders lack the entire MHC and that histoincompatibility reactions are triggered by-products of minor or weak *H* alloantigens. This explanation, however, does not fit all the data. In the mouse, alloantigenic products of minor *H* loci vary significantly with respect to the rapidity of allograft rejection that they can evoke (Hildemann, 1970; Graff and Bailey, 1973). Recently it was proposed that: (1) like those of the mouse, the minor *H* systems of salamanders are of unequal "strength," and (2) within the framework of subacute and chronic rejection, one system is relatively strong (DeLanney and Blackler, 1969; Cohen and Collins, 1977). In a genetic, functional, and phylogenetic sense, this postulated system could be the predominant *H* locus (i.e., a "major" minor *H* locus) of the species. As such, it might exhibit homology with class I regions (Cohen, 1976). Some data support this concept; other data do not.

### *1. The Multiple Donor–One Host Paradigm*

This postulate that salamanders have a predominant *H* locus leads to certain testable predictions. First, incompatibility at a predominant *H* locus should invariably result in graft rejection. Second, compatibility at this locus but incompatibility at all other minor *H* loci should favor prolonged or even indefinite survival, perhaps as a result of tolerance induction. Third, incompatibility at all loci should result in the observed range of acute to chronic rejection times.

Some data support these predictions and suggest polymorphism at the locus (Tournefier *et al.*, 1969); other data, which also support the concept, argue for minimal polymorphism (Plytycz, 1977). Tournefier *et al.* (1969) mated Spanish newts (*Pleurodeles waltlii*) to produce $F_1$ animals that served as recipients of multiple skin grafts from several different donors. As seen in Table I, such grafts

**Table I. Evidence for a Predominant *H* Locus with Three or Four Alleles[a]**

*Pleurodeles waltlii:* intrasibling grafts (94 allografts: 24 hosts)

Observed: 22% (21/94) survived > 200 days
34% (32/94) rejected 15–20 days
44% (41/94) rejected 21–130 days

Predicted results[b] if number of alleles are:

| Three alleles | | Four alleles |
|---|---|---|
| Parental genotypes *ab* × *bc* | | Parental genotypes *ab* × *cd* |
| 37.5% | prolonged survival | 25% |
| 12.5% | rapid rejection | 25% |
| 50.0% | slow rejection | 50% |

[a]Adapted from a study by Tournefier *et al.* (1969).
[b]Prediction assumes a gene-dose effect (i.e., rapid rejection occurs only when donor and host differ by both alleles at the postulated predominant *H* locus). When one allele is shared, rejection is more chronic; when both are shared, survival is even more prolonged.

could be classified into those that survived more than 200 days, those that were rejected chronically (21-130 days), and those that were rejected relatively rapidly (15-20 days). If we assume that rapidity of rejection reflects a gene-dose effect (Galton, 1967; Lapp and Bliss, 1967), then the percentage of grafts in each of the aforementioned classes is consistent with a minimum of three to four alleles at a predominant *H* locus segregating in the sibship. This interpretation also assumes that survival of a single graft is not sharply affected by placing multiple grafts of different genotypes on a single host. The most critical objection to this interpretation of a predominant *H* locus is that the parental *Pleurodeles* were apparently derived from a laboratory-raised colony that may have been partially inbred. If so, the parentals could have been identical at several *H* loci, including the postulated predominant one. Thus, the observed survival of 22% of the intrasibling grafts would only mean that one-quarter of the sibs were homozygous at one more *H* locus than their parents.

There are additional experimental data with partially inbred strains of axolotls in which a 1:2:1 segregation of alleles at a single predominant *H* locus is sufficient to explain the genetic basis of the survival patterns of $F_2$ grafts on parentals (DeLanney *et al.*, 1975; DeLanney, 1978). That the axolotls used to develop these inbred strains perhaps originated from a geographically isolated Mexican population (DeLanney, 1978), however, again limits this interpretation. Clearly, what is called for are definitive genetic experiments involving outbred parentals from different locations, and an intrasibling-grafting protocol that involves just one graft per host.

### 2. *The One Donor–Multiple Host Paradigm*

Although the breeding study and segregation analyses just suggested currently offer the most direct way to prove the existence of a predominant *H* locus, the animal husbandry involved in successfully rearing a sibship makes this experiment an arduous and time-consuming one. For the moment we must rely on other protocols to provisionally support or reject this concept. In the one donor–multiple host paradigm, each member of a panel of hosts receives a single skin graft from the same donor. If sufficient numbers of donors are used, one can, in principle, screen a population of animals to reveal a variety of genetic relationships (provided that the criteria of rapidity and chronicity of graft rejection are reliable). I will review, in some detail, two such studies.

The first study argues for the existence of a minimally polymorphic predominant *H* locus; the second suggests considerable allelic diversity. In the first study, Plytycz (1977) recorded individual graft survival times of from 5 to more than 70 days for the European alpine newt, *Triturus alpestris.* This is, of course, the typical rejection pattern that has been described for other species of salamanders. More informative were data involving newts from the same pond (Table II). Two of the three donors used provided skin that was rejected with

**Table II. One Donor–Multiple Host Experiment with *Triturus alpestris*[a]**

| Donor | Postulated predominant *H*-locus genotype of donor | Number of hosts | MST (days) | Percentage grafts rejected: Acutely (5–11 days) | Percentage grafts rejected: Chronically (20–>70 days) |
|---|---|---|---|---|---|
| #1 | *ab* | 20 | 43 | 0.0 | 100.0 |
| #2 | *bb* | 17 | 34 | 17.6 | 82.4 |
| #3 | *aa* | 22 | 8 | 77.3 | 22.7 |

[a]Data from Plytycz (1977).

chronic MSTs (34 and 43 days). Skin from the third donor in this population, however, was rejected acutely (5–10 days) by 17 of the 22 recipients (Fig. 2; Table II). The remaining 5 hosts (Fig. 2) rejected their grafts from this donor between 20 and 31 days after grafting. To explain this unusually high incidence (77%) of acute reactivity, Plytycz proposed that donor number 3 possessed a strong antigen foreign to the 17 recipients that rejected rapidly but shared by those 5 animals that rejected slowly. (For the latter combinations, then, chronic rejection would only be the outcome of weak histoincompatibility interactions). Plytycz subjected her hypothesis to experimental analysis by selecting one of the hosts that rejected donor number 3's skin slowly and used it as a donor of

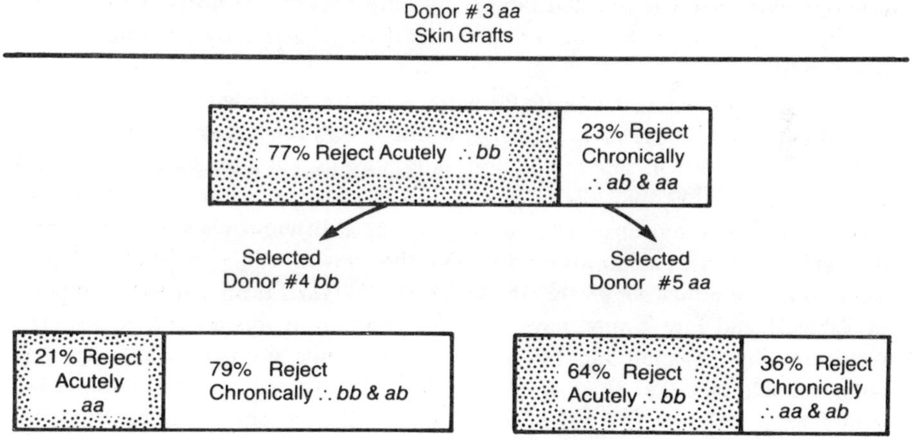


Figure 2. Analysis of the immunogenetic basis of skin-allograft rejection by application of the one donor–multiple host protocol to newts (*T. alpestris*) from a single population. The data are from a study by Plytycz (1977); the genotype assignments at the postulated predominant *H* locus (*aa*, *ab*, *bb*) are my responsibility. Twenty-two hosts received a graft from donor #3; 14 hosts received a graft from donor #4; 19 hosts received a graft from donor #5. See text for full description and interpretation.

skin grafts (Fig. 2; donor number 5) that were placed on a new panel consisting of 19 newts from the same pond. She reasoned that if animal number 5 had originally rejected skin from donor number 3 slowly because it shared a "strong" H alloantigen(s) with that donor, then its skin should, in turn, be rejected rapidly by the significant proportion of animals in the new panel that lacked the antigen. Indeed, the fact that some 64% of the new hosts did reject these transplants rapidly (5-10 days) while 36% rejected slowly (26-52 days) supported her proposition. Similarly, she reasoned that the hosts that had rejected skin from donor number 3 rapidly did so because they lacked the antigen in question. Thus, skin from one of these recipients (donor number 4; Fig. 2) should be rejected slowly by *all* members of a new panel of animals from the same population. Since the MST of grafts in this new combination was 28 days, Plytycz felt that her hypothesis was again supported. However, she failed to discuss her observation that although 11 of 14 recipients of skin grafts coming from donor number 4 did reject relatively chronically (14-56 days), the remaining three newts rejected skin from the same donor acutely (7-11 days). The point is that if donor number 4 really lacked this postulated strong antigen, then the group that rejected vigorously should not have existed.

There is another inconsistency in this study. Were Plytycz's interpretation correct, then the strong allele in question should be carried by some 23 to 36% of the animals in this pond (i.e., those that rejected slowly). This frequency, however, is inconsistent with data obtained from another one-donor-multiple-host panel (donor number 2; Table II) in the original study. Donor number 2 provided skin that was rejected rapidly by only 18% of the hosts. Thus, on the one hand the allele seems rare; on the other it seems shared by some 82% of the population.

It is still possible to reconcile Plytycz's interesting data with the existence of a predominant *H* locus in *T. alpestris*, if one makes the following two assumptions. First, at least in this population, polymorphism at a predominant *H* locus is reflected by only two alleles (i.e., *a* and *b*). Second, acute rejection occurs only when donor and host are homozygous for a different allele (i.e., the gene-dose effect). If these assumptions are valid, then newts in this population (Fig. 2, Table II) were either *aa*, *ab*, or *bb*. To obtain Plytycz's results, donor number 3 in Table II and Fig. 2 must have been homozygous at this locus (i.e., *aa*). The recipients that rejected rapidly would be *bb*, while the chronically rejecting animals could be either *ab* or *aa*. Donor number 5 selected from this latter group would have to be *aa* to explain why 64% of the recipients of grafts from this animal rejected rapidly (*bb* hosts) and 35% rejected slowly (*aa* and *ab*). Donor number 4 selected from the rapidly rejecting sample would then have the *bb* genotype. Since some two-thirds to three-quarters of the entire population would also be *bb* (as judged from the results that divided the original recipients into two groups), the percentage of animals in the subgroups would be consistent with the genotypes assigned to them in Fig. 2.

Although this simple explanation fits the data, the use of additional animals that received skin from donor number 3 as donors of skin for new panels of recipients, to verify either Plytycz's or my hypothesis, was not carried out. Nevertheless, it is interesting that this one locus–two allele model is consistent with data obtained from the other two panels of animals from the same pond. Thus, in the situation in which donor number 2 provided skin that was rejected acutely by only 18% of the recipients (Table II), this donor would be assigned the genotype *bb*. Since, according to my analysis, this is the relatively common genotype in the population, then it is to be expected that only 18% of the panel's members (those that were *aa*) were stimulated to reject rapidly. Since donor number 1 from this population provided skin that was destroyed chronically by all hosts (Table II), it would be a heterozygous animal.

While the gene-dose effect is well documented in transplantation biology (Galton, 1967; Lapp and Bliss, 1967), the notion that a predominant *H* locus has only two alleles is a novel one. Even if Plytycz's (1977) population data can be squeezed into a model involving three alleles, the locus would still be minimally polymorphic. If serological and more traditional genetic studies were to support this notion of a minimally polymorphic predominant *H* locus, and if this *H* locus proves to be ancestral to the class I region loci of endotherms by biochemical criteria, it would certainly argue against a duplicated state of class I gene loci at this level of phylogeny. Equally important, it would add a new dimension to speculations concerning the selective advantage of polymorphism at such loci (Klein, 1979). Before investigators expend the intellectual energy making such speculations, however, they should be aware that the minimal hypothesis of a single locus and two alleles does not easily fit data from a one-donor–multiple-host study currently under way in my laboratory. This study involves 10 different newt donors (*Notophthalmus v. viridescens*) and from 12 to 16 animals in each of the 10 panels of recipients. All animals were collected at the same time from the same pond (in Livingston County, New York), and all were experimented upon at the same time. The overall pattern of rejection of the 153 grafts from all 10 donors is seen in Fig. 3. The MST for these grafts was approximately 35 days; individual rejection times ranged from 16 to 60 days (at 23°C). For purposes of this chapter, observations were terminated at day 60, a time when about 28% of all grafts were still partially to fully viable. As seen in Table III, all but 1 donor provided skin that was rejected over the entire range (16 > 60 days). However, the *percentage* of grafts rejected within a given number of days postoperatively appeared to vary (in some instances, significantly) as a function of the particular donor used. Thus, 4 of 10 donors each provided skin to their respective panel recipients that was rejected with the overall survival pattern typical for the species (Fig. 3B). In contrast, another 4 donors provided skin that, by and large, appeared to enjoy a somewhat more prolonged survival (Fig. 3C). In this group, an average of only 3% of the transplants was rejected before 21 days, while an average of more than 40% was

**Table III. One Donor–Multiple Host Experiment with *Notophthalmus viridescens***

| Days postgrafting | Cumulative percentage of grafts rejected at various intervals after grafting | | | | | | | | | |
|---|---|---|---|---|---|---|---|---|---|---|
| | Donor #1 (16)[a] | Donor #2 (12) | Donor #3 (16) | Donor #4 (16→14) | Donor #5 (16→15) | Donor #6 (16→15) | Donor #7 (14→12) | Donor #8 (16) | Donor #9 (14→13) | Donor #10 (16) |
| 16–20 | 25 | 25 | 6 | 6 | 6 | 13 | 0 | 6 | 0 | 6 |
| 21–25 | 33 | 38 | 25 | 13 | 33 | 13 | 14 | 13 | 0 | 13 |
| 26–30 | 75 | 81 | 44 | 36 | 33 | 25 | 29 | 19 | 7 | 13 |
| 31–35 | 83 | 100 | 63 | 43 | 67 | 73 | 29 | 38 | 14 | 13 |
| 36–40 | 83 | | 81 | 50 | 67 | 80 | 39 | 44 | 35 | 13 |
| 41–45 | 92 | | 81 | 71 | 67 | 87 | 39 | 50 | 50 | 25 |
| 46–50 | 92 | | 88 | 79 | 80 | 87 | 46 | 56 | 57 | 31 |
| 50–60[b] | 92 | | 88 | 79 | 80 | 87 | 75 | 63 | 57 | 31 |
| Survival pattern: | Subacute | | | Typical | | | | Prolonged | | |

[a]Number in parentheses is the number of grafts per donor scored; when two numbers are given, host(s) died during the experiment.
[b]Study concluded at day 60, when from 0–69% of the grafts were partially to fully viable.

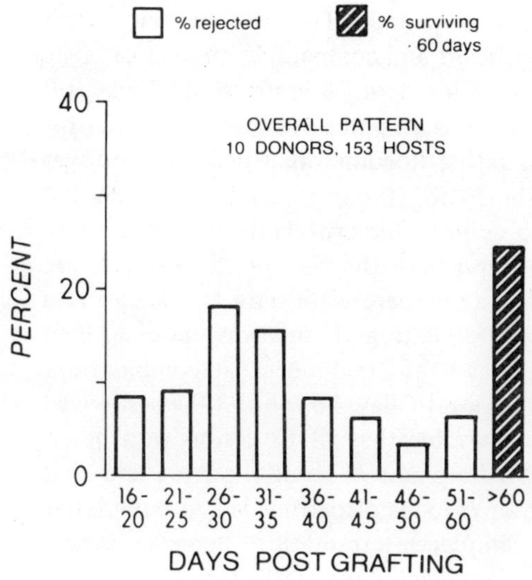


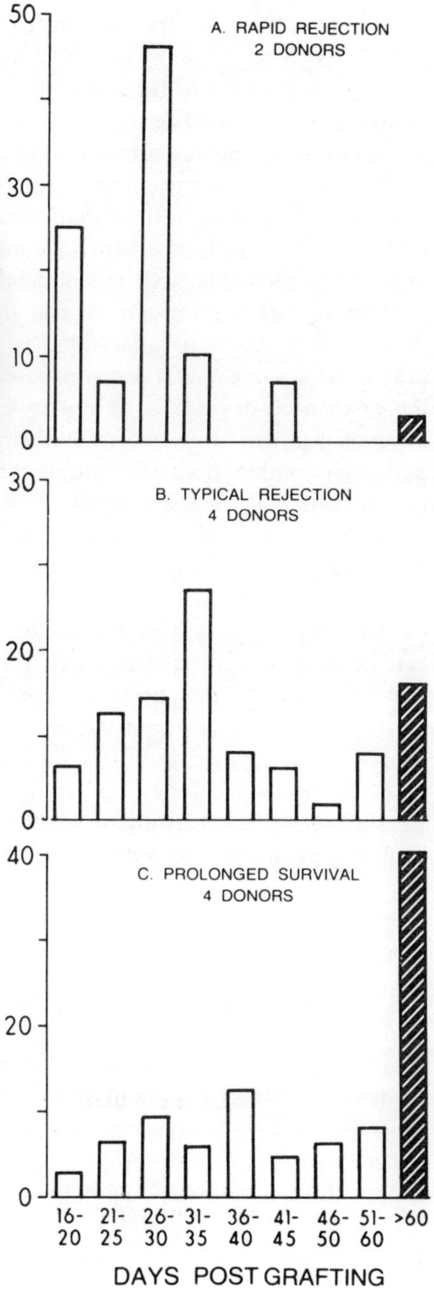


Figure 3. Application of the one donor–multiple host protocol to newts (*N. viridescens*) from one population. Ten animals served as donors; from 12–16 animals received a single graft from each donor. This is a graphic expression of the raw data presented in Table III. The overall survival pattern of the 153 grafts (on 153 hosts) derived from 10 donors is shown on the left. Two of these donors (panel A) provided skin that was rejected relatively rapidly; 4 donors (panel B) provided skin that was rejected in the typical fashion of the species (see "overall pattern" histogram); and 4 donors (panel C) provided skin grafts that enjoyed relatively prolonged survival.

still viable at the time the experiment was concluded. The last two donors each provided skin that was rejected by a significant and comparable number of hosts (25%) in the subacute fashion (Fig. 3A). Only 1 of 28 grafts studied was still surviving by day 60. These preliminary data again point out that, at least in this species of salamander, acute rejection is rather uncommon. When rejection was rapid, it was still more chronic than the 5- to 10-day survival times recorded under comparable conditions (and using comparable criteria for destruction) by Plytycz (1977) with *T. alpestris*. More important, the *Notophthalmus* data are difficult to reconcile with the possibility that there were only two alleles at a predominant *H* locus segregating in this population. If this was the case, then it becomes difficult to understand why, in 9 of 10 donor–host combinations (Table III), some grafts were rejected prior to day 20 while others survived longer than 60 days. It is, of course, conceivable that all 10 donors were heterozygous for the same alleles at this predominant *H* locus (i.e., *ab*) and that particular combinations of multiple minor *H*-locus disparities led to cumulative interactions and subacute rejection. A simpler interpretation, however, is that the wide range of survival times of skin from each donor reflects polymorphism at a predominant *H* locus and/or considerable antigenic diversity associated with multiple minor *H* loci.

Unfortunately, one of the donors in this experiment whose skin had triggered a significantly greater number of relatively rapid rejections than seen in the other panels died before it could be used to reciprocally exchange skin grafts with the other donor whose skin was reacted to in the same way. Such a procedure will prove useful in the future in uncovering what may be similar antigenic profiles among population members, in providing interesting animals for third-party test grafting, in identifying animals for breeding and segregation analyses, and in carrying out MLR-locus-typing protocols (discussed in Section B).

### 3. *Interpopulation Grafting*

Significant insight into the genetic basis of rejection of skin by salamanders has been derived from evaluating the survival of first-set, second-set, and third-party test grafts transplanted within and between members of several populations. One such study involving the reciprocal exchange of grafts (Cohen and Hildemann, 1968) argues that if such a predominant *H* locus exists, then its presence may be masked by a complex interplay of allelic diversity, antigen sharing, cumulative interactions of multiple minor *H* loci, and a balance between suppressive and cytotoxic immune responses. Newts from population B rejected one another's first-set grafts chronically (Table IV). Unexpectedly, but fortuitously, newts from population A rejected intrapopulation grafts much more rapidly. Nearly 40% of the population A allografts were destroyed by day 20; another 30% were rejected by day 25 (Table IV). If we assume that the large number of population-A animals that rejected rapidly did so because they dif-

**Table IV. Median Survival Times, 95%-Confidence Limits, Standard Deviations, and Ranges of Intra- and Interpopulation Allograft Survival in *Notophthalmus v. viridescens* from Two Geographically Distant Ponds**[a]

| Donor–host combination | Number of grafts scored | MST (days) | 95%-confidence limits (days) | S.D. (days) | Range of individual graft survival (days) |
|---|---|---|---|---|---|
| Pond A ⟷ pond A | 131 | 22.0 | 20.7–23.4 | 8.4 | 8–79 |
| Pond B ⟷ pond B | 52 | 41.4 | 34.9–49.1 | 28.2 | 15–>300[b] |
| Pond A → pond B | 18 | 42.0 | 31.6–55.9 | 28.8 | 19–>350[c] |
| Pond B → pond A | 19 | 44.8 | 36.7–56.5 | 23.7 | 16–>350[d] |

[a] Statistical determinations from Litchfield's (1949) nomographic method. This study from Cohen and Hildemann (1968).
[b] Seven grafts survived >300 days with full to partial viability.
[c] One graft survived >350 days with partial viability.
[d] Three grafts survived >350 days with full to partial viability.

fered from one another by one or more relatively "strong" alleles (antigens) at a predominant *H* locus, and that such diversity was lacking in population B, then we would expect the rapid rejection of A grafts on B newts. However, graft rejection in this interpopulation combination was chronic (Table IV). If we assume that population B animals rejected chronically because they shared the same alleles at the postulated predominant *H* locus, but that these "strong" alleles were present in a lower frequency in population A, then grafts from population B animals to population A animals should reflect this disequilibrium by exhibiting a high incidence of rapid rejection. Chronic rejection, however, also characterized the fate of interpopulation grafts exchanged in this direction. Only 5% of the grafts in each interpopulation combination were destroyed before 20 days. The *intra*population data, like those previously presented, argue that if there is a predominant *H* locus, it is multiallelic. The *inter*population data, however, are inconsistent with a predominant *H* locus–if differences at this locus are to be causally associated and solely responsible for acute and subacute reactions. The data, however, do support the notion that disparities at multiple minor *H* loci can synergize to effect relatively rapid rejection in salamanders, as well as in mice (Graff *et al.*, 1966). Thus, the high incidence of acute rejection in pond A vis-à-vis pond B could be accounted for by allele frequencies of several loci and by the additive effects of multiple minor *H*-locus differences.

Unpublished interpopulation studies, as well as those sited above (Cohen and Hildemann, 1968), involving animals from additional ponds and using the third-party-test grafting protocol (Hildemann and Hass, 1961), have pointed out that the degree of chronicity encountered in any population is, in part, a statement of the extent to which some alloantigens are effectively shared between donor and host. Typical survival times of 35 to 50 days speak to a moderate degree of antigen sharing; more prolonged survival reflects increased sharing; and more rapid rejections are invariably associated with minimal, if any, antigen sharing.

### *4. The Immune Response Capacity Story*

Most transplantation studies in my laboratory involve the common eastern spotted newt, *Notophthalmus viridescens viridescens.* On several occasions, however, I have had the opportunity to investigate alloimmunity in two other subspecies, namely *N. v. dorsalis* and *N. v. louisianensis.* In each of these subspecies, subacute rejection was commonly recorded. For example, the MST of about 140 *dorsalis* allografts transplanted on several different occasions was 20 days, with individual survival end points being recorded as early as 12 days post-transplantation (Cohen, 1973; Baldwin and Cohen, 1972). In contrast, a parallel study of grafts transplanted to *N.v. viridescens* resulted in an MST of about 40 days, with individual survival times ranging from 17 to greater than 200 days. Several hypotheses can be advanced to explain the more rapid rejection by the *dorsalis* subspecies. One possibility is that *dorsalis* is a "better responder" to alloantigens than *viridescens.* Another is that *dorsalis* has a single multiallelic predominant *H* locus (in addition to minor *H* loci) whose antigenic products are "strong," while the *viridescens* subspecies has the same gene locus but lacks polymorphism. A third possibility is that rapid rejection in *dorsalis* results from a cumulative interaction of products of multiple minor *H* loci, while *viridescens*, again, shows minimal polymorphism at these loci. To test the latter two possibilities, skin grafts were exchanged between the subspecies. If polymorphism at a predominant *H* locus is restricted in *viridescens* but not in *dorsalis*, *viridescens* should reject *dorsalis* vigorously, while *dorsalis* should reject *viridescens* chronically (provided, of course, that the allelic products of this

**Table V. Inter- and Intrasubspecific Skin Transplantation within Two Subspecies of *Notophthalmus viridescens*[a]**

| Number of grafts | Host | Donor | MST (range) (days)[b] | Percentage grafts destroyed: By 20 days | Percentage grafts destroyed: After 50 days | Percentage grafts surviving >150 days |
|---|---|---|---|---|---|---|
| 37 | *viridescens* | *viridescens* | 41.0 (20->200) | 5.4 | 18.9 | 18.9 |
| 30 | *dorsalis* | *dorsalis* | 23.5 (14->150) | 50.0 | 6.7 | 3.4 |
| 30 | *dorsalis* | *viridescens* | 18.3 (15-77) | 73.3 | 21.6 | 0.0 |
| 28 | *viridescens* | *dorsalis* | 38.3 (21->200) | 0.0 | 6.7 | 21.6 |

[a]Control and experimental animals from same shipment; data from Cohen (1973).
[b]MSTs calculated nomographically (Litchfield, 1949).

postulated predominant *H* locus are present in both subspecies). The actual data were contrary to this expectation (Table V). *Dorsalis* rejected *viridescens* grafts with the rapidity with which they rejected *dorsalis* grafts, and *viridescens* rejected *dorsalis* grafts with the chronicity with which they rejected *viridescens* allografts. Thus it was provisionally proposed that *dorsalis* is a better responder than *viridescens.* What this means in terms of physiological and/or genetic systems is totally open to speculation.

### B. The Mixed Lymphocyte Reaction (MLR)

When individuals from two outbreeding endothermic vertebrates of the same species are cocultured, a strong two-way stimulation-response reaction occurs, which is characterized by blast-cell transformation and cell proliferation (Bach and Hirschhorn, 1964). Invariably, disparities at class II loci of the MHC of chickens, mice, rats, man, and other warm-blooded species are always equated with intense reactivities. In the face of MHC compatibility, however, stimulation of chicken, rat, and human lymphoid cells in mixed-leukocyte culture (MLC) is either undetectable by current techniques (Miggiano *et al.*, 1974, Thorsby, 1974; Cramer *et al.*, 1974), or else significantly less than that recorded when MHC disparities prevail (Colley and DeWitt, 1969). In the mouse, where immunogenetic definition of the strains providing the allogeneic cells is more precise, a less black-and-white picture emerges. In the face of MHC compatibility, stimulation in MLC ranges from that which is comparable to control syngeneic cultures, through weak responses, to strong stimulation indexes that are similar to those obtained in the presence of MHC incompatibilities (Dutton, 1966; Häyry and Defendi, 1970; Rychilikova and Ivanyi, 1969; Mangi and Mardiney, 1971; Peck and Click, 1973). The degree of stimulation is very much dependent on the culture conditions that are involved. Regardless of whether weak or even strong stimulation can occur as a response to multiple minor *H* loci or to gene products of the *Mls* locus (Festenstein, 1976; Festenstein *et al.*, 1977), it *always* occurs with an MHC difference (e.g., with cells from outbred endotherms).

Numerous studies with the frog *Xenopus laevis* by Du Pasquier *et al.* (1975, 1977) and in my laboratory (Hailparn and Cohen, 1977) have revealed that the MLR is genetically and functionally linked to strong histoincompatibility reactions. As with skin grafting, MLC studies with outbreeding salamanders paint an entirely different picture. The MLR has been studied in four urodele genera, *Ambystoma* (Collins, 1976; DeLanney *et al.*, 1975; Collins and Cohen, 1976), *Necturus* (Collins, 1976), *Cynops* (Cohen, unpublished), and *Notophthalmus* (Collins, 1976; Cohen and Horan, 1977), with microculture techniques. When animals are paired, and reciprocal one-way MLCs are performed (with irradiated stimulators), a significant MLR occurs about 50% of the time. When stimulation is positive, stimulation indexes range from 1.5 to 4.0 ($\bar{x} = {\sim}2$).

Thymectomy studies have pointed out that the cells involved in allograft rejection in at least two species of salamander (Cohen, 1969*b*; Tournefier, 1973) are thymus-dependent. Studies with mice have pointed out that lymphocytes primarily responsible for target-cell destruction and responding in MLC are different (Bach *et al.*, 1977). Thus, at least one explanation for these apparently sporadic MLRs in salamanders (and the minimal proliferation observed) could be that urodeles have a homologue of the class II region but lack the population of cells that recognize and respond to the relevant determinant. Arguments supporting the possibility of a real difference between T cells of salamanders and those of frogs and higher vertebrates are detailed elsewhere (Cohen, 1976; Ruben and Edwards, Chapter 3, this volume). One important difference is that, unlike cells from several species of frogs, salamander lymphocytes respond poorly, if at all, to the T-cell mitogens, PHA and Con A. They respond well, however, to LPS (Collins and Cohen, 1976; Collins, 1976).

Another possible explanation for the poor and seemingly sporadic MLRs, which must be taken very seriously, is that salamanders have the appropriate responding cells but that the laboratory's *in vitro* conditions fail to support the proliferative response of cells to alloantigens as well as to PHA and Con A (as measured by blast-cell counts or by incorporation of tritiated thymidine). It is relatively meaningless to point out that the culture conditions we use for salamanders routinely result in excellent proliferative responses of frog cells to both mitogens and alloantigens. It is more important to note that we have tried to modify our culture procedures in a variety of ways (Collins, 1976; Collins and Cohen, 1976; Cohen, unpublished). These include: varying cell densities, culturing lymphoid cells from different tissue, feeding cultures, providing different media with different nutritional supplements, adding macrophages, purifying cells on nylon wool columns, incubating at different temperatures and taking cells from animals that have themselves been kept at different temperatures (Cohen and DeLanney, unpublished). Recently we have added either homologous serum or pooled *Xenopus* serum to our 1% fetal calf serum, since Du Pasquier *et al.* (1977) reported for *Xenopus* that some batches of homologous serum can effectively suppress background counts per minute (cpm) as well as increase stimulated cpm. In several MLC experiments with *Notophthalmus* or *Cynops* spleen cells, addition of *Xenopus* or *Cynops* serum did indeed depress background cpm, but it also depressed stimulated cpm so that analyses of either stimulation indexes or of stimulation-minus-control cpm revealed no increased magnitude of reactivity or increased incidence of positive responses.

Another recent unpublished study from my laboratory also argues against technical problems as the critical limiting factor. I wondered whether the relative "absence" of PHA-reactive cells might serve as a marker for the relative "absence" of cells reactive to alloantigens in the same organ from the same animal. This, however, did not appear to be the case. First, spleen cells from *Bombina*, a primitive discoglossid frog that rejects skin allografts chronically (Richards and

Cohen, unpublished), are also unresponsive to alloantigens (in a limited series involving only splenocytes). Unlike salamanders, but very much like other anurans, however, spleen cells from *Bombina* responded quite vigorously to PHA and Con A. Second, salamander splenocytes that do react to PHA may or may not proliferate in MLC. This was determined by selecting one newt and incubating its splenocytes with several concentrations of PHA-P. At the same time, but in separate cultures, splenocytes from the same animal were cocultured with irradiated stimulator cells from a panel of other newts. If no MLR was repeatedly observed when no PHA reactivity was noted (or vice versa), then the postulates that a technical problem was manifest, that some cell was indeed limiting, and/or that there was some unknown humoral or physiological regulatory system in operation would become more attractive. However, the data in Table VI revealed that the failure of splenocytes to respond to PHA did not mean that cells in the same preparation were not alloantigen-reactive. Thus, the PHA-reactive cell and the alloreactive cell appear to be real but separate entities. Whether such cells are thymus-dependent is currently being determined.

The data in Table VI do not confront the issue of why positive MLCs are typically characterized by only a twofold stimulation. It is still possible that in some way the cells themselves are limiting the reaction, either numerically or by their state of differentiation (an evolutionarily interesting possibility, indeed). Even if we are dealing with a limitation of the culture system, however, the technical (or physiological) situation does not appear to affect PHA and alloantigen-reactive cells in the same way.

**Table VI. Detection of a Proliferative Response to PHA Does Not Predict MLR**

| Responses in a one-way MLC by responder cells that display: | | | |
|---|---|---|---|
| No PHA reactivity[a] | | Positive PHA reactivity | |
| Responder newt | MLC response with cells from each stimulator newt | Responder newt | MLC response with cells from each stimulator newt |
| #1 | (–) (–) (+)[b] | # 8 | (–) (–) (–) |
| #2 | (–) (+) (+) | # 9 | (+) (+) (+) |
| #3 | (+) | #10 | (+) |
| #4 | (+) (+) (+) (+) | #11 | (+) (+) (+) (+) (–) |
| #5 | (+) (+) (+) (+) | #12 | (+) (+) (+) (+) (–) |
| #6 | (–) (–) (–) (–) | #13 | (+) (+) (+) (+) (–) |
| #7 | (–) (–) (–) (–) | #14 | (–) (–) (–) (–) |

[a] Splenocytes ($0.5 \times 10^5$) cultured for 7 days with 0.39–3.12 μl PHA-P/ml.
[b] Each symbol [(+) or (–)] indicates the result of a one-way MLC involving irradiated stimulator cells (6000 R) from a different newt. Positive MLR reflects a stimulation index (SI) >1.40. Mean positive SIs were 1.9 and 2.1 for MLC and PHA, respectively.

### *1. One Genetic Explanation for the MLR*

The data summarized in Table VI are more important in another regard. They suggested a testable hypothesis concerning the immunogenetic basis of the responses of salamander lymphocytes in MLC, and they offered an explanation of why, when MLCs were carried out just in reciprocal combinations, positive reactions appeared to be sporadic or random events. Basically, the data (Table VI) point out that when splenocytes from a newt responded to irradiated stimulators from one animal, they responded to stimulators from others. Similarly, when splenocytes from an animal failed to respond to stimulators from one newt, the same responder cells did not respond to stimulators from other newts. At first glance, it appeared that we were dealing with a responder–nonresponder situation. A closer examination of the data in Table VI, however, reveals critical exceptions. Thus, a positive MLC of one responder (Table VI, number 11 or 13) to stimulator cells from 4 different newts did not mean a positive response with a fifth stimulator population. These observations suggested that stimulatory alloantigens were under genetic control. They further suggested the formal hypothesis that the MLR in *Notophthalmus* is under the control of a single gene locus that has but two codominant alleles. If this hypothesis is valid (and we assume that, like the MLR in other species, differences involving only one allele are sufficient to effect a positive MLC), then of the three possible MLR-locus genotypes present in a population (*aa*, *bb*, *ab*), the genotype of any animal responding in MLC must be either *aa* or *bb*.

One beauty of this simple one gene locus–two allele model is that it is testable. First, one can carry out matrix analyses of one-way MLCs in which cells from each member of a panel of from 4 to 6 newts (depending upon the number of available cells) serve as both irradiated stimulators and normal responders when placed in culture with cells from all other panel members. Our analysis of 92 one-way MLCs involving 27 newts from one population (5 matrices) and 42 one-way MLCs with 10 newts from another population (2 matrices) allowed us to assign to each animal MLR-locus genotypes that were virtually completely consistent with the model of restricted MLR-locus polymorphism. Indeed, only 5% of the 134 MLCs failed to agree with the genotypes suggested by the other MLCs. In the examples of such matrices presented in Figs. 4 and 5, the numbers running in a diagonal from upper left to lower right are the control background cpm resulting from culturing responder cells with irradiated autologous cells. As seen in Fig. 4, 2 newts typed as *aa*, 2 as *ab*, and 2 as *bb*. These genotype assignments were made as follows: Cells from animals number 3, number 5, and number 6 responded positively. Therefore, according to the model, they had to be homozygous. Since cells from number 5 and number 6 were mutually nonstimulatory, they were considered to be homozygous for the same allele. Cells from number 3 and number 4 were also mutually nonstimulatory, but since they stimulated cells from number 5 and number 6, they

| Code number (and proposed MLR-locus genotypes) of responders | Code number (and proposed MLR-locus genotypes) of irradiated stimulators: #1 (*ab*) | #2 (*ab*) | #3 (*bb*) | #4 (*bb*) | #5 (*aa*) | #6 (*aa*) |
|---|---|---|---|---|---|---|
| (*ab*) #1 | *582 ± 105* | 1.17 | 1.03 | ND | 1.27 | 1.34 |
| (*ab*) #2 | 1.21 | *589 ± 50* | 1.25 | ND | 1.11 | 1.27 |
| (*bb*) #3 | 1.97 | 2.17 | *197 ± 12* | ND | 1.95 | 1.58 |
| (*bb*) #4 | ND | ND | ND | *650 ± 49* | ND | ND |
| (*aa*) #5 | 1.69 | 1.59 | 1.80 | 1.42 | *409 ± 16* | 1.27 |
| (*aa*) #6 | 1.45 | 1.54 | 1.98 | 2.05 | 1.33 | *261 ± 21* |

Figure 4. MLR locus genotyping of Allegheny pond *Notophthalmus viridescens:* matrix 1. Spleen cells from each newt served as both irradiated stimulators and normal responders in one-way MLC with cells from other animals from the same population. The numbers in italics running diagonally from upper left to bottom right are the control counts per minute (cpm) ± S.E. of responder cells ($2.5 \times 10^4$) plus an equal number of irradiated autologous cells cultured in 200 $\mu$l of medium. All other numbers are stimulation indexes (SI) calculated according to the formula

$$\text{SI} = \frac{(\text{CPM responder cells} + \text{cpm irradiated stimulator cells})}{(\text{CPM responder cells} + \text{cpm irradiated autologous cells})}$$

Cultures harvested after 5 days; methods detailed elsewhere (Cohen and Horan, 1977). Stimulation indexes $\geqslant$1.4 were judged to be positive, according to the calculation for the coefficient of variation (S.D./mean). ND, Not determined.

had to be homozygous for the other allele. Cells from the remaining two animals could stimulate responder cells but they did not respond to cells from any animal in the panel. Thus they were considered to be heterozygous. A similar example of typing by matrix analysis is seen in Fig. 5. In this example, there is one discordant point. Although number 17 and number 19 typed as heterozygotes, number 17 did display a small but significant stimulation when cultured with irradiated cells from number 19.

The ideal way to perform a matrix analysis would be to carry out the experiment with cells from a panel of animals one day and then to repeat the experiment with the same animals on another day. Technically, this is not possible with these newts. They have little more than 30 $\mu$l of blood. Lymphocytes are found only in the spleen, liver, kidney, and atrophied thymus, and the spleen contains only $5\text{-}15 \times 10^5$ cells (Cohen and Horan, 1977). Given that we culture at a density of $2.5 \times 10^5$ cells/ml in 200 $\mu$l of medium, and that we clearly prefer a minimum of triplicate determinations for each point, it is easy to see why the appropriate design fits paper better than reality. As an alternative, I attempted a kinetic analysis of MLR. In this study, animals came from a pond that was different from the one used to generate the data in Figs. 4 and 5. Of

| Code number (and proposed MLR-locus genotypes) of responders | Code number (and proposed MLR-locus genotypes) of irradiated stimulators | | | | |
|---|---|---|---|---|---|
| | #16(*ab*) | #17(*ab*) | #18(*bb*) | #19(*ab*) | #20(*aa*) |
| (*ab*) #16 | *179 ± 21* | 1.32 | 0.53 | 0.50 | 1.37 |
| (*ab*) #17 | 1.13 | *431 ± 89* | 1.08 | 1.50* | 1.36 |
| (*bb*) #18 | 1.75 | 2.62 | *106 ± 9* | 2.44 | 5.59 |
| (*ab*) #19 | 0.82 | 1.30 | 1.32 | *310 ± 3* | 1.06 |
| (*aa*) #20 | 2.60 | 2.73 | 2.03 | 1.73 | *307 ± 86* |

Figure 5. MLR locus genotyping of Allegheny pond *Notophthalums viridescens:* matrix 3. Animals were from the same population as those typed in Fig. 4. Stimulation index is considered positive when ⩾1.4*, discordant. See text and legend for Fig. 4 for further details.

the 6 animals in this new matrix, the single newt that appeared to be homozygous on day 5 was also the only one that responded when replicate cultures were harvested 2 days later. Similarly, the unresponsiveness of the other newts on day 5 was maintained on day 7.

As I mentioned, the animals that provided the data generated in Figs. 4 and 5 and those animals that were used in the aforementioned kinetic study came from different populations. In each population, then, the single-locus–two-allele model seemed to be substantiated. In another recent experiment, MLC matrices were set up with animals from both populations in interpopulation as well as intrapopulation combinations. Although the data are quite preliminary, they support the idea that the same MLR-locus alleles are common to animals of both populations. That is, an animal from one population that was typed by an intrapopulation MLC as a homozygote or a heterozygote responded to and stimulated cells from animals in the second population, as would be predicted by the model.

I would be remiss if I did not point out that although these and other unpublished data fit rather well with this one locus–two allele model, it may be possible to fit the same data to a model involving more alleles. To do so, one has to postulate a gene-dose effect in which a two-allele difference is necessary for an MLR; that certain MLR-locus alleles are associated with better stimulation than others; and that cells of a certain genotype fail to respond, even with a two-allele difference. For the present, however, I prefer to be a disciple of Occam and adopt the simpler alternative, at least as a working model. It is obvious that this model must be tested genetically. One way to do this is to select pairs of field-collected salamanders whose lymphocytes are either mutually stimulatory (*aa* and *bb*) or mutually nonstimulatory, breed them (splenectomized animals live long lives), and then examine the segregation pattern of MLR in the $F_1$ and backcross progeny. Even if these and other experiments reveal that allelic polymorphism is greater than currently proposed, it now seems evident that the MLR is not a random event. Rather, there is a genetic system involved, and there are lymphocytes capable of recognizing and proliferating in response to these alloantigens in our culture system. Other issues that must still be resolved include what type of lymphocyte is reactive (e.g., a T cell homologous with one but not another population of murine T cells of a specific Ly phenotype) and why positive MLC responses (as measured by incorporation of tritiated thymidine) rarely exceed three times that of the controls.

### 2. *Is MLR "Linked" to Allograft Rejection?*

If salamanders have a MHC, then by definition antigens eliciting the MLR and relatively rapid graft rejection (as well as other markers) should be coded for by the same or closely linked genes. Unfortunately, nobody has mated outbreeding salamanders and examined the $F_1$ progeny for associations of MLR and rapid rejection. Similarly, nobody has yet systematically and thoroughly exploited histocompatible partly inbred strains of *Pleurodeles* (Charlemagne and Tournefier, 1974) or axolotls (DeLanney, 1978). We have shown that neither intrastrain nor irradiated parental-plus-$F_1$ MLCs are stimulatory (DeLanney *et al.*, 1975), but analyses of interstrain MLC combinations are only just beginning. Thus, there are virtually no data demonstrating either the presence or the absence of a genetic linkage between MLR and acute or at least relatively rapid graft rejection in any salamander, or in any ectothermic vertebrate other than *Xenopus.* On the other hand, several studies do suggest that MLR and allograft reactivity are *not* functionally linked. Such a functional association would be anticipated were we dealing with products of the same locus or of linked loci. In one such study, we splenectomized several pairs of newts and at the same time reciprocally exchanged first-set skin grafts between members of each pair. The spleen cells were then cultured in reciprocal one-way MLC. Splenectomy at the time of grafting failed to demonstrably affect first- or second-set rejection times (Cohen and Horan, 1977). If the one locus–two allele model of MLR in this species is correct, then a MLR-locus genotype can be assigned to each animal of the pair, according to whether mutual stimulation, mutual nonstimulation, or unidirectional stimulation occurred. As summarized in Table VII, the rapidity of allograft rejection was not correlated with the detection of a positive MLC (i.e., with the proposed MLR-locus genotype of donor and host) or the magnitude of the MLR. Thus, the MLR locus does not appear to be a "moderately strong" *H* locus, for if it were, survival of skin exchanged between pairs of newts whose cells were mutually stimulatory in MLC should have been curtailed relative to survival of grafts exchanged between a pair of MLC-nonreactive newts. It remains to be determined whether this lack of concordance will be sustained when MLCs are carried out in situations in which reciprocal allografts survive for more than 100 days or less than 20 days. In view of data revealing that human

**Table VII. Lack of Relationship between MLR-Locus Disparity and Rapidity of Allograft Rejection**

| MLR-locus relationship between donors of responding cells + donors of irradiated stimulators | Survival times (days) of individual grafts |
|---|---|
| MLR-locus identical | |
| *aa* + *aa* or[a] | 22, 25, 26, 27, 27, 37 |
| *bb* + *bb* or | |
| *ab* + *ab* | |
| MLR-locus disparate | |
| 1. *aa* + *ab* or | 29, 34 |
| *bb* + *ab* | |
| 2. *ab* + *aa* or | 31, 35 |
| *ab* + *bb* | |
| 3. *aa* + *bb* or | 19, 25, 26, 27, 27, 29 |
| *bb* + *aa* | 31, 32 |

[a]Data do not permit a distinction to be made among these three possibilities.

skin grafts exchanged between class II region disparate individuals are rejected significantly more rapidly than those exchanged between class II identical subjects (Jonker *et al.*, 1979*a*,*b*), our data suggesting no such relationship between MLR-locus disparity and graft survival in salamanders may mean that the MLR locus is not linked (in the genetic sense) to the postulated predominant *H* locus (or to any *H* system) of the species. If this point can be verified by the necessary grafting and breeding studies, it would provide compelling evidence for a lack of complete MHC homology at this level of vertebrate evolution.

Another line of evidence also suggests that the MLR locus is not linked to any *H* system. In the frog *Xenopus* (Hailparn and Cohen, 1977) and in the rabbit and other mammals (Milthor *et al.*, 1979; Wilson *et al.*, 1967), immunization of animals with a first-set skin allograft can (but need not always) alter the kinetics and magnitude of the MLR (relative to nonimmune controls) when cells from the immune animal are cultured with stimulator lymphocytes from the MHC-incompatible skin graft donor (but not from a third party). Recent studies with the newt *Notophthalmus* again reveal that the salamander is very different from the frog. A kinetic study of MLR, partly summarized in Table VIII, pointed out that after 2 days in culture only 2 of 12 reciprocal MLCs were positive. By 3 days, 4 more positive MLCs appeared. To determine whether prior immunization would alter MLR kinetics, we harvested responder cells from animals that had rejected a skin graft, and cultured them for 2 days with

**Table VIII. Early Kinetics of 1-Way MLR with Spleen Cells from *Notophthalmus viridescens*[a]**

| Days in culture | | | |
|---|---|---|---|
| Day 2 | | Day 3 | |
| CPM ± S.E.[b] | SI[c] | SI | CPM ± S.E. |
| 621 ± 54 | 0.92 | 0.99 | 991 ± 56 |
| 2263 ± 61 | 1.00 | 1.07 | 2161 ± 217 |
| 297 ± 33 | 1.06 | 0.82 | 550 ± 56 |
| 694 ± 32 | 1.00 | 1.31 | 1311 ± 67 |
| 1663 ± 66 | 0.85 | 1.33 | 2670 ± 134 |
| 344 ± 13 | 1.14 | 0.98 | 348 ± 29 |
| 4371 ± 874 | 1.13 | 1.95 | 525 ± 50 |
| 242 ± 15 | 0.95 | 1.63 | 619 ± 43 |
| 1867 ± 20 | 1.15 | 1.76 | 1246 ± 73 |
| 1208 ± 13 | 1.01 | 1.43 | 1561 ± 268 |
| 677 ± 51 | 1.76 | 3.42 | 869 ± 32 |
| 416 ± 35 | 1.97 | 2.20 | 698 ± 57 |

[a]Data on days 2 and 3 are for the same stimulator–responder combination.
[b]CPM of responder cells + irradiated (6000R) allogeneic stimulator cells.
[c]SI = (CPM of responder cells + irradiated stimulator cells)/(CPM of responder cells + irradiated autologous cells). SI ⩾ 1.4 is positive.

the appropriate stimulator cells from the graft donor. To determine whether the magnitude of the positive MLC responses was affected by *in vivo* immunization, we performed a similar experiment (different animals), but harvested the cells after 7 days in culture. The data summarized in Table IX point out that the immune state of the responder newt altered neither the kinetics nor the magnitude of the MLR. Fortunately for the viability of the one locus–two allele model, prior immunization also failed to convert a nonresponding combination to a positive response, as judged by the comparable incidence of positive MLCs in combinations involving responders from putatively immune and nonimmune animals. Not shown in Table IX is that there also appears to be no simple relationship between the rapidity of first-set rejection (degree of histoincompatibility) and the time the spleens were harvested for MLC after first-set rejection (possible sequestration of MLR-memory cells) with either the positivity of an MLC or the relative magnitude of such a positive reaction (Cohen and Horan, 1977).

The roles of class II region products in cell collaboration and MHC-restricted recognition of antigen are becoming better defined in murine systems. If salamanders lack the class II homologue, then their immune responses should be

**Table IX. Lack of Effect of Skin-Allograft Rejection on Kinetics and Magnitude of 1-Way MLR**

| Days in culture | Immune status | Percentage positive MLC (positive/total) | Stimulation indexes |
|---|---|---|---|
| 2 | Immune | 25% (3/12) | 2.5, 2.8, 3.4 |
| | Nonimmune | 17% (2/12) | 1.8, 2.0 |
| 7 | Immune | 47% (7/15) | 1.4, 1.8, 2.7, 3.1, 3.1, 3.6, 4.8 |
| | Nonimmune | 43% (6/14) | 1.5, 1.6, 2.7, 3.3, 3.6, 4.4 |

quite different from those of higher vertebrates or even from the frog. This indeed appears to be the case. For example, attempts to detect antibodies in sera of salamanders immunized with antigens that are classically thymus-dependent in mice (diverse serum proteins, ferritin, horseradish peroxidase) are usually unsuccessful. Urodeles, however, do make antibodies to bacteria, phages, and erythrocytes, which in mice elicit a thymus-independent IgM response. Although larval thymectomy alters the ability of salamanders to reject allografts (Cohen, 1969*b*; Tournefier, 1973), it does not appear to alter their ability to produce most respectable serum-antibody titers to heterologous erythrocytes or to *Salmonella* H antigen (Tournefier and Charlemagne, 1975). In mice, production of IgG to these antigens is thymus-dependent. Finally, if one recalls that in mice T-B cooperation seems most important for IgG production, these results with urodeles may not be surprising, since only IgM has been detected in normal or immune sera from several salamander species (Houdayer and Fougereau, 1972; Marchalonis and Cohen, 1973; Tournefier and Charlemagne, 1975). Ruben and Edwards (this volume) have reviewed T-B cooperation from a phylogenetic perspective. They point out striking differences between carrier–hapten phenomena in frogs and salamanders. Although they do present evidence for cell collaboration in the newt, there is no indication that such a collaborative interaction involves T as well as B cells. It is intriguing that in some protocols, helper reactivity can be explained by polyfunctional specificity of antigen-binding cells rather than by cell cooperation (Ruben and Selker, 1975; Ruben and Edwards, 1978).

## IV. CONCLUDING COMMENTS

In my introduction to this chapter, I arbitrarily (and somewhat facetiously) divided the investigators interested in MHC phylogeny into three classes. Class I investigators, it will be remembered, speculated that all vertebrates must (should) have the MHC, since this gene complex appears to be essential for a functional immune system, and all vertebrates have immune systems. Class II investigators were faced with the responsibility of gathering hard data to determine the validity of this hypothesis. Although considerably more data must still be collected before one can determine conclusively whether salamanders do or do not have a MHC, the studies just described rather strongly suggest that the negative hypothesis may be correct—that is, that salamanders lack the MHC in so far as it has been defined for mammals.

Even if salamanders lack the complete MHC, they could still have ancestral homologues of gene loci within this complex. For example, if the postulated predominant *H* locus of salamanders is ever substantiated genetically, serologically, and biochemically, then an ancestor of the class I region of the MHC in an extant vertebrate might be documented as well. Arguments supporting the existence of such a locus in invertebrates such as sponges, coelenterates, and tunicates have been presented elsewhere (Du Pasquier, 1974), as has the possibility that such a genetic system forms the cornerstone of MHC phylogeny by convergent gene evolution (Cohen, 1976, 1979). It is also possible that the putative MLR locus of the salamander could be ancestral to the class II region of the MHC, even if this locus is neither genetically nor functionally linked to the salamander's predominant *H* system. One could imagine, for example, a scenario in which evolution of the MHC in the Amphibia involved first the chance bringing together into the same linkage group of two loci from distant portions of the same chromosome or from different chromosomes (translocation) and then the maintenance of this association because of the selective survival advantage it offered the species. On the other hand, this scenario may never have been acted out, since it is well known that lymphocytes from mice that differ only by minor *H* loci or by the nonhistocompatibility *Mls* locus (Festenstein, 1976) can stimulate and respond in MLC. That is, the MLR locus of salamanders may be completely unrelated to the class II region of the MHC.

Salamanders are not unique among vertebrates with respect to the absence of traditional markers of the MHC (e.g., acute rejection, strong MLC). It is unknown whether this means that vertebrates such as hagfish, sharks, lizards, and turtles (Fig. 1) are similar to salamanders with respect to the apparent lack of the complete MHC homologue. If they are, and if the MLR locus of salamanders *is not* ancestral to the class II region of mice and men, then the concept of convergent evolution of the MHC remains reasonable (Cohen, 1976, 1979). If, however, the MLR locus of salamanders is ancestral to, respectively, the *I* and *D* regions of the mouse and human MHC, then convergent evolution involving repetitive translocations becomes more unlikely. In this regard it becomes intriguing to consider briefly what little relevant data there are concerning the immunogenetics of *in vivo* and *in vitro* alloimmunity among the Crocodilia (Fig. 1). Several years ago I determined that skin-allograft rejection among young caimans was chronic (Cohen, 1971*b*). Very recently, Cuchens and Clem (1979) studied MLR and mitogen reactivities of peripheral blood leukocytes from alligators. In contrast to studies with salamanders, stimulation indexes of alligator lymphocytes cultured with lectins and alloantigens were respectably high. However, two-way MLCs of cells from 8 animals collected from different sites in Florida revealed 5 of the 28 possible combinations to be nonstimulatory (i.e., MLC combinations 1 + 2, 1 + 4, 1 + 10, 2 + 10, and 4 + 10 were nonresponsive; combination 2 + 4 was weakly positive). (Unfortunately, the cultures were harvested only on day 5 and a replicate using the same animals has not been attempted). On the one hand, these preliminary data suggest the phylogenetic emergence of a requisite set of reactive T cells in the crocodilians, and on the other, a striking lack of polymorphism of gene loci associated with *in vivo* and *in vitro* manifestations of alloimmunity. Suffice it to say that at this point the approach of class III immunologists to understanding the evolutionary history of the MHC is limited more by the number of investigators working from this perspective than by the number of experiments that must be carried out.

## ACKNOWLEDGMENTS

Research cited from the author's laboratory was supported by U.S. Public Health Service Grant HD 07901 and by Research Career Development Award AI-70736. The technical assistance of Ms. Mary Horan in the execution of some of the unpublished experiments cited in this paper is greatly appreciated.

## V. REFERENCES

Bach, F. H., and Hirschhorn, K., 1964, Lymphocyte interaction: a potential histocompatibility test *in vitro*, *Science* **142**:813.

Bach, F. H., Kuperman, O. J., Sollinger, H. W., Zarling, J. M., Sondel, P. M., Alter, B. J., and Bach, M. L., 1977, Cellular immunogenetics and LD-CD collaboration, *Transpl. Proc.* 9:859.

Baldwin, W. M. III, and Cohen, N., 1972, Immunosuppression of subacute skin allograft rejection in the newt *Diemictylus v. dorsalis* by alloantigenic pretreatment with kidney and liver implants, *Folia Biol.* **18**:181.

Barnstable, C. J., Jones, E. A., and Crumpton, M. J., 1978, Isolation, structure, and genetics of HLA-A, -B, -C and -DRW (Ia) antigens, *Br. Med. Bull.* **34**:241.

Charlemagne, J., and Tournefier, A., 1974, Obtention of histocompatible strains in the urodele *Pleurodeles waltlii* Michah (Salamandridae), *J. Immunogenet.* **1**:125.

Cohen, N., 1968, Chronic skin graft rejection in the *Urodela.* I. A comparative study of first- and second-set allograft reactions, *J. Exp. Zool.* **167**:37.

Cohen, N., 1969*a*, Chronic skin graft rejection in the *Urodela.* II. A comparative study of xenograft rejection, *Transplantation* 7:332.

Cohen, N., 1969*b*, Immunogenetic and developmental aspects of tissue transplantation immunity in urodele amphibians, in: *Biology of Amphibian Tumors: Recent Results in Cancer Research* (M. Mizell, ed.), pp. 153–168, Springer-Verlag, Berlin.

Cohen, N., 1971*a*, Amphibian transplantation reactions: A review, *Am. Zool.* **11**:193.

Cohen, N., 1971*b*, Reptiles as models for the study of immunity and its phylogenesis, *J. Am. Vet. Med. Assoc.* **159**:1662.

Cohen, N., 1973, Predictable variability in the response of two newt subspecies (*D. v. viridescens* and *D. v. dorsalis*) to first-set allografts, *Folia Biol.* **19**:169.

Cohen, N., 1976, Phylogeny of the major histocompatibility complex: theoretical implications of studies with urodele amphibians, in: *Phylogeny of Thymus and Bone Marrow-Bursa Cells* (R. K. Wright and E. L. Cooper, eds.), pp. 169–182, Elsevier North-Holland, Amsterdam.

Cohen, N., 1979, Evolution of the major histocompatibility complex in vertebrates: A saga of convergent gene evolution? *Transplant. Proc.* **11**:1118.

Cohen, N., and Collins, N. H., 1977, Major and minor histocompatibility systems of ectothermic vertebrates, in: *The Major Histocompatibility System in Man and Animal* (D. Götze, ed.), Springer-Verlag, Berlin.

Cohen, N., and Hildemann, W. H., 1968, Population studies of allograft rejection in the newt, *Diemictylus viridescens*, *Transplantation* **6**:208.

Cohen, N., and Horan, M., 1977, Lack of correlation between rapidity of newt allograft rejection and the frequency and magnitude of stimulation in the mixed lymphocyte reaction, in: *Developmental Immunobiology* (J. B. Solomon and J. D. Horton, eds.), pp. 259–266, Elsevier North-Holland, Amsterdam.

Cohen, N., and Rich, L. C., 1970, Exceptionally prolonged survival of allogeneic heart implants in untreated and previously skin grafted salamanders, *Am. Zool.* **10**:536.

Cohen, N., Baldwin, W. M. III, and Manickavel, V., 1975, Phylogeny of functional humoral transplantation immunity: Comparative studies in amphibians and rodents, *Adv. Exp. Med. Biol.* **64**:411.

Colley, D. G., and DeWitt, C. W., 1969, Mixed lymphocyte blastogenesis in response to multiple histocompatibility antigens, *J. Immunol.* **102**:107.

Collins, N. H., 1976, Mitogenic and mixed lymphocyte culture reactivities of lymphoid cells from three urodele species: Perspectives on the evolution of immunity, Ph.D. thesis, University of Rochester, Rochester, N.Y.

Collins, N. H., and Cohen, N., 1976, Phylogeny of immunocompetent cells. II. *In vitro* behavior of lymphocytes from the spleen, blood and thymus of the urodele, *Ambystoma mexicanum*, in: *Phylogeny of Thymus and Bone Marrow-Bursa Cells* (R. K. Wright and E. L. Cooper, eds.), pp. 143–152, Elsevier North-Holland, Amsterdam.

Cooper, E. L., 1976, *Comparative Immunology*, Prentice-Hall, Englewood Cliffs, N.J.

Cramer, C. V., Shonnard, J. W., and Gill, T. J. III, 1974, Genetic studies in inbred rats. II. Relationship between the major histocompatibility complex and mixed lymphocyte reactivity, *J. Immunogen.* **1**:421.

Cuchens, M. A., and Clem, L. W., 1979, Phylogeny of lymphocyte heterogeneity. III. Mitogenic responses of reptilian lymphocytes, *Dev. Comp. Immunol.* **3**:287.

DeLanney, L. E., 1978, Immunogenetic profile of the axolotl: 1977, *Am. Zool.* **18**:289.

DeLanney, L. E., and Blackler, K., 1969, Acceptance and regression of a strain specific lymphosarcoma in Mexican axolotls, in: *Biology of Amphibian Tumors: Recent Results in Cancer Research* (M. Mizell, ed.), pp. 399–408, Springer-Verlag, Berlin.

DeLanney, L. E., Collins, N. H., Cohen, N., and Reid, R., 1975, Transplantation immunogenetics and MLC reactivities of partially inbred strains of salamanders (*A. mexicanum*): Preliminary studies, *Adv. Exp. Biol. Med.* **64**:315.

Démant, P., 1973, *H-2* gene complex and its role in alloimmune reactions, *Transpl. Proc.* **15**:162.

Du Pasquier, L., 1974, The genetic control of histocompatibility reactions: phylogenetic aspects, *Arch. Biol.* **85**:91.

Du Pasquier, L., Chardonnens, X., and Miggiano, V. C., 1975, A major histocompatibility complex in the toad, *Xenopus laevis* (Daudin), *Immunogenetics* **1**:482.

Du Pasquier, L., Miggiano, V. C., Kobel, H. R., and Fischberg, M., 1977, The genetic control of histocompatibility reactions in natural and laboratory-made polyploid individuals of the clawed toad *Xenopus*, *Immunogenetics* **5**:129.

Dutton, R. W., 1966, Spleen cell proliferation in response to homologous antigen: Studies in congenic resistant strains of mice, *J. Exp. Med.* **123**:665.

Festenstein, H., 1976, The Mls system, *Transpl. Proc.* **8**:339.

Festenstein, H., Bishop, C., and Tanlon, B. A., 1977, Location of Mls locus on mouse chromosome 1, *Immunogenetics* **5**:357.

Galton, M., 1967, Factors involved in the rejection of skin transplanted across a weak histocompatibility barrier: gene dosage, sex of recipient, and nature of expression of histocompatibility genes, *Transplantation* **5**:154.

Götze, D., 1977, *The Major Histocompatibility System in Man and Animals*, Springer-Verlag, Berlin.

Graff, R. J., and Bailey, D. W., 1973, The non-*H-2* histocompatibility loci and their antigens, *Transpl. Rev.* **15**:26.

Graff, R. J., Silvers, W. K., Billingham, R. E., Hildemann, W. H., and Snell, G. D., 1966, The cumulative effect of histocompatibility antigens, *Transplantation* **4**:605.

Hailparn, E., and Cohen, N., 1977, Allograft rejection alters the kinetics and magnitude of the mixed lymphocyte reaction in *Xenopus laevis*, *Am. Zool.* **17**:892.

Häyry, P., and Defendi, V., 1970, Allograft immunity *in vitro*. II. Induction of DNA-synthesis in mixed cultures of mouse peripheral lymphocytes from inbred strains differing at non-*H-2* loci, *Transplantation* **9**:410.

Hildemann, W. H., 1970, Components and concepts of antigenic strength, *Transpl. Rev.* **3**:5.

Hildemann, W. H., and Haas, R., 1961, Histocompatibility genetics of bullfrog populations, *Evolution* **15**:267.

Houdayer, M., and Fougereau, M., 1972, Phylogénie des immunoglobulines: La réaction immunitaire de l'axolotl, *Ambystoma mexicanum*. Cinétique de la réponse immunitaire et caractérisation des anticorps, *Ann. Inst. Pasteur* **123**:4.

Jonker, M., Hoogeboom, J., van Leeuwen, A., Koch, C. T., van Oud Alblas, D. B., and van Rood, J. J., 1979*a*, The influence of matching for HLA-DR antigens on skin graft survival, *Transplantation* in press.

Jonker, M., Hoogeboom, J., van Leeuwen, A., Koch, C. T., van Oud Alblas, D. B., Persijn, G., Frederiks, E., and van Rood, J. J., 1979*b*, Experimental skin grafting in man, *Transpl. Proc.* **11**:607.

Klein, J., 1977, Evolution and function of the major histocompatibility system: facts and speculations, in *The Major Histocompatibility System in Man and Animals* (D. Götze, ed.), pp. 339–378, Springer-Verlag, Berlin.

Klein, J., 1979, The major histocompatibility complex of the mouse, *Science* **203**:516.

Kobel, H. R., and Du Pasquier, L., 1977, Strains and species of *Xenopus* for immunological research, in *Developmental Immunobiology* (J. B. Solomon and J. D. Horton, eds.), pp. 299–306, Elsevier North-Holland, Amsterdam.

Lachman, P. J., and Hobart, M. J., 1978, Complement genetics in relation to HLA, *Br. Med. Bull.* **134**:247.

Lapp, W. S., and Bliss, J. Q., 1967, The effects of allelic dosage and graft size on skin graft survival across a weak histocompatibility barrier, *Immunology* **12**:103.

Litchfield, J. T., Jr., 1949, A method for rapid graphic solution of time per cent effect curves, *J. Pharm. Exp. Ther.* **97**:399.

Mangi, R. J., and Mardiney, M. R., Jr., 1971, The mixed lymphocyte reaction: Detection of single histocompatibility loci and the correlation to skin graft survival in mice, *Transplantation* **11**:369.

Manickavel, V., and Cohen, N., 1975, Does chronic rejection elicited by weak histocompatibility antigens in mice and salamanders result from active enhancement? *Transpl. Proc.* **7**:451.

Manning, M. J., and Turner, R. J., 1976, *Comparative Immunobiology*, Blackie and Sons, Glasgow.

Marchalonis, J. J., 1977, *Immunity in Evolution*, Edward Arnold Ltd., London.

Marchalonis, J. J., and Cohen, N., 1973, Isolation and partial characterization of immunoglobulin from a urodele amphibian (*Necturus maculosus*), *Immunology* **24**:395.

Meo, T., Krasteff, T., and Shreffler, D. C., 1975, Immunochemical characterization of murine H-2 controlled Ss protein through the identification of its human homologue as the fourth component of complement, *Proc. Natl. Acad. Sci. USA* **72**:4536.

Miggiano, V. C., Birgen, F., and Pink, J. R. L., 1974, The mixed leukocyte reaction in chicken: Evidence for control by the major histocompatibility complex, *Eur. J. Immunol.* **4**:397.

Milthor, P. P., Belanges, R., and Richter, M., 1979, The cells involved in cell-mediated and transplantation immunity in the normal outbred rabbit. I. The accelerated response in the one-way MLR of rabbit WBC from skin allograft recipients, *Immunology* **36**:25.

Möller, G. (ed.), 1978, *Acquisition of the T Cell Repertoire*, *Immunological Reviews*, Vol. 42, Munksgaard, Copenhagen.

Peck, A. B., and Click, 1973, Immune responses *in vitro*. III. Differentiation of H-2 and non-H-2 alloantigens of the mouse by a dual mixed leukocyte culture, *Transplantation* **16**:331.

Plytycz, B., 1977, Strong histocompatibility antigens in Urodela amphibians (*Triturus alpestris*/*T. vulgaris*), *Folia Biol.* **23**:72.

Ruben, L. N., and Edwards, B. F., 1978, Visualization of bispecific antigen-binding in immunized splenic lymphocytes of the newt, *Triturus viridescens*, *Dev. Comp. Immunol.* **2**:175.

Ruben, L. N., and Selker, E. U., 1975, Polyfunctional antigen-binding specificity in hapten-carrier responses of the newt, *Triturus viridescens*, *Adv. Exp. Med. Biol.* **64**:387.

Rychilikova, M., and Ivanyi, P., 1969, Mixed lymphocyte cultures and histocompatibility antigens in mice, *Folia Biol.* **15**:126.

Shreffler, D. C., David, C. S., Passmore, H. C., and Klein, J., 1971, Genetic organization and evolution of the mouse H-2 region: A duplication model, *Transpl. Proc* **3**:176.

Silver, J., Cecka, J. M., McMillan, M., and Hood, L., 1977, Chemical characterization of products of the *H-2* complex, *Cold Spring Harbor Symp. Quant. Biol.* **41**:369.

Strominger, J. L., Mann, D. L., Parham, P., Robb, R., Springer, T., and Terhorst, C., 1977, Structure of HLA-A and B antigens isolated from cultured human lymphoblasts, *Cold Spring Harbor Symp. Quant. Biol.* **41**:323.

Thorsby, E., 1974, The human major histocompatibility system, *Transpl. Rev.* **18**:51.

Tournefier, A., 1973, Développement des organes lymphoides chez l'Amphibien Urodèle *Triturus alpestris* Laur.: Tolérance des allogreffes après la thymectomie larvaine, *J. Embryol. Exp. Morphol.* **29**:383.

Tournefier, A., and Charlemagne, J., 1975, Antibodies against salmonella and SRBC in urodele amphibians: Synthesis and characterization, *Adv. Exp. Med. Biol* **64**:161.

Tournefier, A., Charlemagne, J., and Houillon, C., 1969, Évolution des homogreffes cutanées chez l'amphibien urodèle *Pleurodeles waltlii* Michah: Résponse immunitaire primaire et secondaire, *C. R. Acad. Sci.* **268**:456.

Wilson, D. B., Silvers, W. K., and Nowell, P. C., 1967, Quantitative studies on the mixed lymphocyte interaction in rats. II. Relationship of the proliferative response to the immunological status of the donors, *J. Exp. Med.* **126**:655.

*Chapter 6*

# *Membrane Immunoglobulins of Vertebrate Lymphocytes*

**Gregory W. Warr**

*Cancer Biology Program*
*NCI Frederick Cancer Research Center*
*Frederick, Maryland 21701*

## I. INTRODUCTION

Since the days when Metchnikoff (1892) investigated the comparative biology of phagocytes, immunology has been increasingly biased toward studies in humans and (with some passing gestures to "relevance") the very convenient model systems offered by the common laboratory rodents. Whether or not the rodents are the proper objects of such immunological anthropomorphism can be argued, but it is clear that a concentration on the immune system of a few species of animal has been at the expense of a wider scientific development of the discipline. It is indisputable that all living vertebrates possess defense mechanisms that conform to any of our definitions of adaptive immunity: Stated simply, they possess the ability to respond, by means of humoral antibodies and cellular mechanisms, to an appropriate (antigenic) foreign stimulus, with a response that shows both specificity and memory (Hildemann, 1972, 1974; Cooper, 1976; Marchalonis, 1977*a*; Warr and Marchalonis, 1978). This being so, it would seem reasonable that any theory of immune recognition should take into account the presumption that all vertebrates are linked by their evolutionary history, and therefore might be expected to share certain common or simple patterns of organization in their immune systems.

This review, therefore, represents an attempt to analyze the available comparative data on one of the membrane structures by which vertebrate lymphocytes recognize and respond to antigens. I will attempt to consider such problems as the universal role of immunoglobulin (Ig) as a receptor, and the occurrence, detection, quantitation, and characterization of lymphocyte-surface Igs. In view of the gaps in our knowledge of many aspects of the immunobiology of the so-called lower classes of vertebrates, it is almost inevitable that many of the interpretations offered here will prove to be oversimplifications. However, as much of current murine cellular immunology constitutes a bewildering array of factors and ever-increasing numbers of lymphocyte subpopulations, and is consequently susceptible only to the most convoluted interpretations, perhaps a comparative approach may offer some readily testable hypotheses.

## II. A NOTE ON METHODS FOR THE DEMONSTRATION OF MEMBRANE IMMUNOGLOBULINS

Although a detailed description and discussion of techniques for investigating lymphocyte-membrane Igs would be out of place in a review such as this, I nevertheless hope that a brief description of some of the problems in this area will enable the reader to make a more critical appraisal of the available information.

Without exception, all methods for the demonstration of lymphocyte-membrane Ig involve the use of antibodies to Igs (i.e., antiglobulin reagents) (Warner, 1974; Warr and Marchalonis, 1977*a*). These antiglobulin reagents can be coupled with identifiable tracer groups—such as fluorochromes (Cebra and Goldstein, 1965; Raff, 1970; Johnson *et al.*, 1978; Nairn, 1969), enzymes (Avrameas and Guilbert, 1971), isotopes (Jones *et al.*, 1970; Nossal *et al.*, 1972), and macromolecules (An *et al.*, 1972; Biberfeld *et al.*, 1971)—and used to demonstrate surface Ig *in situ* in the lymphocyte membrane, by the use of appropriate light or electron-microscopic techniques coupled with, when appropriate, such methods as fluorescent-light illumination and autoradiography. In addition, antiglobulin reagents can be used to detect Igs in isolated or solubilized extracts of membranes by such techniques as radioimmunoassay (Rabellino *et al.*, 1971; Jensenius and Williams, 1974) or immune diffusion in agar (Misra *et al.*, 1976). Finally, antiglobulin reagents can be used as affinity reagents to isolate the lymphocyte-membrane Igs for further characterization analysis (Marchalonis and Cone, 1973; Vitetta and Uhr, 1973; Warner, 1974; Warr and Marchalonis, 1977*a*). Because of the small amounts of protein associated with a lymphocyte membrane, this process frequently involves isolating Igs from solubilized extracts of cells that have had their membrane proteins externally labeled by a variety of radioisotopic methods (Carraway, 1975; Marchalonis, 1977*b*).

There are problems of interpretation of results obtained by many of these methods. For example, although the easiest method for demonstrating surface

Igs is the direct binding of (usually fluorochromated) antiglobulin reagents, this direct method, or derivatives of it using several layers ("sandwiches") of antiglobulin reagents, is the one with the greatest likelihood of producing erroneous results. First, if the antiserum contains antibodies reactive with non-Ig membrane components, or antibodies that cross-react with Ig and non-Ig membrane antigens, a spurious positive reaction may be obtained. Such cross-reactions have been reported with carbohydrate antigens and antisera to IgM (Merler *et al.*, 1974: Yamaga *et al.*, 1978*a,b*; Mattes and Steiner, 1978), and a very small percentage of antisera made against kappa light chains showed reactivity with $\beta_2$ microglobulin (Gottlieb *et al.*, 1977).

Second, with the direct-binding assay there is not only a risk of detecting passively adsorbed serum Ig bound to Fc receptors on the lymphocyte membrane, but also the risk of detecting receptors on the cell membrane reactive with the Fc portion of the antiglobulin reagents themselves (Winchester *et al.*, 1975). These problems can be overcome to a certain extent by carrying out careful controls to establish that lymphocyte-surface Igs are endogenously produced (Preud'homme and Seligmann, 1972), and by enzymically removing the Fc portion of the antiglobulin antibody to eliminate the possibility of its being bound to an Fc receptor (Winchester *et al.*, 1975).

A third, and not widely recognized, problem in the use of direct antiglobulin binding methods in the study of lymphocyte-surface Igs is that, while surface-Ig molecules may be present in the membrane, for a number of reasons they are inaccessible to direct binding by antiglobulin reagents.

An example of this phenomenon not involving Ig can be found in the case of histocompatibility antigens, where sometimes, although the molecules cannot be detected easily by direct-binding assays, they are present in an appreciable amount in extracts of the membrane (Molnar *et al.*, 1973). However, two examples closer to the point at issue can be taken from studies of lymphocyte-surface Igs. The first question is concerned with surface Ig on mammalian thymocytes and thymus-derived (T) lymphocytes. Most (but not all) antisera to Ig raised in mammalian species fail to stain these T cells (Warner, 1974). However, antisera to Ig raised in birds will react with putative Ig molecules on mammalian T cells (Hämmerling *et al.*, 1976*a*; Szenberg *et al.*, 1977; Jones *et al.*, 1976; Marchalonis *et al.*, 1977*b*, 1978). Furthermore, molecules with the antigenic and physicochemical characteristics of Ig can be detected in lysates of T-cell membranes (Marchalonis and Cone, 1973; Marchalonis, 1975; Haustein *et al.*, 1975; Haustein and Goding, 1975; Hämmerling *et al.*, 1976*b*; Misra *et al.*, 1976; Gabison *et al.*, 1977; Chavin, 1974; Cone and Brown, 1976; Cone, 1976; Cone *et al.*, 1977; Moroz and Lahat, 1974; Szenberg *et al.*, 1977; Boylston and Mowbray, 1974; Warr *et al.*, 1978*b*).

A second example can be found in the case of the "null" lymphocyte. This

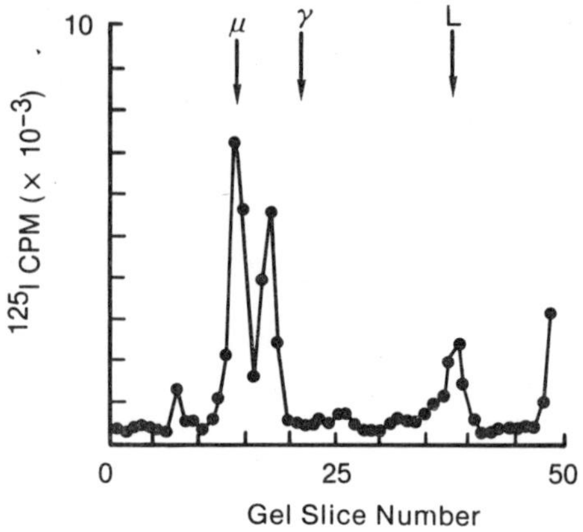


Figure 1. Surface Ig of murine "null" lymphocytes. Null cells were isolated from suspensions of splenocytes from NIH Swiss athymic (nude) mice by passage twice through a column of rabbit antibody to mouse IgM coupled with Sepharose-6B Macrobeads. The effluent cells were all negative for membrane fluorescence with rabbit antisera to mouse heavy or light immunoglobulin chains. Following surface radioiodination of the "null" lymphocytes (Marchalonis *et al.*, 1971) and lysis of the cells in nonionic detergent, surface Igs were isolated by binding to rabbit antibodies to IgM coupled with Sepharose-4B (Haustein and Warr, 1976) and analyzed by SDS-polyacrylamide-gel electrophoresis under reducing conditions, as described by Haustein *et al.* (1975). The mobility of μ, γ, and L chains of murine standard immunoglobulins is indicated by arrows.

cell, isolated from blood and peripheral lymphoid organs of mice and humans (Kiessling *et al.*, 1975; Chess *et al.*, 1975; Greenberg *et al.*, 1973), lacks typical markers of T cells, such as the Thy-1 (formerly Θ) surface antigen (in mice), and also lacks the typical B-cell marker of membrane Ig detectable by the usual fluorescent antibody techniques. However, these cells bear Ig detectable by some antiglobulin-binding methods (Haegert, 1978), including those using the avian antiglobulin reagents mentioned above; in addition, null cells can be shown to possess substantial amounts of typical B-cell Igs, both by radioimmunoassay and by analysis of membrane extracts of surface-radioiodinated cells (Warr *et al.*, 1978*a*). Fig. 1 illustrates the membrane Ig of null cells as characterized by polyacrylamide-gel electrophoresis. A comparison with Fig. 2 shows that null-cell Ig looks, when analyzed in this manner, identical to that of B cells. These results are in marked contrast to those obtained by just a conventional immunofluorescent examination of Ig exposed on the membrane of the intact lymphocyte.

The obvious conclusion to be drawn from these observations is that some lymphocytes (e.g., null and T cells) bear membrane Igs, but that these are occluded in the membrane in such a manner that only the N-terminal antigen-binding portion is exposed, and hence are unavailable for reaction with many antiglobulin reagents that recognize antigenic determinants elsewhere on the molecule.

Bearing in mind these problems in interpretation of results, I shall in the next section review briefly reports bearing on the demonstration of membrane Ig in the vertebrates. I will attempt to review them critically, and then draw con-

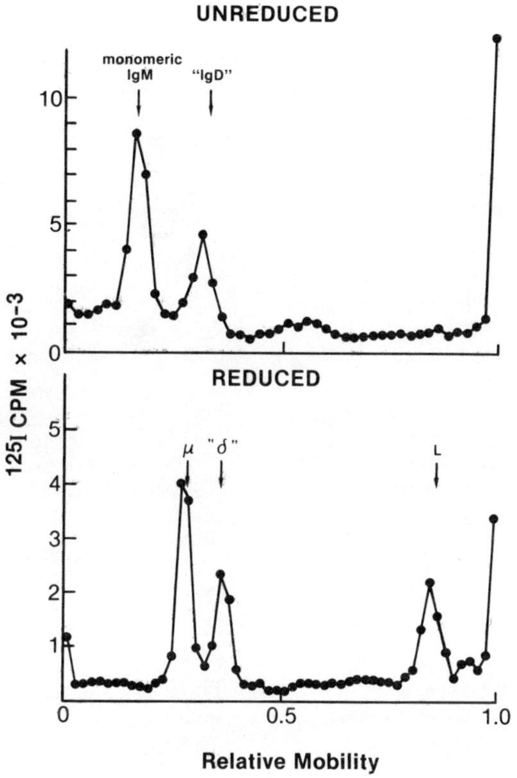


Figure 2. Surface Ig of murine B cells. The splenocytes obtained from CBA mice were surface-radioiodinated and lysed in detergent, and the labeled surface Igs were isolated, as described in the caption to Fig. 1. The surface Igs were analyzed under reducing and nonreducing conditions by SDS-polyacrylamide-gel electrophoresis, as described by Haustein *et al.* (1975). The observed peaks are identified as monomeric IgM, "IgD," or their constituent polypeptide chains, $\mu$, $\gamma$, and L. This figure is taken from the unpublished data of the author.

clusions, before considering the question of the functional role of these molecules in lymphocyte activation.

## III. SURFACE IMMUNOGLOBULINS OF VERTEBRATE LYMPHOCYTES

Table I summarizes some of the reports on the occurrence of lymphocyte-surface Igs in vertebrates. It can be seen that there is a considerable variation in the amount of information available for the various classes of vertebrates, and though I have tried to be comprehensive in my survey, the mammals (and, to a lesser extent, the birds) have by the sheer number of reports in the literature prevented the attainment of this goal.

Whereas Table I lists percentages of cells in various organs positive for surface Ig (generally by immunofluorescence or autoradiography), Table II presents a breakdown of some of these figures by Ig isotype. The data in Tables I and II can be considered in terms of a number of questions, outlined below.

**Table I. Immunoglobulin-Bearing Lymphocytes[a]**

| | Percentage positive cells | References |
|---|---|---|
| Mammalia | | |
| Human | | |
| Peripheral blood | 5–34 | Warner, 1974; Preud'homme and Seligmann, 1974; Froland and Natvig, 1972; Ross *et al.*, 1973; Gajl-Peczalska *et al.*, 1972; Paraskevas *et al.*, 1971; Papamichail *et al.*, 1971 |
| Spleen | 21–39 | |
| Lymph nodes | 9–52 | |
| Bone marrow | 36–51 | |
| Thoracic-duct lymph | 2 | |
| Thymus | 2 | |
| Thymus | 16–24[b] | Jones *et al.*, 1976 |
| Mouse | | |
| Peripheral blood | 11–34 | Raff *et al.*, 1970; Nossal *et al.*, 1972; Osmond and Nossal, 1974; Bankhurst and Warner, 1971; Paraskevas *et al.*, 1971; Takahashi *et al.*, 1971; Jones *et al.*, 1971; Lee *et al.*, 1971; Rabellino *et al.*, 1971; Yakulis *et al.*, 1972; Yamana *et al.*, 1973; Goding and Layton, 1976 |
| Spleen | 24–50 | |
| Lymph nodes | 7–30 | |
| Bone marrow | 8–42 | |
| Thoracic-duct lymph | 14–30 | |
| Thymus | 0–4 | |
| Thymus | 95–100[b] | Nossal *et al.*, 1972; Hämmerling *et al.*, 1976*a*; Szenberg *et al.*, 1977; Santana *et al.*, 1974 |
| Rabbit | | |
| Peripheral blood | 24–85 | Coombs *et al.*, 1970; An and Sell, 1973; Pernis *et al.*, 1970; Jones *et al.*, 1970 |
| Spleen | 39–48 | |
| Lymph nodes | 16–21 | |
| Bone marrow | 13 | |
| Thymus | 0–1 | |
| Aves | | |
| Chicken | | |
| Peripheral blood | 18–40 | Kincade *et al.*, 1971; Hudson and Roitt, 1973; Rouse *et al.*, 1973; Rabellino and Gray, 1971 |
| Spleen | 26–40 | |
| Bursa of Fabricius | 78–93 | |
| Amphibia | | |
| Salamander (*Pleurodeles waltlii*) | | |
| Spleen | 65–85 | Charlemagne and Tournefier, 1975 |
| Thymus | 98 | |
| Toad (*Xenopus laevis*) | | |
| Gut-associated lymphoid tissue | 51–68 | Jurd, 1977 |
| Peripheral blood | 25–82 | Jurd and Stevenson, 1976; DuPasquier *et al.*, 1972; DuPasquier, 1976 |
| Spleen | 40–92 | |
| Thymus | 9–70[c] | |
| Pisces | | |
| Skate (*Raja naevus*) | | |
| Peripheral blood | 80 | Ellis and Parkhouse, 1975 |
| Spleen | 80 | |
| Thymus | 82 | |

**Table I. (Cont'd)**

| | Percentage positive cells | References |
|---|---|---|
| Teleostii[d] | | |
| Peripheral blood | 25–90 | Clem *et al.*, 1977; Emmrich *et al.*, 1975; Ellis and Parkhouse, 1975; Etlinger *et al.*, 1977; Warr *et al.*, 1976*b*, 1977; DeLuca *et al.*, 1978 |
| Spleen | 25–99 | |
| Head nephros | 85–100 | |
| Thymus | 95–100 | |

[a] Values given are the range of those reported. Techniques of immunofluorescence, autoradiography, and antiglobulin rosetting were used in the studies cited here.
[b] Using conditions of greater sensitivity than usual or antisera raised in chickens.
[c] This value varies with developmental age (DuPasquier *et al.*, 1972; Du Pasquier, 1976; Jurd and Stevenson, 1976).
[d] Pooled data for *Carassius auratus*, *C. carassius*, *Cyprinus carpio*, *Salmo gairdneri*, and *Lepomis macrochirus*.

## A. Universality of Lymphoid Heterogeneity in the Vertebrates

Most immunologists would agree that the paradigm of lymphoid heterogeneity is the division into T- and B-cell types, as originally described in both avian and mammalian species (Thorbecke *et al.*, 1978; Warner *et al.*, 1962; Miller, 1972), but subsequently most thoroughly studied in the latter. Evidence is accumulating that the division of lymphocytes into functional T- and B-cell types was an ancient evolutionary event in vertebrate history, probably preceding the divergence of the teleost fish from the stem line of vertebrate evolution. This topic has been reviewed previously (Marchalonis *et al.*, 1977*a*; Warr and Marchalonis, 1978; Warr *et al.*, 1976*a*), and also forms the subject of one of the reviews in this book (Ruben and Edwards, 1978). Suffice it to say here that this evidence has come from both structural and functional studies of (1) the anatomical partition of mitogen responses and antibody production, (2) hapten–carrier effects in the antibody response, (3) thymus ablation and reconstitution, (4) use of thymus-dependent and -independent antigens, (5) physical separation of lymphocyte subpopulations, and (6) studies on the physicochemical properties of lymphocyte-surface Igs. For the purposes of this chapter, I will accept the premise that functional T- and B-type heterogeneity occurs in vertebrates from teleosts to man, and that some valid parallels between corresponding lymphoid organs (such as thymus and spleen) can be drawn in diverse vertebrate taxa.

## B. B-Cell-Surface Ig

B cells can generally be considered to be the precursors of high-rate antibody-producing (plasma) cells. In mammals and birds, B cells are generally considered

**Table II. Lymphocyte-Membrane Immunoglobulins: Class Distribution**

| | Class of Ig | Percentage of total Ig positive cells[a] | References |
|---|---|---|---|
| Mammalia | | | |
| Human | | | |
| Peripheral blood | IgG | 3–54 | Gajl-Peczalska *et al.*, 1972; Froland and Natvig, 1972; Grey *et al.*, 1971; Papamichail *et al.*, 1971; Winchester *et al.*, 1975; Coombs *et al.*, 1969; Pernis *et al.*, 1971 |
| | IgM[b] | 25–90 | |
| | IgA | 3–46 | |
| | IgE | 2–14 | |
| | IgD[b] | 14–92 | Winchester *et al.*, 1975; Knapp *et al.*, 1973; Rowe *et al.*, 1973 |
| Mouse | | | |
| Spleen | IgG | 2–66 | Nossal *et al.*, 1972; Bankhurst and Warner, 1971; Abney *et al.*, 1976; Takahashi *et al.*, 1971; Jones *et al.*, 1971; Goding and Layton, 1976; Goding *et al.*, 1976; Parkhouse *et al.*, 1976; Lamelin *et al.*, 1972; Grey *et al.*, 1972 |
| | IgM[b] | 48–88 | |
| | IgA | 6–76 | |
| | IgD-like[b] | 72–86 | |
| Rabbit | | | |
| Peripheral blood | IgM | 23–80 | Coombs *et al.*, 1970; Pernis *et al.*, 1970 |
| | IgG | 8–80 | |
| Aves | | | |
| Chicken | | | |
| Peripheral blood | IgM | 33–63 | Hudson, 1975; Kincade *et al.*, 1971 |
| | IgY | 32–68 | |
| | IgA | 5–6 | |
| Bursa of Fabricius | IgM | 27 | |
| | IgY | 58 | |
| | IgA | 6 | |
| Spleen | IgM | 45 | |
| | IgY | 57 | |
| | IgA | 2 | |

| | | | |
|---|---|---|---|
| Reptilia–Immunofluorescence data unavailable | | | |
| Tortoise (*Agrionemys horsfieldii*) | | | |
| Peripheral blood, Spleen | IgM and IgY | Observed by analysis of radioiodinated membrane extracts | Fiebig and Ambrosius, 1975 |
| Alligator | | | |
| Peripheral blood | IgM, IgY? | Observed by analysis of radioiodinated membrane extracts | Cuchens *et al.*, 1975 |
| Amphibia | | | |
| Toad (*Xenopus laevis*) | | | |
| Gut-associated lymphoid tissue | IgM | 92–95 | Jurd and Stevenson, 1976; Jurd, 1977 |
| | IgY | 1–8 | |
| Peripheral blood | IgM | 93–99 | |
| | IgY | 1–7 | |
| Spleen | IgM | 94–99 | |
| | IgY | 1–6 | |
| Thymus | IgM | 80–100 | |
| | IgY | <1–20 | |
| Pisces–In both chondrichthyean and teleostean fish the only known serum and lymphocyte-surface Ig is IgM | | | Clem *et al.*, 1977; Warr *et al.*, 1976*b*; Warr and Marchalonis, 1977*b*; Fiebig and Ambrosius, 1975 |

[a] As assessed by immunofluorescence, autoradiography, and antiglobulin-rosetting techniques. Values have been calculated from data in the cited literature.
[b] Up to 85% or more of these cells are doubles for IgM and IgD.

to be those lymphocytes bearing surface Ig readily detectable by fluorescence studies using antiglobulin reagents raised in mammalian species. Exceptions to this rule have been reported in mammals (see Section III.D), and this rule breaks down completely in the urodele amphibians and fish, in which apparently all lymphocytes can be positive for surface Ig using mammalian-derived antiglobulin sera (Table I). However, confining ourselves initially to the mammals, the results of immunofluorescent analyses of B cells are highly variable with respect to both the numbers of Ig-positive cells in an organ and the isotypes of Ig expressed by these cells (Tables I and II). For example, in man these have been reported to include IgM, IgG, IgD, IgA, and IgE (all the serum isotypes, in fact). One view held by a number of investigators (Winchester *et al.*, 1975; Goding *et al.*, 1977; Goding, 1978; Vitetta and Uhr, 1975, 1977) is that many of these reports, especially the earlier ones, are erroneous, and might well be discounted until verified in the light of our present knowledge about Fc receptors and the passive adsorption of antibodies to cells (see above). One current view, to which I subscribe, is that the major isotypes of surface Ig in man, mouse, and probably rat are the monomeric ($\mu_2L_2$) form of IgM and IgD, or an IgD-like molecule (Abney and Parkhouse, 1974; Melcher *et al.*, 1974; Parkhouse *et al.*, 1976; Ruddick and Leslie, 1977; Goding *et al.*, 1977; Goding, 1978; Vitetta and Uhr, 1975, 1977; Warr and Marchalonis, 1977*a*). It should also be noted that many lymphocytes bearing IgM in these species are also positive for IgD. Up to 85% or more of IgM-positive lymphocytes are doubles, and these cells in addition show haplotype exclusion and identical variable regions on both IgM and IgD (Goding *et al.*, 1977; Goding, 1978; Abney *et al.*, 1976). Fig. 2 illustrates the mobilities, on sodium dodecyl sulfate–polyacrylamide gel electrophoresis, of the intact murine B-cell-surface IgM and IgD-like molecule, and the mobilities of their constituent heavy and light chains. Other isotypes of Ig, such as IgA, IgE and IgG, probably do occur as endogenously produced membrane molecules, but at a much lower frequency than was previously thought. Although IgD or an equivalent has been identified in primates (Martin *et al.*, 1976), mice (Table II), and rats (Ruddick and Leslie, 1977), it has not yet been demonstrated in other mammals, birds, or the poikilothermic vertebrates. While it may be a reasonable presumption that IgD or an equivalent will be proved to exist as a lymphocyte-surface Ig in mammals and possibly birds, as yet no widespread search for its existence has been undertaken in the poikilothermic-vertebrate classes. Studies by Jurd and Stevenson (1976) and Jurd (1977), however, suggest that in one amphibian species (*Xenopus laevis*) the only lymphocyte-surface Igs appear to be IgM and the low-molecular-weight IgY (sometimes referred to as IgG). Thus we are left with the tentative conclusion that the only phylogenetically universal lymphocyte-membrane Ig is IgM. Interestingly enough, in all cases in which its structure has been examined it has been discovered that lymphocyte-surface IgM is in the monomeric form, despite the fact that the monomer is the least frequently observed serum form of

IgM in the vertebrates, where dimers, tetramers, pentamers, and hexamers have all been reported in the circulation (Litman, 1976; Marchalonis, 1977*a*). In vertebrates where serum-Ig isotypes other than IgM have been reported, these have also been identified on the membrane of B (or putative B) cells. This includes IgA in the rat (Williams and Gowans, 1975), IgA and IgY in the chicken, and IgY in amphibians (Jurd and Stevenson, 1976; Jurd, 1977) and reptiles (Fiebig and Ambrosius, 1975; Cuchens *et al*., 1975). IgM is the only isotype of Ig reported in the serum and on the cells of teleost and chondrichthyean fish, although the possibility of a subclass distinction between lymphocyte and serum IgM in these forms has not yet been thoroughly investigated. Nothing is known of lymphocyte-surface Igs in the Agnatha.

Some evidence exists showing that B-cell-surface Ig differs from serum forms in a number of properties. The clearest examples of this are (1) the fact that membrane IgM is always monomeric rather than the typical polymer found in serum (Marchalonis and Cone, 1973; Vitetta and Uhr, 1973; Warr *et al.*, 1976*b*) and (2) the restriction of the murine IgD to the surface of the lymphocyte. This molecule, as far as is known, does not possess a serum conterpart present in detectable amounts.

Other reports suggest that B-cell-membrane IgM can differ from the serum form in (1) the apparent molecular weight of the $\mu$ chain, (2) detergent solubility, and (3) buoyant density of the molecule (Melcher *et al.*, 1975; Melcher and Uhr, 1976, 1977; Warr and Marchalonis, 1977*b*).

The concept that membrane Ig is distinct from the similar secreted form is an attractive one, from a teleological viewpoint. It would be satisfying if the insertion of an Ig into the hydrophobic environment of the lymphocyte membrane were accompanied by changes in the primary structure of the molecule to adapt it to the milieu. However, there is no clear evidence that surface Ig is intimately associated with the hydrophobic regions of the plasma membrane. In addition, the finding that both mouse and human B-lymphocyte-surface $\mu$ chains have the same C-terminal amino acid (tyrosine) as the secreted $\mu$ chains (McIlhinney *et al.*, 1978) strongly suggests that the membrane $\mu$ chains do not possess an extra hydrophobic C-terminal tail. However, we cannot yet exclude the possibility that there is an *insertion* of a hydrophobic stretch near the C-terminal end of the $\mu$ chain, and until we have a more detailed knowledge of the molecular structure of lymphocyte-surface Igs it would be best to reserve judgment on this issue. The alternative hypothesis for association of membrane Ig with the lymphocyte surface is that it interacts with a second membrane protein that has properties similar to those of an Fc receptor. Both hypotheses are compatible with the suggestion that lymphocyte-surface Ig interacts functionally with another membrane protein ("transducer") to transmit a triggering signal to the interior of the cell upon union with antigen (Marchalonis *et al.*, 1977*a*; Marchalonis, 1976; Decker and Marchalonis, 1978; Krolick and Sercarz, 1977).

### C. T-Cell-Surface Ig

For the purposes of this review, I will consider primarily surface Ig of thymocytes, rather than the truly thymus-derived peripheral (T) cells, in order to simplify the issues. As far as I am aware, nothing that I will say about Ig of thymocytes is inapplicable to the peripheral T cell, although it should be borne in mind that the functional heterogeneity of T cells may be reflected in a heterogeneity of receptor molecules (Lonai *et al.*, 1978).

The subject of T-cell Ig is still controversial for a number of reasons. First, until recently T-cell Ig in mammalian species could not easily be demonstrated *in situ* with the use of antiglobulin reagents. Second, the physicochemical properties of T-cell Ig, and/or the manner in which it associates with the plasma membrane, makes its routine isolation, quantitation, and characterization a difficult technical undertaking. Other, more comprehensive reviews of this topic are available (Marchalonis, 1975, 1976; Cone, 1977), and I propose to consider here only some of the more recent developments in this area, and to summarize our current knowledge.

### D. Direct Demonstration of T-Cell Ig

Antisera raised in one species of mammal to the serum Igs of another mammal fail to react with the Ig determinants in the membrane of thymocytes and T cells. This statement is not absolutely correct (Santana *et al.*, 1974; Burckhardt *et al.*, 1974), but it describes accurately enough the most commonly encountered situation. Ig determinants on the surface of mammalian T cells can, however, be readily demonstrated with the use of antisera raised in birds (Jones *et al.*, 1976; Hämmerling *et al.*, 1976*a*; Szenberg *et al.*, 1977) or (in mammals) raised to the idiotypic determinants (the antigen-binding $NH_2$-terminal region) of the Ig molecule (Binz *et al.*, 1975; Binz and Wigzell, 1977; McKearn *et al.*, 1974). The immunofluorescent demonstration of murine T-cell Ig using avian reagents is shown in Fig. 3. These observations, coupled with the numerous reports demonstrating surface Ig on thymocytes of fish and amphibians by direct-binding assays using mammalian-raised antisera, allow us to propose a hypothesis about the display of T-cell Ig and its *in situ* recognition by antiglobulin reagents. Stated simply, I would suggest [or rather, revive suggestions (Marchalonis and Cone, 1973)] that T-cell Ig is inserted in the membrane (or occluded in its display) in such a manner that only the $NH_2$-terminal antigen-binding region is exposed. This situation would not interfere with the antigen-binding function of the Ig, and it helps to explain why many antiglobulin reagents fail to stain T cells. The latter point follows from the fact that many commonly used antisera recognize primarily constant-region determinants on the Ig molecule. Antisera reacting with T-cell Ig *in situ* can thus be raised by immunizing deliberately to produce antibody to the

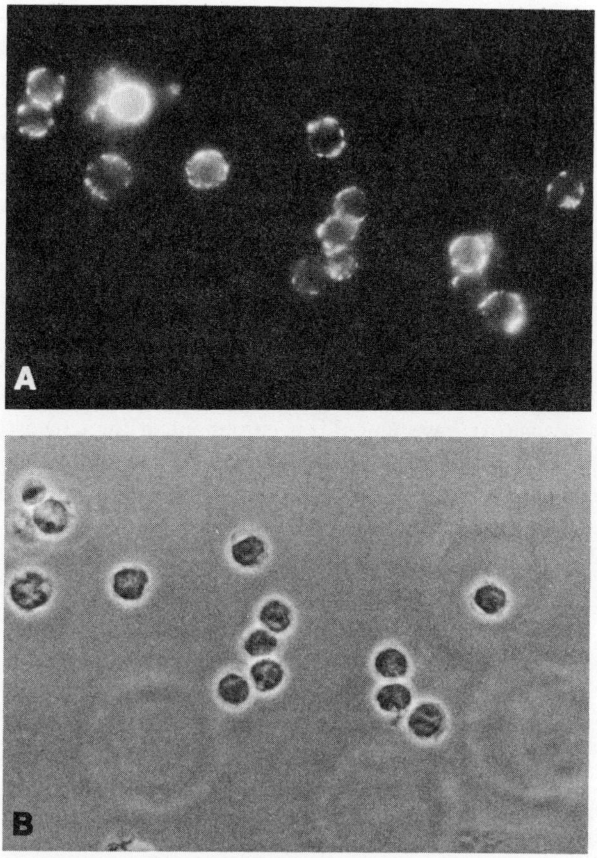


Figure 3. Direct immunofluorescent demonstration of murine T-cell-membrane Ig. BALB/c thymocytes were incubated either with chicken antibody to the (Fab′)$_2$ fragment of mouse IgG, or with normal chicken IgY, and then with fluorescein-conjugated goat antichicken gamma globulin antibodies (Szenberg *et al.*, 1977; Marchalonis *et al.*, 1977*b*). The cells reacted with normal-fowl IgY failed to show membrane fluorescence, but those reacted with chicken antibody to the (Fab′)$_2$ fragment of mouse IgG showed typical bright fluorescence under ultraviolet illumination (A). A bright-field view of the same field is also shown (B). Figure courtesy of C. Bucana and L. Hoyer.

antigen-combining site (as in the case of the antiidiotype antibody) or by immunizing across a wide phylogenetic distance, in which case, one might predict that determinants common to the antigen-binding regions (perhaps "framework" residues) would be recognized. In fact, some avian antibodies raised to the (Fab′)$_2$ fragment of mouse IgG are predominantly reactive with determinants shared with other isotypes of Ig, and are virtually lacking in $\gamma$ heavy-chain specific reactions (Warr *et al.*, 1978*b*).

Before considering other aspects and properties of T-cell Ig, I wish to include here a cautionary note about interpreting direct demonstrations of T-cell Ig by fluorescent or similar techniques. There are now several reports that antiglobulin sera can contain minor (or in some cases major) activities directed against non-Ig cell-membrane constituents, e.g., carbohydrates (Mattes and Steiner, 1978; Merler *et al.*, 1974; Yamaga *et al.*, 1978*a,b*) or $\beta_2$ microglobulin (Gottlieb *et al.*, 1977). Although these cross-reactions occur in only some antisera (Gottlieb *et al.*, 1977), they must obviously be taken into account in interpreting all serological demonstrations of Ig, on both T and B cells. Apart from the appropriate serological controls, which most careful investigations would include, the clearest way to exclude this sort of cross-reaction as an explanation for a putative demonstration of Ig on a lymphocyte surface is to obtain some physicochemical (as opposed to serological) characterization of the molecules recognized. A large number of investigators have met this requirement in their investigations of T-cell Ig (see below), although the nature of these polypeptide chains will probably remain a matter of dispute until finer structural information, including primary amino-acid sequence data, becomes available.

In the following consideration of the accumulating body of information on the molecular structure of T-cell Ig, I will make no further mention of non-Ig cross-reactions present in antisera, since this problem is particularly acute only in terms of serological analyses, and loses much of its relevance when the analyses of reactions are appropriately carried out at a molecular level.

### E. Molecular Properties of T-Cell Ig

In the mammals, T-cell Ig differs from its B-cell counterpart in a number of properties. Whereas B-cell Ig typically consists, in the mouse, of IgM and IgD, only one type of Ig is found on T cells. This molecule shows several interesting features. (1) The heavy chain shows, on polyacrylamide-gel electrophoresis in the presence of sodium dodecyl sulfate, a mobility faster than $\mu$ (Haustein *et al.*, 1975; Haustein and Goding, 1975) and an apparent molecular mass of between 65,000 and 70,000 daltons. This is illustrated in Fig. 4, which also shows the T-cell Ig light chain, which possesses a mobility typical of murine light chains. (2) The T-cell Ig molecule frequently exists in a form in which the light chains are not covalently bound (by disulfide bridges) to the heavy chains (Moseley *et al.*, 1977; Moroz and Lahat, 1974; Cone and Brown, 1976). This observation may explain some failures to detect light chains on T-cell Ig when heavy-chain-specific reagents are used (Binz and Wigzell, 1976, 1977). It should also be noted that noncovalent associations of light and heavy chains have been observed in the secreted Igs (especially IgA) of man, mouse, and chickens (Jerry *et al.*, 1970; Warner and Marchalonis, 1972; Vaerman *et al.*, 1974). A representation of the covalent structure of T-cell Ig is shown in Fig. 5, where the heavy chains are

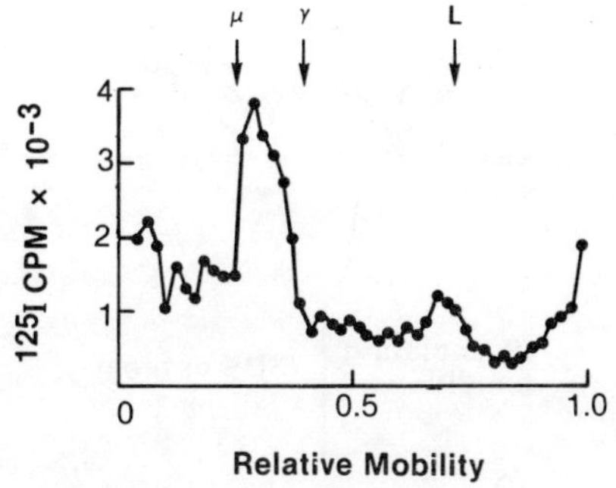


Figure 4. Immunoglobulin of the murine T-lymphoma WEHI-7. Radioiodinated immunoglobulins present in culture fluid in which the monoclonal T-lymphoma WEHI-7 had been grown were isolated by binding to a solid-phase immunoadsorbent of Sepharose 4B-conjugated rabbit antibodies to mouse IgM (Moseley *et al.*, 1977), and analyzed by SDS-polyacrylamide-gel electrophoresis under reducing conditions, as described by Moseley *et al.* (1977) and Haustein *et al.* (1975). Mobilities of standard murine μ, γ, and L chains are indicated by arrows. Further details of experimental protocols are to be found in the cited references.

shown covalently linked as a dimer, with light chains noncovalently associated. (3) T-cell Ig differs from that of B cells in its requirements for solubilization from the lymphocyte membrane. Notably, nonionic detergents above critical micelle concentration (as typically used for solubilization of B-cell membranes before isolation of Ig by reaction with anti-Ig reagents) are inefficient at solubilizing T-cell Ig in a form that makes it available for isolation by standard methods (Cone and Marchalonis, 1974). It has been suggested that occlusion of T-cell Ig within detergent micelles occurs under these conditions (Cone, 1976; Cone and Brown, 1976; Cone *et al.*, 1977).

In summary, T-cell Ig appears in the mammals to be composed of heavy and light chains, and to differ from B-cell and serum Ig in terms of its covalent structure, its interaction with the lymphocyte membrane, and its interaction with nonionic detergents; in addition, it is antigenically probably of a new isotype for both heavy (Binz *et al.*, 1976) and light chains. Although assumption-free methods for the quantitation of membrane Ig have not been used, it seems that T cells bear less membrane Ig than do B cells, although the degree of difference is a matter of controversy (Jensenius and Williams, 1974; Grey *et al.*, 1971, 1972; Jensenius, 1976; Haustein *et al.*, 1975; Boylston, 1973).

In vertebrate classes other than the mammals, T-cell Ig has not been exhaustively studied. However, the surface Igs of thymocytes from three teleost fish—the goldfish (*Carassius auratus*), carp (*Cyprinus carpio*), and bream (*Lepomis macrochirus*)—have been isolated and their constituent heavy and light chains described (Warr *et al.*, 1976*b*; Clem *et al.*, 1977; Fiebig and Ambrosius, 1975). In Fig. 6 is shown a comparison of the constituent polypeptide chains of goldfish splenocyte- and thymocyte-membrane Igs. Interesting parallels between the properties of thymocyte Ig in mammals and some teleost fish have been reported, in terms of physicochemical properties, such as apparent molecular weight of the heavy chain and problems with solubilization, especially with the

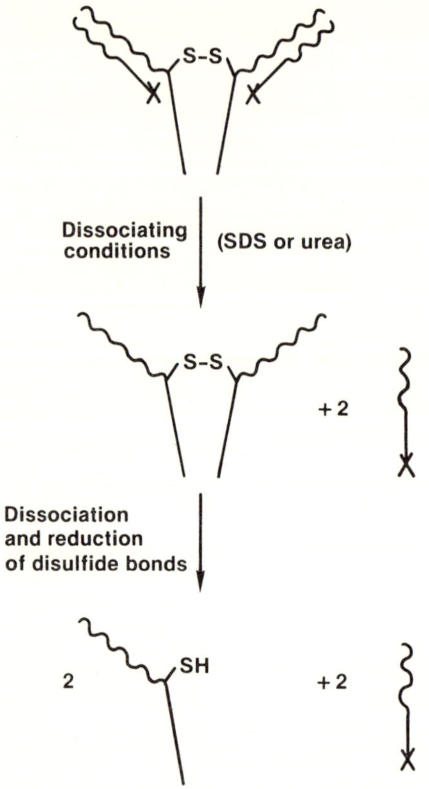


Figure 5. A model of the structure of murine T-cell Ig and its reactions upon exposure to dissociating and reducing conditions. In the native state, it shows a disulfide-(S—S) bonded heavy-chain dimer, with noncovalently associated light chains. Variable portions of the polypeptides are represented diagrammatically as wavy lines (~~), the constant portions as straight lines (—). The X at the C terminal end of the light chain represents the lack of covalent disulfide bonding between heavy and light chains. The exact nature of this block, and the presence or absence of free SH groups on heavy and light chains, is not known.

use of nonionic detergents (Warr *et al.*, 1976*b*); but whether this apparent degree of similarity is universal remains to be determined.

## IV. FUNCTION OF LYMPHOCYTE-SURFACE IMMUNOGLOBULINS

The concept that surface Ig is implicated in the primary recognition of antigen by lymphocytes, of both T and B types in mammals and putative T and B types in the birds and ectothermic vertebrates, is supported by the observations that antiglobulin reagents (1) inhibit antigen binding and (2) inhibit some (but not all) lymphocyte functions. This evidence, some of which is controversial, has been reported or reviewed elsewhere (Warner, 1974; Marchalonis, 1975).

The studies on antigen-binding lymphocytes in the ecothermic vertebrates, including inhibition of antigen binding by antiglobulin reagents, are listed in Table III. In addition to these studies, further presumptive evidence of a receptor

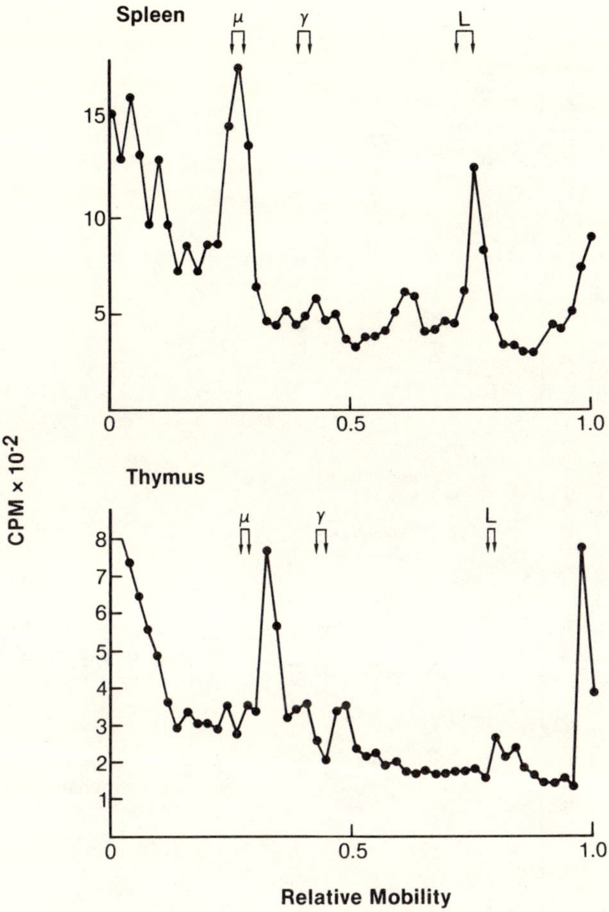


Figure 6. Surface Ig of goldfish thymocytes and splenocytes. Surface Ig was isolated from extracts of membrane-radioiodinated goldfish splenocytes and thymocytes by immune precipitation, as described by Warr *et al.* (1976*b*) and Warr and Marchalonis (1977*b*). Analysis under reducing conditions was by SDS-polyacrylamide-gel electrophoresis. The mobilities of standard mammalian μ, γ, and L polypeptide chains are indicated by arrows. Further details of experimental protocols can be found in the cited references.

role of surface Ig in lower vertebrates comes from a report showing that in both the goldfish and crucian carp, Ig determinants on the membrane of antigen-binding cells codistribute with the bound antigen (DeLuca *et al.*, 1978). Although this phenomenon was observed with cells from thymus, spleen, and head nephros, it does not formally *prove* the Ig nature of the antigen receptor. Like the studies demonstrating inhibition of antigen binding by antiglobulin reagents, a possibility (albeit unlikely) exists that the surface Ig is merely in very close

**Table III. Antigen-Binding Lymphocytes in the Poikilothermic Vertebrates**

| | Antigens | Animals immunized | Lymphoid organ | Frequency of binding cells in unimmunized animals (percentage) | Inhibition by antiglobulin | References |
|---|---|---|---|---|---|---|
| Grass frog (*Rana pipiens*) | Sheep and horse erythrocytes, trinitrophenyl hapten | Yes | Thymus, spleen | 0.04 | Yes | Edwards *et al.*, 1975; Ruben and Edwards, 1977 |
| Toad (*Xenopus laevis*) | Sheep and horse erythrocytes, trinitrophenyl hapten | Yes | Spleen | – | NT[a] | Ruben and Edwards, 1977 |
| Toad (*Bufo marinus*) | Flagellin of *Salmonella adelaide*, horse | Yes | Spleen | – | NT | Azzolina, 1975 |
| | erythrocytes | Yes | Spleen | 0.005 | Yes | Cone and Marchalonis, 1972 |
| Newt (*Triturus viridescens*) | Trinitrophenyl hapten, horse erythrocytes | Yes | Spleen | – | NT | Ruben and Edwards, 1977 |
| Goldfish (*Carassius auratus*) | Flagellin of *S. adelaide* | Yes | Spleen | – | NT | Azzolina, 1975, 1978 |
| | Horse erythrocytes, trinitrophenyl hapten | Yes | Spleen, thymus, head nephros | – | Yes | Ruben *et al.*, 1977 |
| | Keyhole limpet hemocyanin, myoglobin, horse spleen ferritin | No | Spleen, thymus, head nephros | 0.3–3.4 | NT | DeLuca *et al.*, 1978 |
| Crucian carp (*Carassius carassius*) | Keyhole limpet hemocyanin, myoglobin, horse spleen ferritin | No | Spleen, thymus, head nephros | 0.7–5.0 | NT | DeLuca *et al.*, 1978 |

[a] NT, not tested.

proximity to the true antigen receptor. Suffice it to state here that it is reasonable to assume that if Ig exists on the surface of lymphocytes, both B and T, it might be presumed to have a functional role. In qualification of this teleological statement, I would point out that the mere presence of antigen-binding Ig on B and T lymphocytes, and evidence of modification of antigen-driven lymphocyte functions by antiglobulin reagents, although suggestive, is not conclusive in proving that surface Ig is a functional receptor for antigen.

Formal demonstration of an antigen-receptor role for any molecule in the lymphocyte membrane should include evidence not only that the molecule in question can bind antigen, but also that such binding leads to functional activation of the cell. Unfortunately, at the moment we have no clear idea, at a molecular level, of how union of antigen with its receptor at the lymphocyte surface leads to activation, division, and differentiation of the cell. At the first step of the process, we are uncertain as to which external stimuli, besides binding of receptor and ligand, are necessary for activation. For B cells, it has been suggested variously that antigen binding to receptor is a tolerogenic signal, and that a second signal (from "associative antibody") is needed for triggering (Bretscher and Cohn, 1970), or else that a single inherent nonspecific (mitogenic) stimulus from an antigen can trigger the B cell, the receptor serving merely to bind and concentrate the antigen at the lymphocyte surface (Coutinho and Möller, 1974). In view of the fact that antiglobulin reagents can stimulate B cells to mitogenesis (presumably by binding to surface Ig and mimicking the action of antigen) with facility in some species, but with difficulty in mice (reviewed by Decker and Marchalonis, 1978), it would seem likely that efficient B-cell triggering requires not only a combination of surface Ig with antigen, but also that further stimuli (of the various sorts discussed above) may (or may not) be needed, depending on species and circumstance. Similarly, there is a great deal of information available on the requirements for T-cell triggering (primarily in the mouse), but it is not possible, at present, to give a simple statement of the interactions necessary at the T-cell surface for activation to occur. In some situations in which T cells are recognizing antigen associated with a cellular target, there is an apparent requirement for identity at subregions of the mouse major histocompatibility complex (MHC) between target and reactive T cell (Shearer *et al.*, 1975; Zinkernagel and Doherty, 1977). This restriction is by no means universal, as reported for a number of experimental systems in man and mouse (Burton *et al.*, 1977; Jondal *et al.*, 1975; Ting and Law, 1977; Whitelaw *et al.*, 1977). In addition, it is difficult to fit classical T-cell-mediated allogeneic killing into this conceptual framework. Furthermore, there is confusion as to whether T cells (1) have antigen receptors with a predilection for recognizing altered or modified self MHC antigens (Shearer *et al.*, 1975), (2) have two receptors, one for antigen, and one for self MHC antigens (Zinkernagel *et al.*, 1978), or (3) can learn to recognize antigen on foreign MHC antigens during a primary response (Miller and Vadas, 1977*a,b*).

This reviewer's opinion is that T cells recognize most antigens by means of an immunoglobulinlike receptor, as outlined above, and that the phenomena of MHC restriction and cell collaboration in T-cell responses (Miller and Vadas, 1977*a,b*; Paul *et al.*, 1977; Feldmann *et al.*, 1977) reflect secondary recognition phenomena, and perhaps also physiological interactions not directly relevant to the binding of receptor to ligand, but very relevant to the question of lymphocyte activation, as discussed in Chapter 1 of this volume. As such, these factors that are probably involved secondarily in lymphocyte activation will not be discussed further here. Neither do I propose to discuss here the biochemical changes that occur in the cell following union of antigen with receptor (receptor redistribution, influx of divalent cations, changes in the levels of cyclic nucleotides), which may also be presumed to play some role in activation. For reviews of these phenomena, the reader is referred to Ling and Kay (1975), Wedner and Parker (1976), Cooper (1973), and Edelman (1976).

I propose to consider, instead, the question of whether or not we can discern any correlation between the structure and the function of lymphocyte-surface Igs. Put simply, is the diversity of functional responses in lymphocytes in any way correlated with structural diversity of surface Ig types? Although this is an interesting question, there is no reason *per se* for us to assume that the direction of lymphocyte responses is determined solely by, or even correlates with, the isotype of Ig expressed on the plasma membrane. The only hypothesis of this nature that has received substantial experimental attention is the proposition that mammalian (mostly murine) B-cell responses to antigen, e.g., in terms of tolerance (no response, inactivation) or activation, correlates with or is related to the isotypes of surface Ig. Quite a large number of reviews on this topic have been published in recent years, most of them dealing with the question of the function of the recently discovered murine IgD (for example, see *Immunological Reviews*, 1977).

There is evidence that the relative amount of IgD on the surface of B cells in adult mice correlates with responsiveness to two different types of thymus-independent antigens (Mosier *et al.*, 1977). One of these subpopulations of B cells appears earlier in ontogeny than the other (Mosier *et al.*, 1977), and can apparently by distinguished on the basis of a number of phenotypic characters, in addition to differential expression of IgM and IgD. Evidence is still lacking that the differences in surface-Ig expression on these cell types is causally related to their functional immune responses.

A further or alternative role for B-cell surface Igs is that they determine the ease of tolerization of the cell. For example, the acquisition of IgD during ontogeny correlates with an increased resistance to tolerance induction in some species, notably the mouse, but not in others, e.g., the rat (Cuchens and Leslie, 1977). The hypotheses dealing with this idea, and the experimental systems that have been used in examining them, are quite complex and ingenious, and the reader interested in the details is referred to several recent reviews (Goding *et al.*, 1977; Vitetta and Uhr, 1977; Goding, 1978; Parkhouse and Cooper, 1977). It would be fair to conclude that at present the function of IgD still remains largely unknown, but that data on its function are accumulating and it may soon be possible, we hope, to assign to it a definitive role.

Although the function of other cell-surface Ig isotypes in the mouse is also unclear, it seems that some of the IgG-bearing cells form part of the antigen-specific B-cell memory pool (Okumura *et al.*, 1976).

On a wider phylogenetic scale, the investigation of lymphocyte-surface Igs has not extended to studies of the molecular mechanisms of triggering. However, as mentioned above, surface Ig has been implicated in the binding of antigen by all lymphocytes, including putative T cells, as assessed by (1) inhibition of antigen binding with the use of antiglobulin reagents and (2) codistribution of antigen and surface Ig on the membrane of antigen-binding cells.

## V. CONCLUDING COMMENTS

There is good evidence that Ig, or a structurally related molecule, serves as the receptor for primary binding of antigen by all lymphocytes in all vertebrates.

Monomeric IgM appears to be universally present as an antigen receptor on those lymphocytes that form the antibody-secreting series (B cells in birds and mammals). In addition, a second major class of lymphocyte-surface Ig (IgD) appears in primates and some rodents. The presence of IgD on lymphocytes in other mammals, birds, and poikilothermic vertebrates has not been investigated thoroughly enough to permit any definitive conclusions to be drawn regarding its occurrence and significance.

Thymocytes and T cells apparently bear Ig receptors whose heavy chains are likely to be of a new and unique class, and some controversy still exists about whether or not these heavy chains are also associated with light chains in the T-cell Ig (Rajewsky and Eichmann, 1977; Binz and Wigzell, 1976, 1977; Moseley *et al.*, 1977; Marchalonis, 1975; Cone, 1977; Cone and Janeway, 1977).

Although there appear to be considerable differences among surface Igs of different types of lymphocytes (as exemplified by T and B cells), the following issues remain unresolved:

1. The nature of structural differences between cell-surface and secreted Igs, and their relevance for the association of the Ig with the lymphocyte membrane.
2. The molecular mechanisms by which the reaction of lymphocyte-surface Ig with an antigen results in the transmembrane passage of a signal triggering the cell to divide and/or differentiate.

3. Whether or not there is a simple correlation between the isotype of surface Ig, and its functional role (e.g., the postulated triggering function of IgD).

There seems good reason for us to hope that in the next few years these problems will be resolved.

ACKNOWLEDGMENT

Research on this subject was sponsored by the National Cancer Institute under contract number N01-C0-75380 with Litton Bionetics, Inc.

## VI. REFERENCES

Abney, E. R., and Parkhouse, R. M. E., 1974, Candidate for immunoglobulin D present on murine B lymphocytes, *Nature* **252**:600.

Abney, E. R., Hunter, I. R., and Parkhouse, R. M. E., 1976, Preparation and characterisation of an antiserum to the mouse candidate for immunoglobulin D, *Nature* **259**:404.

An, T., and Sell, S., 1973, Increased numbers of rabbit blood lymphocytes with a1 allotypic determinants demonstrated by double-coating indirect rosette formation, *Immunology* **24**:277.

An, T., Miuai, K., and Sell, S., 1972, Electron microscopic localization of rabbit immunoglobulin allotype b4 on blood lymphocytes by an indirect ferritin immune complex labeling technique, *J. Immunol.* **108**:1271.

Avrameas, S., and Guilbert, B., 1971, A method for quantitative determination of cellular immunoglobulins by enzyme-labelled antibodies, *Eur. J. Immunol.* **1**:394.

Azzolina, L. S., 1975, Differentiation of antigen-binding cells in the teleost *Carassius auratus* and in the anuran *Bufo marinus, Haematologica* **60**:409.

Azzolina, L. S., 1978, Antigen recognition and immune response in goldfish *Carassius auratus* at different temperatures, *Dev. Comp. Immunol.* **2**:77.

Bankhurst, A. D., and Warner, N. L., 1971, Surface immunoglobulins on mouse lymphoid cells, *J. Immunol.* **107**:368.

Biberfeld, P., Biberfeld, G. and Perlmann, P., 1971, Surface immunoglobulin light chain determinants on normal and PHA-stimulated human blood lymphocytes studied by immunofluorescence and electronmicroscopy, *Exp. Cell. Res.* **66**:177.

Binz, H., and Wigzell, H., 1976, Shared idiotypic determinants on B and T lymphocytes reactive against the same antigenic determinants. V. Biochemical and serological characteristics of naturally occurring soluble antigen-binding T-lymphocyte-derived molecules, *Scand. J. Immunol.* **5**:559.

Binz, H., and Wigzell, H., 1977, Antigen-binding, idiotypic T-lymphocyte receptors, in: *Contemporary Topics in Immunobiology,* Vol. 7: *T Cells* (O. Stutman, ed.), pp. 113–177, Plenum Press, New York.

Binz, H., Bächi, T., Wigzell, H., Ramseier, H., and Lindenmann, J., 1975, Idiotype positive T cell visualized by autoradiography and electronmicroscopy, *Proc. Natl. Acad. Sci. USA* **72**:3210.

Binz, H., Wigzell, H., and Bazin, H., 1976, T-cell idiotypes are linked to immunoglobulin heavy chain genes, *Nature* **264**:639.

Boylston, A. W., 1973, Theta antigen and immunoglobulin on a tissue-cultured mouse lymphoma, *Immunology* **24**:851.

Boylston, A. W., and Mowbray, J. F., 1974, Surface immunoglobulin of a mouse T cell lymphoma, *Immunology* **27**:855.

Bretscher, P., and Cohn, M., 1970, A theory of self-nonself discrimination, *Science* **169**:1042.

Burckhardt, J. J., Guggisberg, F., and von Fellenberg, R., 1974, Thymus immunoglobulin receptors: ontogenic development, response to antigenic stimulation and their possible role in the regulation of "aggressive" immune reactions, *Immunology* **26**:521.

Burton, R. C., Chism, S. E., and Warner, N. L., 1977, *In vitro* induction of tumor-specific immunity. III. Lack of requirement for *H-2* compatibility in lysis of tumor targets by T cells activated *in vitro* to oncofetal and plasmacytoma antigens, *J. Immunol.* **118**:971.

Carraway, K. L., 1975, Covalent labeling of membranes, *Biochim. Biophys. Acta* **415**:379.

Cebra, J. J., and Goldstein, G., 1965, Chromatographic purification of tetramethylrhodamine-immune globulin conjugates and their use in the cellular localization of rabbit γ-globulin peptide chains, *J. Immunol.* **95**:230.

Charlemagne, J., and Tournefier, A., 1975, Cell surface immunoglobulins of thymus and spleen lymphocytes in urodele amphibian *Pleurodeles waltlii* (Salamandridae), *Adv. Exp. Med. Biol.* **64**:251.

Chavin, S. I., 1974, Membrane associated immunoglobulin in pig thymocytes, *Biochem. Biophys. Res. Commun.* **61**:432.

Chess, L., Levine, H., MacDermott, R. P., and Schlossman, S. F., 1975, Immunologic functions of isolated human lymphocyte subpopulations. VI. Further characterization of the surface Ig negative, E. rosette negative (null cell) subset, *J. Immunol.* **115**:1483.

Clem, L. W., McLean, W. E., Shankey, V. T., and Cuchens, M. A., 1977, Phylogeny of lymphocyte heterogeneity. I. Membrane immunoglobulins of teleost lymphocytes, *Dev. Comp. Immunol.* **1**:105.

Cone, R. E., 1976, Factors influencing the isolation of membrane immunoglobulins from T and B lymphocytes. I. Detergent effects and iodination conditions, *J. Immunol.* **116**: 847.

Cone, R. E., 1977, The search for the T cell antigen receptor, *Progr. Immunol.* **3**:47.

Cone, R. E., and Brown, W. C., 1976, Isolation of membrane associated immunoglobulins from T lymphocytes by nonionic detergents, *Immunochemistry* **13**:571.

Cone, R. E., and Janeway, C., 1977, The T cell receptors (workshop summary), in: *Immune System: Genetics and Regulation* (E. E. Sercarz, L. A. Herzenberg, and C. F. Fox, eds.), pp. 175–178, Academic Press, New York.

Cone, R. E., and Marchalonis, J. J., 1972, Cellular and humoral aspects of the influence of environmental temperature on the immune response of poikilothermic vertebrates, *J. Immunol.* **108**:952.

Cone, R. E., and Marchalonis, J. J., 1974, Surface proteins of thymus-derived and bone-marrow-derived lymphocytes: selective isolation of immunoglobulin and the theta antigen by nonionic detergents, *Biochem. J.* **140**:345.

Cone, R. E., Hoessli, D., and Rosenstein, R. W., 1977, Analysis of detergent-extracted immunoglobulins of T and B lymphocytes by ultracentrifugation and column chromatography, *Immunochemistry* **14**:345.

Coombs, R. R. A., Feinstein, A., and Wilson, A. B., 1969, Immunoglobulin determinants on the surface of human lymphocytes, *Lancet* **2**:1157.

Coombs, R. R. A., Gurner, B. W., Janeway, C. A., Wilson, A. B., Gell, P. G. H., and Kelus, A. S., 1970, Immunoglobulin determinants on the lymphocytes of normal rabbits. I. Demonstration by the mixed antiglobulin reaction of determinants recognized by anti-γ, anti-μ anti-Fab and anti-allotype sera, anti-As4 and anti-Asb, *Immunology* **18**:417.

Cooper, E. L., 1976, *Comparative Immunology*, Prentice-Hall, Englewood Cliffs, N.J.

Cooper, H. L., 1973, Effects of mitogens on the mitotic cycle: A biochemical evaluation of lymphocyte activation, in: *Drugs and the Cell Cycle* (A. M. Zimmerman, G. M. Padille, and I. L. Cameron, eds.), pp. 137–194, Academic Press, New York.

Coutinho, A. and Möller, G., 1974, Immune activation of B cells: Evidence for one nonspecific triggering signal not delivered by Ig receptors, *Scand. J. Immunol.* **3**:133.

Cuchens, M. A., and Leslie, G. A., 1977, B-cell function in rats treated as neonates and adults with anti-IgD and anti-IgM, in: *Developmental Immunobiology* (J. B. Solomon and J. D. Horton, eds.), pp. 197–204, Elsevier North-Holland, New York.

Cuchens, M., McLean, E. and Clem, L. W., 1975, Lymphocyte heterogeneity in fish and reptiles, in: *Phylogeny of Thymus and Bone Marrow-Bursa Cells* (R. K. Wright and E. L. Cooper, eds.), pp. 205–213, Elsevier North-Holland, New York.

Decker, J. M., and Marchalonis, J. J., 1978, Molecular events in lymphocyte activation: Role of nonhistone chromosomal proteins in regulating gene expression, in: *Contemporary Topics in Molecular Immunology*, Vol. 7 (R. A. Reisfeld and F. P. Inman, eds.), pp. 365–413, Plenum Press, New York.

DeLuca, D., Warr, G. W., and Marchalonis, J. J., 1978, Phylogenetic origins of immune recognition: Lymphocyte surface immunoglobulins and antigen-binding in the genus *Carassius* (Teleostii), *Eur. J. Immunol.* **8**:525.

DuPasquier, L., 1976, Amphibian models for study of the ontogeny of immunity, in: *Comparative Immunology* (J. J. Marchalonis, ed.), pp. 390–418, Blackwell, Oxford.

DuPasquier, L., Weiss, N. and Loor, F., 1972, Direct evidence for immunoglobulins on the surface of thymus lymphocytes of amphibian larvae, *Eur. J. Immunol.* **2**:366.

Edelman, G. M., 1976, Surface modulation in cell recognition and growth, *Science* **192**:218.

Edwards, B. F., Ruben, L. N., Marchalonis, J. J., and Hylton, C., 1975, Surface characteristics of spleen cell–erythrocyte rosette formation in the grass frog *Rana pipiens, Adv. Exp. Med. Biol.* **64**:397.

Ellis, A. E., and Parkhouse, R. M. E., 1975, Surface immunoglobulins on the lymphocytes of the skate, *Raja naevus, Eur. J. Immunol.* **5**:726.

Emmrich, F., Richter, R. F., and Ambrosius, H., 1975, Immunoglobulin determinants on the surface of lymphoid cells of carps, *Eur. J. Immunol.* **5**:76.

Etlinger, H. M., Hodgins, H. O., and Chiller, J. M., 1977, Evolution of the lymphoid system. II. Evidence for immunoglobulin determinants on all rainbow trout lymphocytes and demonstration of mixed leukocyte reaction, *Eur. J. Immunol.* **7**:881.

Feldmann, M., Beverley, P., Erb, P., Howie, S., Kontiainen, S., Maoz, A., Mathie, M., McKenzie, I., and Woody, J., 1977, Current concepts of the antibody response: Heterogeneity of lymphoid cells, interactions, and factors, *Cold Spring Harbor Symp. Quant. Biol.* **41**:113.

Fiebig, H., and Ambrosius, H., 1975, Cell surface immunoglobulin of lymphocytes in lower vertebrates, in: *Phylogeny of Thymus and Bone Marrow-Bursa Cells* (R. K. Wright and E. L. Cooper, eds.), pp. 195–203, Elsevier North-Holland, New York.

Froland, S. S., and Natvig, J. B., 1972, Surface-bound immunoglobulin on lymphocytes from normal and immunodeficient humans, *Scand. J. Immunol.* **1**:1.

Gabison, D., Bergman, Y., Haimovich, J., and Berke, G., 1977, Immunoglobulins detected in cell populations involved in graft rejection, *Transpl. Proc.* **9**:741.

Gajl-Peczalska, K. J., Biggar, W. D., Park, B. H., and Good, R. A., 1972, B lymphocytes in DiGeorge Syndrome, *Lancet* **1**:1344.

Goding, J. W., 1978, Allotypes of IgM and IgD receptors in the mouse: A probe for lymphocyte differentiation, in: *Contemporary Topics in Immunobiology*, Vol. 8 (N. L. Warner and M. D. Cooper, eds.), pp. 203–237, Plenum Press, New York.

Goding, J. W., and Layton, J. E., 1976, Antigen-induced co-capping of IgM and IgD-like receptors on murine B cells , *J. Exp. Med.* **144**:852.

Goding, J. W., Warr, G. W., and Warner, N. L., 1976, Genetic polymorphism of IgD-like cell surface immunoglobulin in the mouse, *Proc. Natl. Acad. Sci. USA* **73**:1305.

Goding, J. W., Scott, D. W. and Layton, J. E., 1977, Genetics, cellular expression and function of IgD and IgM receptors, *Immunol. Rev.* **37**:152.

Gottlieb, A. B., Englehard, E., and Kunkel, H. G., 1977, A cross-reaction between $\beta_2$-microglobulin and $\kappa$-light chain, *J. Immunol.* **119**:2001.

Greenberg, A. H., Hudson, L., Shen, L., and Roitt, I., 1973, Antibody dependent cell-mediated cytotoxicity due to a "null" lymphoid cell, *Nature New Biol.* **242**:111.

Grey, H. M., Rabellino, E., and Pirofsky, B., 1971, Immunoglobulins on the surface of lymphocytes. IV. Distribution of hypogammaglobulinemia, cellular immune deficiency and chronic lymphatic leukemia, *J. Clin. Invest.* **50**:2368.

Grey, H. M., Colon, S., Campbell, P., and Rabellino, E., 1972, Immunoglobulins on the surface of lymphocytes. V. Quantitative studies on the question of whether immunoglobulins are associated with T cells in the mouse, *J. Immunol.* **109**:776.

Haegert, D. G., 1978, Observations on the number of immunoglobulin-bearing lymphocytes in human peripheral blood with the mixed antiglobulin rosetting reaction and direct immunofluorescence, *J. Immunol.* **120**:124.

Hämmerling, U., Mack, C., and Pickel, H. G., 1976*a*, Immunofluorescence analysis of Ig determinants on mouse thymocytes and T cells, *Immunochemistry* **13**:525.

Hämmerling, U., Pickel, H. G., Mack, C., and Masters, D., 1976*b*, Immunochemical study of an immunoglobulin-like molecule of murine T lymphocytes, *Immunochemistry* **13**:533.

Haustein, D., and Goding, J. W., 1975, Surface immunoglobulin heavy chains of murine splenocytes and thymocytes are different, *Biochem. Biophys. Res. Commun.* **65**:483.

Haustein, D., and Warr, G. W., 1976, Use and abuse of Sepharose-conjugated antibodies for the isolation of lymphocyte-surface immunoglobulins, *J. Immunol. Meth.* **12**:323.

Haustein, D., Marchalonis, J. J., and Harris, A. W., 1975, Immunoglobulin of T lymphoma cells: biosynthesis, surface representation and partial characterization, *Biochemistry* **14**:1826.

Hildemann, W. H., 1972, Phylogeny of transplantation reactivity, in: *Transplantation Antigens: Markers of Biological Individuality* (B. D. Kahan and R. A. Reisfeld, eds.), pp. 3–73, Academic Press, New York.

Hildemann, W. H., 1974, Some new concepts in immunological phylogeny, *Nature* **250**:116.

Hudson, L., 1975, Immunoglobulin-bearing lymphocytes of the chicken. I. Heavy chain commitment and organ distribution, *Eur. J. Immunol.* **5**:694.

Hudson, L., and Roitt, I. M., 1973, Immunofluorescent detection of surface antigens specific to T and B lymphocytes in the chicken, *Eur. J. Immunol.* **3**:63.

*Immunological Reviews*, Immunoglobulin D: Structure, Synthesis, Membrane Representation and Function, Vol. 37, 1977.

Jensenius, J. C., 1976, Evidence against T-cell immunoglobulin from radioimmunoassay on serum and cells from bursectomized chickens, *Immunology* **30**:145.

Jensenius, J. C., and Williams, A. F., 1974, Total immunoglobulin of rat thymocytes and thoracic duct lymphocytes, *Eur. J. Immunol.* **4**:98.

Jerry, L. M., Kunkel, H. G., and Grey, H. M., 1970, Absence of disulfide bonds linking the heavy and light chains, a property of genetic variant of gamma A-2 globulins, *Proc. Natl. Acad. Sci.* **65**:557.

Johnson, G. D., Holborow, E. J., and Dorling, J., 1978, Immunofluorescence and immunoenzyme techniques, in: *Handbook of Experimental Immunology*, Vol. 1 (D. M. Weir, ed.), pp. 15.1–15.30, Blackwell, Oxford.

Jondal, M., Svedmyr, E., Klein, E., and Singh, S., 1975, Killer T cells in a Burkitts' lymphoma biopsy, *Nature* **255**:405.

Jones, G., Marcusson, E. C., and Roitt, I. M., 1970, Immunoglobulin, allotypic determinants on rabbit lymphocytes, *Nature* **227**:1051.

Jones, G., Torrigiani, G., and Roitt, I. M., 1971, Immunoglobulin determinants on mouse lymphocytes, *J. Immunol.* **106**:1425.

Jones, V. E., Graves, H. E., and Orlaus, E., 1976, The detection of $(Fab')_2$-related surface antigens on the thymocytes of children, *Immunology* **30**:281.

Jurd, R. D., 1977, Secretory immunoglobulins and gut-associated lymphoid tissue in *Xenopus laevis,* in: *Developmental Immunobiology,* (J. B. Solomon and J. D. Horton, eds.), pp. 307–334, Elsevier North-Holland, New York.

Jurd, R. D., and Stevenson, G. T., 1976, Surface immunoglobulins on *Xenopus laevis* lymphocytes, *Comp. Biochem. Physiol.* **53A**:381.

Kiessling, R., Klein, E., Pross, H., and Wigzell, H., 1975, "Natural" killer cells in the mouse. II. Cytotoxic cells with specificity for mouse Moloney leukemia cells: Characteristics of of the killer cell, *Eur. J. Immunol.* **5**:117.

Kincade, P. W., Lawton, A. R., and Cooper, M. D., 1971, Restriction of surface immunoglobulin determinants to lymphocytes of the plasma cell line, *J. Immunol.* **106**:1421.

Knapp, W., Bolhuis, R. L. H., Radl, J., and Higmans, W., 1973, Independent movement of IgD and IgM molecules on the surface of individual lymphocytes, *J. Immunol.* **111**: 1295.

Krolick, K. A., and Sercarz, E. E., 1977, Mouse B cell membrane fluidity from the cradle to the grave, in: *Developmental Immunobiology* (J. B. Solomon and J. D. Horton, eds.), pp. 189–196, Elsevier North-Holland, New York.

Lamelin, J.-P., Lisowska-Berstein, B., Matter, A., Ryser, J. E., and Vassalli, P., 1972, Mouse thymus-independent and thymus-derived lymphoid cells. I. Immunofluorescent and functional studies, *J. Exp. Med.* **136**:984.

Lee, S.-T., Paraskevas, F., and Israels, L. G., 1971, Cell surface associated gamma globulins in lymphocytes. II. The pluropotentiality of mouse spleen lymphocytes, *J. Immunol.* **107**:1583.

Ling, N. R., and Kay, J. E., 1975, *Lymphocyte Stimulation,* North-Holland, Amsterdam.

Litman, G. W., 1976, Physical properties of immunoglobulins of lower species: A comparison with immunoglobulins of mammals, in: *Comparative Immunology* (J. J. Marchalonis, ed.), pp. 239–275, Blackwell, Oxford.

Lonai, P., Ben-Neriah, Y., Steinman, L., and Givol, D., 1978, Selective participation of immunoglobulin V region and major histocompatibility complex products in antigen binding by T cells, *Eur. J. Immunol.* **8**:827.

McIlhinney, R. A. J., Richardson, N. E., and Feinstein, A., 1978, Evidence for a C-terminal tyrosine residue in human and mouse B-lymphocyte membrane $\mu$-chains, *Nature* **272**: 555.

McKearn, T. J., Hamada, Y., Stuart, F. P., and Fitch, F. W., 1974, Antireceptor antibody and resistance to graft-versus-host disease, *Nature* **251**:648.

Marchalonis, J. J., 1975, Lymphocyte surface immunoglobulin, *Science* **190**:20.

Marchalonis, J. J., 1976, Surface immunoglobulins of B and T lymphocytes: Molecular properties, association with the cell membrane, and a unified model of antigen recognition, in: *Contemporary Topics in Molecular Immunology*, Vol. 5 (H. N. Eisen and R. A. Reisfeld, eds.), pp. 125–160, Plenum Press, New York.

Marchalonis, J. J., 1977*a*, *Immunity in Evolution*, Harvard University Press, Cambridge, Mass.

Marchalonis, J. J., 1977*b*, External covalent labels in analytical studies of lymphocyte membrane proteins, *Progr. Immunol.* **3**:23.

Marchalonis, J. J., and Cone, R. E., 1973, Biochemical and biological characteristics of lymphocyte surface immunoglobulin, *Transpl. Rev.* **14**:3.

Marchalonis, J. J., Cone, R. E., and Santer, V. E., 1971, Enzymic iodination: A probe for accessible surface proteins of normal and neoplastic lymphocytes, *Biochem. J.* **124**:921.

Marchalonis, J J., Decker, J. M., DeLuca, D., Moseley, J. M., Smith, P., and Warr, G. W., 1977*a*, Lymphocyte surface immunoglobulins: Evolutionary origins and involvement in activation, *Cold Spring Harbor Symp. Quant. Biol.* **41**:261.

Marchalonis, J. J., Warr, G. W., Bucana, C., Hoyer, L., Szenberg, A., and Warner, N. L., 1977*b*, Demonstration and partial characterization of murine B and T cell surface immunoglobulin using avian antibodies, in: *Immune System: Genetics and Regulation* (E. Sercarz, L. Herzenberg, and C. F. Fox, eds.), pp. 285–295, Academic Press, New York.

Marchalonis, J. J., Bucana, C., Hoyer, L., Warr G. W., Hanna, M. G., Jr., and Szenberg, A., 1978, Visualization of a guinea pig T lymphocyte surface component cross-reactive with immunoglobulin, *Science* **199**:433.

Martin, L. N., Leslie, G. A., and Hindes, R., 1976, Lymphocyte surface IgD and IgM in non-human primates, *Int. Arch. Allergy Appl. Immunol.* **51**:320.

Mattes, M. J., and Steiner, L. A., 1978, Antisera to frog immunoglobulins cross-react with a periodate-sensitive cell surface determinant, *Nature* **273**:761.

Melcher, U., and Uhr, J. W., 1976, Cell surface immunoglobulin. XVI. Polypeptide chain structure of mouse IgM and IgD-like molecule, *J. Immunol.* **116**:409.

Melcher, U., and Uhr, J. W., 1977, Density differences between membrane and secreted immunoglobulins of murine splenocytes, *Biochemistry* **16**:145.

Melcher, U., Vitetta, E. S., McWilliams, M., Lamm, M. E., Phillips-Quagliata, J. M., and Uhr, J. W., 1974, Cell surface immunoglobulin. X. Identification of an IgD-like molecule on the surface of murine splenocytes, *J. Exp. Med.* **140**:1427.

Melcher, U., Eidels, L., and Uhr, J. W., 1975, Are immunoglobulins integral membrane proteins? *Nature* **258**:434.

Merler, E., Gatien, J., and DeWilde, G., 1974, Significance of immunofluorescent staining of lymphocytes with antisera to IgM immunoglobulins, *Nature* **251**:652.

Metchnikoff, E., 1892, *Leçons sur la Pathologie Comparée de l'Inflammation*, G. Masson, Paris.

Miller, J. F. A. P., 1972, Lymphocyte interactions in antibody responses, *Int. Rev. Cytol.* **33**:77.

Miller, J. F. A. P., and Vadas, M. A., 1977*a*, The major histocompatibility complex: Influence on immune reactivity and T-lymphocyte activation, *Scand. J. Immunol.* **6**:771.

Miller, J. F. A. P., and Vadas, M. A.,1977*b*, Antigen activation of T lymphocytes: Influence of major histocompatibility complex, *Cold Spring Harbor Symp. Quant. Biol.* **41**:579.

Misra, D. N., Ladoulis, C. T., Gill, T. J. III, and Bazin, H., 1976, Lymphocyte plasma membranes. V. Immunoglobulins on isolated plasma membranes of the thymic and splenic lymphocytes of the rat, *Immunochemistry* **13**:613.

Molnar, J., Klein, G., and Friberg, S., Jr., 1973, Subcellular localization of murine histocompatibility antigens in tumor cells: Localization of H-2 antigens, *Transplantation* **16**:93.

Moroz, C., and Lahat, N., 1974, Surface immunoglobulin of mouse thymus cells and its *in vitro* biosynthesis, *Cell. Immunol.* **13**:397.

Moseley, J. M., Marchalonis, J. J., Harris, A. W., and Pye, J., 1977, Molecular properties of T lymphoma immunoglobulin. I. Serological and general physicochemical properties, *J. Immunogenet.* **4**:233.

Mosier, D. E., Zitron, I. M., Mond, J. J., Ahmed, A., Scher, I., and Paul, W. E., 1977, Surface immunoglobulin D as a functional receptor for a subclass of B lymphocytes, *Immunol. Rev.* **37**:89.

Nairn, R. C., 1969, *Fluorescent Protein Tracing,* Williams and Wilkins, Baltimore.

Nossal, G. J. V., Warner, N. L., Lewis, H., and Sprent, J., 1972, Quantitative features of a sandwich radioimmunolabelling technique for lymphocyte surface receptors, *J. Exp. Med.* **135**:405.

Okumura, K., Julius, M. H., Tsu, T., Herzenberg, L. H., and Herzenberg, L. A. 1976, Demonstration that IgG memory is carried by IgG-bearing cells, *Eur. J. Immunol.* **6**:467.

Osmond, D. G., and Nossal, G. J. V., 1974, Differentiation of lymphocytes in mouse bone marrow. I. Quantitative radioautographic studies of antiglobulin binding by lymphocytes in bone marrow and lymphoid tissues, *Cell. Immunol.* **13**:117.

Papamichail, M., Brown, J. C., and Holborow, E. J., 1971, Immunoglobulin on the surface of human lymphocytes, *Lancet* **2**:850.

Paraskevas, F., Lee, S. T., and Israels, L. G., 1971, Cell surface associated $\gamma$-globulins in lymphocytes. I. Reverse immune cytoadherence: a technique for their detection in mouse and human lymphocytes, *J. Immunol.* **106**:160.

Parkhouse, R. M. E., and Cooper, M. D., 1977, A model for the differentiation of B lymphocytes with implications for the biological role of IgD, *Immunol. Rev.* **37**:105.

Parkhouse, R. M. E., Hunter, I. R., and Abney, E. R., 1976, Heterogeneity of surface immunoglobulin on murine B lymphocytes, *Immunology* **30**:409.

Paul, W. E., Shevach, E. M., Thomas, D. W., Pickeral, S. F., and Rosenthal, H. S., 1977, Genetic restriction in T-lymphocyte activation by antigen-pulsed peritoneal exudate cells, *Cold Spring Harbor Symp. Quant. Biol.* **41**:571.

Pernis, B., Forni, L., and Amante, L., 1970, Immunoglobulin spots on the surface of rabbit lymphocytes, *J. Exp. Med.* **132**:1001.

Pernis, B., Forni, L., and Amante, L., 1971, Immunoglobulins as cell receptors, *Ann. N. Y. Acad. Sci.* **190**:420.

Phillips, B., and Roitt, I. M., 1973, Evidence for transformation of human B lymphocytes by PHA, *Nature New Biol.* **241**:254.

Preud'homme, J. L., and Seligmann, M., 1972, Anti-human immunoglobulin G activity of membrane-bound monoclonal immunoglobulin M in lymphoproliterative disorders, *Proc. Natl. Acad. Sci. USA* **69**:2132.

Preud'homme, J. L., and Seligmann, M., 1974, Surface immunoglobulins on human lymphoid cells, *Prog. Clin. Immunol.* **2**:121.

Rabellino, E., and Grey, H. M., 1971, Immunoglobulins on the surface of lymphocytes. III. Bursal origin of surface immunoglobulin on chicken lymphocytes, *J. Immunol.* **106**: 1418.

Rabellino, E., Colon, S., Grey, H. M., and Unanue, E. R., 1971, Immunoglobulins on the surface of lymphocytes. I. Distribution and quantitation, *J. Exp. Med.* **133**:156.

Raff, M. C., 1970, Two distinct populations of peripheral lymphocytes in mice distinguishable by immunofluorescence, *Immunology* **19**:637.

Raff, M. C., Sternberg, M., and Taylor, R. B., 1970, Immunoglobulin determinants on the surface of mouse lymphoid cells, *Nature* **225**:553.

Rajewsky, K., and Eichmann, K., 1977, Antigen receptors of T helper cells, in: *Contemporary Topics in Immunobiology*, Vol. 7: *T Cells* (O. Stutman, ed.), pp. 69–112, Plenum Press, New York.

Ross, G. D., Rabellino, E. M., Polley, M. J., and Grey, H. M., 1973, Combined studies of complement receptor and surface immunoglobulin-bearing cells and sheep erythrocyte-rosetting cells in normal and leukemic human lymphocytes, *J. Clin. Invest.* **52**:377.

Rouse, B. T., Wells, R. J. H., and Warner, N. L., 1973, Proportions of T and B lymphocytes in lesions of Marek's disease. Theoretical implications for pathogenesis, *J. Immunol.* **110**:534.

Rowe, D. S., Hug, K., Faulk, W. P., McCormick, J. N., and Gerber, H., 1973, IgD on the surface of peripheral blood lymphocytes of the human newborn, *Nature New Biol.* **242**: 155.

Ruben, L. N., and Edwards, B. F., 1977, Phenotypic restriction of antigen-binding specificity on immunized amphibian spleen cells, *Cell. Immunol.* **33**:437.

Ruben, L. N., Warr, G. W., Decker, J. M., and Marchalonis, J. J., 1977, Phylogenetic origins of immune recognition: Lymphoid heterogeneity and the hapten/carrier effect in the goldfish, *Carassius auratus*, *Cell. Immunol.* **31**:266.

Ruddick, J. H., and Leslie, G. A., 1977, Structure and biologic functions of human IgD. XI. Identification and ontogeny of a rat lymphocyte immunoglobulin having antigenic cross-reactivity with human IgD, *J. Immunol.* **118**:1025.

Santana, V., Wedderburn, N., and Turk, J. L., 1974, Demonstration of immunoglobulin on the surface of thymus lymphocytes, *Immunology* **27**:65.

Shearer, G. M., Rehn, T. G., and Garbarino, C. A., 1975, Cell-mediated lympholysis of trimitrophenyl-modified autologous lymphocytes: effector cell specificity to modified cell surface components controlled by the H-2K and H-2D serological regions of the murine major histocompatibility complex, *J. Exp. Med.* **141**:1348.

Szenberg, A., Marchalonis, J. J., and Warner, N. L., 1977, Direct demonstration of endogenous murine thymus-dependent cell surface immunoglobulin, *Proc. Natl. Acad. Sci. USA* **74**:2113.

Takahashi, T., Old, L. J., McIntyre, K. R., and Boyse, E. A., 1971, Immunoglobulin and other surface antigens of cells of the immune system, *J. Exp. Med.* **134**:815.

Ting, C.-C., and Law, L. W., 1977, Studies of *H-2* restriction in cell-mediated cytotoxicity and transplantation immunity to leukemia associated antigens, *J. Immunol.* **118**:1259.

Vaerman, J. P., Lebacq-Verheyden, A. M., and Heremans, J. F., 1974, Absence of disulfide bridges between heavy and light chains in IgA from chicken bile, *Immunol. Commun.* **3**:239.

Vitetta, E. S., and Uhr, J. W., 1973, Synthesis, transport, dynamics and fate of surface Ig and alloantigens in murine lymphocytes, *Transpl. Rev.* **14**:50.

Vitetta, E. S., and Uhr, J. W., 1975, Immunoglobulin receptors revisited, *Science* **189**:964.

Vitetta, E. S., and Uhr, J. W., 1977, IgD and B cell differentiation, *Immunol. Rev.* **37**:50.

Warner, N. L., 1974, Membrane immunoglobulins and antigen receptors on B and T lymphocytes, *Adv. Immunol.* **19**:67.

Warner, N. L., and Marchalonis, J. J., 1972, Structural differences in mouse IgA myeloma proteins of different allotypes, *J. Immunol.* **109**:657.

Warner, N. L., Szenberg, A., and Burnet, F. M., 1962, The immunological role of different lymphoid organs in the chicken. I. Dissociation of immunological responsiveness, *Aust. J. Exp. Biol. Med. Sci.* **40**:373.

Warr, G. W., and Marchalonis, J. J., 1977*a*, Lymphocyte surface immunoglobulins: Detection, characterization and occurrence in diseases of the lymphoid system, *Crit. Rev. Clin. Lab. Sci.* **7**:185.

Warr, G. W., and Marchalonis, J. J., 1977*b*, Lymphocyte surface immunoglobulin of the goldfish differs from its serum counterpart, *Dev. Comp. Immunol.* **1**:15.

Warr, G. W., and Marchalonis, J. J., 1978, Specific immune recognition by lymphocytes: An evolutionary perspective, *Q. Rev. Biol.* **53**:225.

Warr, G. W., Decker, J. M., and Marchalonis, J. J., 1976*a*, Evolutionary and developmental aspects of T-cell recognition, *Immunol. Commun.* **5**:281.

Warr, G. W., DeLuca, D., and Marchalonis, J. J., 1976*b*, Phylogenetic origins of immune recognition: lymphocyte surface immunoglobulins in the goldfish, *Carassius auratus*, *Proc. Natl. Acad. Sci. USA* **73**:2476.

Warr, G. W., DeLuca, D., Decker, J. M., Marchalonis, J. J., and Ruben, L. N., 1977, Lymphoid heterogeneity in teleost fish: Studies on the genus *Carassius*, in: *Developmental Immunobiology* (J. B. Solomon and J. D. Horton, eds.), pp. 241–248, Elsevier North-Holland, New York.

Warr, G. W., Lee, J. C., and Marchalonis, J. J., 1978*a*, Null cells in the mouse possess membrane immunoglobulin, *J. Immunol.* **121**:1767.

Warr, G. W., Marton, G. M., Szenberg, A., and Marchalonis, J. J., 1978*b*, Reactions of chicken antibodies with mouse serum and T-cell-associated immunoglobulins, *Immunochemistry,* **15**:615.

Wedner, H. J., and Parker, C. W., 1976, Lymphocyte activation, *Progr. Allergy* **20**:195.

Whitelaw, A., Miller, J. F. A. P., and Mitchell, G. F., 1977, Studies on immune responses to parasitic antigens in mice. VI. Delayed type hypersensitivity to blood cells from *Plasmodium berghei*-infected mice, *Cell Immunol.* **32**:216.

Williams, A. F., and Gowans, J. L., 1975, The presence of IgA on the surface of rat thoracic duct lymphocytes which contain internal IgA, *J. Exp. Med.* **141**:335.

Winchester, R. J., Fu, S. M., Hoffman, T., and Kunkel, H. G., 1975, IgG on lymphocyte surfaces: Technical problems and the significance of a third cell population, *J. Immunol.* **114**:1210.

Yakulis, V., Bhoopalam, N., Schade, S., and Heller, P., 1972, Surface immunoglobulins of circulating lymphocytes in mouse plasmacytoma. I. Characteristics of lymphocyte surface immunoglobulins, *Blood* **39**:453.

Yamaga, K. M., Kubo, R. T., and Etlinger, H. M., 1978*b*, Studies on the question of conventional immunoglobulin on thymocytes from primitive vertebrates. I. Presence of anti-carbohydrate antibodies in rabbit anti-trout Ig sera, *J. Immunol.* **120**:2068.

Yamaga, K., Kubo, R. T., and Etlinger, H. M., 1978*b,* Studies on the question of conventional immunoglobulin on thymocytes from primitive vertebrates. II. Delineation between Ig specific and cross-reactive membrane components, *J. Immunol.* **120**:2074.

Yamana, S., Rolland, J. M., and Nairn, R. C., 1973, T and B cells in various lymphoid tissues in mice: membrane immunofluorescence with purified lymphoid cells, *Immunol. Commun.* **2**:25.

Zinkernagel, R. M., and Doherty, P. C., 1977, Major transplantation antigens, viruses, and specificity of surveillance T cells, in: *Contemporary Topics in Immunobiology,* Vol. 7: *T Cells* (O. Stutman, ed.), pp. 179–220, Plenum Press, New York.

Zinkernagel, R. M., Callahan, G. N., Althage, A., Cooper, S., Klein, P. A., and Klein, J., 1978, On the thymus in the differentiation of "H-2 self recognition" by T cells: Evidence for dual recognition, *J. Exp. Med.* **147**:882.

*Chapter 7*

# *Idiotypes, T-Cell Receptors, and T-B Cooperation*

**Charles A. Janeway, Jr.***

*Department of Pathology*
*Immunology Division*
*Yale University School of Medicine*
*New Haven, Connecticut 06510*

## I. INTRODUCTION

Immune responses in mammals, such as the production of antibody or the rejection of foreign (i.e., non-self) tissue grafts, are the result of complex interactions among a variety of different cell types. The hallmarks of the mammalian immune system–specificity, inducibility, memory, and regulation–have been conclusively shown to be associated with lymphocytes (Gowans, 1970). The division of lymphocytes into two major classes, known as T cells (thymus-derived lymphocytes) and B cells (bone-marrow-derived, thymus-independent lymphocytes), has led to an appreciation of the central role of the T cells in virtually all immune responses. This chapter will explore the genetic and environmental influences that govern T-cell specificity and behavior, as well as some interactions by which T cells regulate immune responses.

One of the central mysteries of contemporary immunology has been, and continues to be, the nature of the specific receptor for antigen on T cells. This problem has resisted definitive solution for a number of reasons, all of which relate to the nature of T cells. The foremost reason is the fact that T cells, unlike

*Investigator, Howard Hughes Medical Institute.

Abbreviations used in this chapter: B, Bone-marrow-derived, thymus-independent; BUdR, 5-bromodeoxyuridine; $C_H$, Heavy-chain constant region; DNP, 2,4-dinitrophenyl; Ig, Immunoglobulin; MHC, Major histocompatibility complex; OVA, Egg albumin; SIII, Pneumococcal polysaccharide; T, Thymus-derived; TNP, 2,4,6-trinitrophenyl; $V_H$, Heavy-chain variable region.

antibody-producing B cells, do not make abundant quantities of an antigen-binding soluble receptor. Rather, their activity is mediated either by direct cell-cell contact or by factors that adhere tightly to the surfaces of other cells, such as macrophages. Secondly, to think of T cells as a single class of cells is obviously erroneous, just as ten years ago it became apparent that not all lymphocytes were the same. Different types of T cells may well have quite different types of receptors. Third, the behavior of T cells is apparently strongly influenced by a set of genes encoded for within the major histocompatibility complex (MHC). These genes, known as immune-response, or *Ir*, genes, govern the intensity of many T-cell responses to relatively simple antigens. However, these genes may not code for antigen-specific receptors on T cells. Fourth, assays of T-cell activity involve complex measurements of cellular behavior, rather than simple antigen binding. And finally, related to this, is the fact that many T cells express their activity by regulating the behavior of other cells—T cells, B cells, and macrophages—and thus cannot be examined as isolated, purified populations of cells. All of these properties of T cells have served both to intensify interest in understanding their behavior and to prevent this understanding.

Despite these problems, a great deal has been learned about T-cell receptors in recent years. This information has been obtained at a variety of levels. It is the central goal of this chapter to set out at least those findings that must be taken into account in assembling a workable model for the T-cell receptor. A subsidiary goal of the chapter is to illustrate, with some examples, the regulatory behavior of certain T cells, and to suggest yet greater levels of complexity and further puzzles in their behavior. For this purpose, the interaction of T cells with B cells leading to the production of serum antibody will be examined.

Because of the vast literature in this area, this review cannot be comprehensive, nor comprehensively referenced (see Katz, 1977). Nor can it, because of the controversial nature of its subject, be entirely objective (Kuhn, 1962). Rather, I will seek to highlight what I see as crucial observations that must be explained (or explained away) in synthesizing the information regarding antigen recognition by T cells and their regulatory behavior.

Before proceeding to the T cells themselves, brief reviews will be given of two gene clusters that play crucial roles in determining T-cell receptor structure and specificity. These gene clusters are the immunoglobulin (Ig) genes and the MHC. An understanding of the genetics of these two gene clusters is essential for understanding T-cell antigen recognition, for it is the gene clusters' interaction that gives rise to the specific T-cell system of receptors, and determines which antigens are recognized as self, and which as non-self, during that T-cell's life span. Since most studies of the immune system are now carried out in mice, the mouse will be used as a model. In doing this, I am assuming that findings in other species will be applicable to the murine immune system, an assumption that has so far repeatedly proven correct.

## II. IMMUNOGLOBULIN GENES

All antibody molecules are the products of two of the three clusters of Ig genes. These three clusters encode for heavy chains and for the two types of light chains, kappa and lambda. Each antibody molecule has two heavy chains and two light chains, either kappa or lambda. In each molecule, each pair of chains is identical. Recent work by Tonegawa *et al.* (1977) has shown that at the DNA level, each of these clusters is present in the DNA in two distinct pieces, which are separated by a segment of chromosome susceptible to restriction endonuclease cleavage, except in cells producing the polypeptide chain in question, where the segments of the gene are brought together [although even in producing cells they do not form a DNA sequence that can directly give rise to mRNA for the polypeptide chain (W. Gilbert and S. Tonegawa, personal communication)]. These two segments of an immunoglobulin gene are named the variable and the constant segment. For heavy chains, there are several different constant-region genes, called $C_H$, which encode the invariant parts of the heavy polypeptide chains, giving rise to different classes of Ig molecules, such as IgM, IgG, IgD, etc. There are also thought to be multiple copies of variable-region genes, which determine antibody specificity. It appears that a given variable-region (denoted $V_H$, for heavy-chain variable regions) gene can associate with any of the $C_H$ genes, and furthermore it does so in a sequential fashion in the maturation of a clone or lineage of antibody-forming cells. Thus, a cell can maintain its specificity while changing the class of the antibody it makes. In addition, the expression of a given $V_H$ gene within a cell clone probably prevents the expression of other $V_H$ genes by that cell or its daughter cells, including the $V_H$ genes on the other chromosome, giving rise to two important features of B cells, allelic exclusion and monospecificity (Raff *et al.*, 1973; Jones *et al.*, 1974; Julius *et al.*, 1976). The products of the VH genes are the variable regions of the heavy chains of Ig molecules. Whether V genes for all possible V-region sequences exist in the genome, or, alternatively, whether variability is generated in somatic cells, is not yet known. In the Ig molecule, the heavy-chain variable region folds to bring together along one side of the antigen-binding cleft the so-called hypervariable regions, which in turn appear to determine two crucial properties of the antibody molecule, its specificity and its idiotype. The other side of the cleft is formed by the light-chain variable region, which also contains three hypervariable regions, at least two of which are also intimately involved in producing the antigen-binding site and the idiotype of the molecule (Poljak *et al.*, 1974; Segal *et al.*, 1974).

*Idiotypes*. Idiotypes are defined as unique antigenic specificities of antibodies, specific for a particular antigenic determinant. In mice, several idiotypes have been described. They are inherited in an autosomal dominant fashion linked to CH genes which determine Ig alloantigens known as immunoglobulin allotypes.

However, this appears to be an oversimplification, since light-chain genes are not highly polymorphic in mice. In strains with variant light-chain genes, idiotype can be shown to be governed also by light-chain V genes (Weigert and Potter, 1977; Laskin *et al.*, 1977). Furthermore, as idiotype has been studied in more detail it has been found that the use of anti-idiotypic antisera—or of other criteria of idiotypy, such as fine specificity—to define the presence or absence of structural genes may be subject to a variety of problems resulting either from imprecision of the antisera used or from regulatory genes masquerading as structural genes (Weigert and Potter, 1977). Nonetheless, idiotype as defined with anti-idiotypic antibody has been crucial in elucidating the nature of the T-cell receptor for antigen, as will be discussed below. Thus, an antiserum that reacts specifically with an antibody of appropriate specificity that has been raised in strains carrying the appropriate V genes can be usefully called an antiidiotypic antiserum. An antigen reacting with this serum, however, is not necessarily structurally identical with the antigen used to elicit the antiidiotypic antiserum.

## III. THE MAJOR HISTOCOMPATIBILITY COMPLEX

Immune responses to allogeneic-tissue grafts can be directed at a variety of different cell-surface antigenic determinants. However, early studies in the mouse demonstrated that strong, rapid rejection of grafts was due to alloantigenic differences mapping as a single locus (see Klein, 1975). Subsequent experimentation has shown that this locus, called *H-2* in the mouse, is actually a cluster of genes coding for a variety of cell-surface antigens, and it is now known as the major histocompatibility complex, or MHC. For present purposes, the products of this highly complex chromosomal region can be divided into two types of antigenic determinants, expressed in different polypeptide chains and subserving different functions.

### A. The *K/D* Loci

At either end of the MHC in mice is a locus encoding a 45,000-dalton polypeptide chain that carries strong transplantation antigens found on all somatic cells; these antigens also give rise to most of the antibody in alloantisera. These loci are called *K* and *D* in the mouse. There is recent evidence that the *D* locus may in fact be two closely linked loci, each encoding a 45,000-dalton polypeptide chain carrying alloantigenic determinants (Hansen *et al.*, 1977).

With antisera used against these determinants, it has been found that each *K* or *D* product carries at least one determinant that is unique to it. These determinants are therefore called private specificities. By contrast, there are other determinants that are found on more than one *K* or *D* product, and so are called public specificities. Indeed, the same public specificities can be found on the *K* and the *D* product in a single inbred animal, showing that these two genes arose by gene duplication, as was already suggested by their structural and functional similarity. This homology has now been confirmed by protein sequencing.

### B. The *I* Region

Between the *K* and *D* loci lies a stretch of chromosome containing, along with various other genes, a region called the *I* region. A large number of interesting and probably interrelated traits are controlled by genes in this segment of chromosome.

Initially, the *I* region was defined by the presence of genes regulating the magnitude of the antibody response to certain polypeptide antigens. These immune-response, or *Ir*, genes were mapped in recombinant strains as lying between the *K* and *D* loci. Subsequently it was shown that this same region contained antigens that strongly stimulated proliferation of allogeneic T cells, and also encoded lymphocyte-cell-surface antigenic determinants called Ia (immune-response-associated) antigens carried on a pair of polypeptide chains of 27,000 and 33,000 daltons. Using both *Ir* genes and Ia antigens, further testing of intra-*H-2* recombinant strains has succeeded in demonstrating the existence of at least five distinct subregions within the *I* region itself. Each subregion is marked by a locus controlling at least one Ia antigen, and is delineated by a crossover on either side. It would appear that different subregions control Ia antigens on different types of lymphoid cells. Thus, *I-A* appears to control Ia antigens on B cells and macrophages, while *I-J* is associated primarily with antigenic determinants carried on T cells. Furthermore, a bewildering variety of lymphocyte- and macrophage-derived factors appear to carry Ia-antigenic determinants, in that they react specifically with anti-Ia antibody.

It is important to note that while *K*/*D* molecules are present on all somatic cells, Ia antigens appear to be present primarily or exclusively on lymphocytes or in lymphoid organs, and on macrophages.

## IV. ANTIGEN RECOGNITION BY T CELLS

Before it was recognized that there were T cells and B cells, a central paradox of the immune system was that an animal immunized with a simple chemical ("hapten"), such as 2,4-dinitrophenyl (DNP), coupled with a protein carrier, such as egg albumin (OVA), would make antibody that was highly specific for DNP coupled with any protein, but would give secondary antibody responses only to

DNP-OVA. Thus, while at least part of the antibody was hapten-specific, the response was said to be entirely carrier-specific (Ovary and Benacerraf, 1963). The discovery of T and B cells solved a part of this mystery (Mitchison, 1971), since the B cells that made the antibody turned out to be essentially as hapten-specific as the antibody they produced. In retrospect this is not surprising, since B-cell receptors are cell-bound antibody molecules identical in VH and VL to their ultimate product. However, yet to be satisfactorily explained is the failure of T cells to recognize DNP and to provide a necessary signal to the B cell leading to antibody formation when DNP is coupled with a carrier other than the original immunizing carrier. It is hoped that after a discussion of the experiments outlined below, an approach to answering this question can be attempted.

## A. Recognition of Antigen by T Cells Is Very Precise

Although it has just been stated that T cells do not recognize haptens unless they are coupled with the immunizing carrier, a number of exceptions to this general rule have in fact been discovered. Two involved hapten coupled with lipid-rich carrier molecules (Janeway, 1976). The third major exception involves hapten coupled with isologous immunoglobulin. I will return later to what these exceptions imply. For the present, they allow one to test the precision of T-cell recognition of antigen.

In the experiment illustrated in Table I, guinea pigs were immunized with DNP coupled with mycobacteria of strain H37Ra (DNP-H37), or with mycobacteria alone. Their T cells were subsequently cultured with various nitrophenyl haptens, all coupled with the unrelated carrier ovalbumin. At the same time, the serum antibody from the animal was reacted with DNP-lysine, and this reaction was inhibited by the same nitrophenyl conjugates. It can be seen that T cells can discriminate between different nitrophenyl haptens at least as precisely as do B cells or antibody. Furthermore, the T cells appear to have an extra dimension in their recognition of these compounds, since the interposition of a tripeptide spacer, in the compound called DAG in Table I, has little effect on binding to an antibody or for activating B cells (Janeway, 1975), but abolishes T-cell recognition.

If one examines the same population of DNP-H37-primed T cells for the effect of carrier on this apparently hapten-specific response, one finds that all protein carriers coupled with DNP will lead to a T-cell response. Some synthetic polypeptide carriers coupled with DNP also give responses, while others do not. Finally, the polysaccharide carriers Ficoll and pneumococcal polysaccharide (SIII) coupled with DNP do not activate T cells. Further examination of this system used the technique of antigen-driven 5-bromodeoxyuridine (BUdR) and light suicide, in which responding cells are specifically eliminated and the responses of residual cells can be determined (Table II, Janeway, 1976). DNP-H37-primed T

**Table I. Precision of Hapten Recognition by T Cells**

| Stimulating antigen (100 μg/ml) | Stimulation (CPM, E-C) after priming | | Inhibition of antibody binding to DNP-lysine ($I_{50}$, b hapten × $10^{-8}$M) |
|---|---|---|---|
| | H37 | DNP-H37 | |
| 0 | (1216) | (2520) | – |
| PPD | 28819 | 22086 | – |
| OVA | 0 | 0 | – |
| $DNP_6$-OVA | 144 | 14331 | 105 |
| $DAG_7$-OVA | 0 | 0 | 18.6 |
| $oNP_{0.5}$-OVA | 607 | 0 | >3300 |
| $pNP_1$-OVA | 1723 | 8263 | 36.4 |
| $TNP_{14}$-OVA | 1767 | 6347 | 310 |
| 2,6-$DNP_4$-OVA | 531 | 2613 | 25000 |
| ε-DNP-L-lysine | – | – | 10.7 |

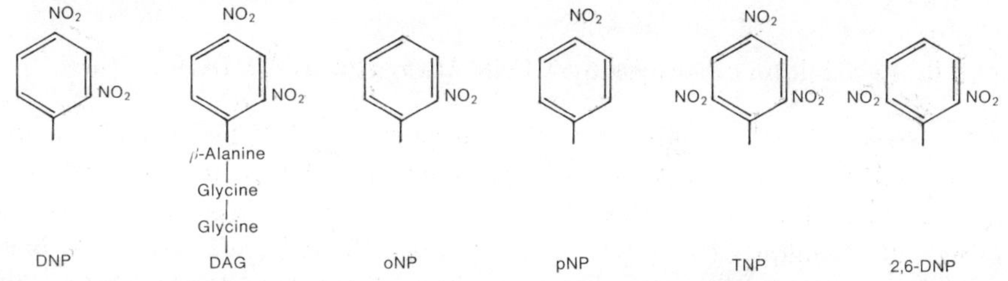


cells responding to DNP on one carrier are partially or entirely distinct from T cells responding to the same DNP hapten coupled with another carrier (Janeway and Paul, 1976). This is not owing to cooperating cells, one specific for carrier and the other for hapten, since carrier alone has no effect, neither stimulating a proliferative response nor leading to suicide of the response to the hapten on that carrier (Janeway, unpublished results). Thus, T cells responding to the hapten DNP not only can discriminate the hapten itself from closely related structures, but also discriminate between the various carrier molecules. Whether this indicates a receptor site specific for each of these antigenic moieties, as originally proposed (Janeway, 1976), or a completely different process, will be discussed later.

Barcinski and Rosenthal (1977) have provided another striking example of the discriminatory power of T cells by examining the cells' responses to various insulin molecules; in this system, single amino-acid interchanges can be detected by T cells. Thus, the recognition of foreign antigens by T cells is as precise as that by B cells or by antibody. For convenience, I will use the term introduced by Thomas *et al.* (1977) in referring to experimentally introduced antigens as "nominal antigens." By this I mean foreign, non-MHC antigens.

Table II. T Cells Reactive to DNP Also Show Carrier Specificity

| Stimulating antigen | Stimulation of BUdR- and light-treated precultured PELs[a] | | | | |
|---|---|---|---|---|---|
| | 0 | PPD[b] | $DNP_{12}$-L-GAT[c] | $DNP_{14}$-L-$GLA^{30}$[d] | $DNP_{13}$-L-GLAT[e] |
| None | (265) | (685) | (731) | (274) | (243) |
| PPD | [59,729] | 1.5 | 95.4 | 68.1 | 82.5 |
| $DNP_{12}$-L-GAT | [8,160] | 60.1 | 9.4 | 45.6 | 5.7 |
| $DNP_{14}$-L-$GLA^{30}$ | [11,446] | 46.2 | 50.4 | 1.3 | 3.7 |
| $DNP_{13}$-L-GLAT | [12,883] | 57.1 | 74.8 | 22.2 | 4.2 |

[a] Data as percentage of response in the control culture, left-hand column, expressed as CPM, thymidine incorporation.
[b] PPD, purified protein derivative of H37.
[c] GAT, glutamic acid, alanine, tyrosine polymer.
[d] $GLA^{30}$, glutamic acid, lysine, alanine polymer.
[e] GLAT, glutamic acid, lysine, alanine, tyrosine polymer.

## B. Recognition of Antigen by T Cells Always Involves MHC Structures

It has long been recognized that T-cell responses to allogeneic stimuli are primarily directed at foreign MHC antigens. A strikingly high percentage of T cells respond to a given MHC difference, a finding made by several authors, using a variety of techniques (Simonsen, 1974; Wilson, 1974; Ford *et al.*, 1975; Binz and Wigzell, 1977). This crucial finding will be discussed at length later in this chapter. Cytotoxic-effector T cells respond to *K/D* structures primarily, while proliferating T cells are primarily responsive to *I*-region structures. However, only in the last five years has it been recognized that T-cell responses to nominal antigens also involve recognition of *self* MHC antigens. A great deal is known about the phenomenology of this process, but the most important questions remain to be elucidated. These are: Does the T cell carry two receptors or receptor sites, one specific for the nominal antigen and one specific for self-MHC antigens, both of which must bind antigen in order for activation to occur? And what is the nature of the antigenic complex formed by the nominal antigen and the MHC antigen on the surface of self cells prior to, or during, T-cell activation? We will leave these questions for now to examine certain critical findings in this area, now commonly called MHC restriction, since responses by T cells primed to the nominal antigen proceed only if the antigen is presented on MHC-identical cells, and since the locus governing this restriction has been amply demonstrated to be the MHC.

### 1. *MHC Restriction of Cytotoxic Effector Cells*

Cytotoxic effector cells immunized to a wide variety of antigens will kill syngeneic, but not allogeneic, target cells bearing the nominal antigen. The locus responsible for this restriction is mapped to *K* and/or *D* in various systems. Furthermore, as in allogeneic killing, private specificities are the dominant factor in this restriction. The nominal antigens in these systems include viruses, haptens, and tumor and minor (i.e., non-MHC) histocompatibility antigens.

Initially it was thought that the effector and the target cells had to share an MHC antigen in order for lysis to occur. However, experiments using $F_1$ T cells immunized with parental cells modified with nominal antigen showed that such cells would lyse modified cells of the immunizing parent only. Thus, sharing of an MHC structure between effector and target cell was not sufficient for lysis to occur. This was carried one step further by several investigators (Pfizenmaier *et al.*, 1976; von Boehmer and Haas, 1976; Zinkernagel, 1976) who injected parental bone-marrow cells into lethally irradiated $F_1$ recipients. In this experimental system the T cells found several months later in the recipient derived from the donor. They originated as bone-marrow precursors and matured in the recipient's thymus. T cells derived from such animals all bore the donor's MHC antigens and were tolerant of the MHC antigens of the other parental strain. They could be immunized to modified (allogeneic) cells derived from the other parental strain, and would specifically lyse modified cells of that parent, while not lysing modified syngeneic cells. Thus it was shown that it was critical that the immunizing cell carry the same MHC antigens as the target cell for lysis to occur, but the T cell and the target could, in this case, differ at the MHC.

Recently, Zinkernagel *et al.* (1978*a*,*b*) and Bevan (1978) have advanced these chimera experiments to demonstrate that $F_1$ stem cells transferred to a lethally irradiated parental-strain mouse will give rise to T cells that behave like parental-strain cells, and will not respond to or lyse modified cells of the other parental strain, although they are tolerant of its alloantigens. Furthermore, Zinkernagel *et al.* (1978*a*) and Bevan (personal communication) have shown that the site where this restricting process takes place is the thymus.

This author has performed an analogous set of experiments, but using mature T cells from normal $F_1$ animals. The approach was to suicide the cells with BUdR and light during their primary response to modified parental cells. If the T cells were precommitted to recognize the nominal antigen (in this case, the hapten 2,4,6-trinitrophenyl, or TNP) associated with one or the other parent's MHC antigens, then suicide with TNP-modified parental cells should be specific for that parent alone, and such cells should respond normally to TNP-modified stimulator cells derived from the other parent. That this was indeed the case is seen in Table III. Furthermore, when such cells were depleted of alloreactive T cells, the residual cells responded well to TNP-modified parental cells, but did not manifest TNP-specific responses to TNP-modified allogeneic cells, as shown in Table IV (Janeway *et al.*, 1978).

Thus, both the chimera experiments and the suicide experiments strongly suggest that T cells are precommitted to recognize particular self-MHC antigens, and that this precommitment is induced by the thymus during differentiation of the developing T cell.

**Table III. Selective BUdR and Light Suicide of (AXB) $F_1$ T Cells Specific for TNP-Parental Targets**

| Suiciding cell | Stimulating cell | Target cell | Relative % cytotoxicity[a] |
|---|---|---|---|
| TNP-A | TNP-A | TNP-A | 15.5 ± 4.7 |
| TNP-B | TNP-A | TNP-A | 81.2 ± 8.4 |
| TNP-A | C | C | 133.4 ± 9.4 |

[a]Calculated as the ratio of specific $^{51}Cr$ release with suicided cells as responders compared with freshly cultured $F_1$ cells as responders; mean and standard error, $n = 5$.

**Table IV. Suicide of (AXB) $F_1$ Cells with Allogeneic (C) Cells Does Not Permit Responses to TNP-C**

| | | % Specific $^{51}Cr$ release on targets[a] | | |
|---|---|---|---|---|
| Suiciding stimulator | Second stimulator | TNP-A | C | TNP-C |
| Fresh responders | C | – | 25.4 ± 3.0 | 24.8 ± 2.7 |
| C | C | – | 2.8 ± 0.2 | 6.7 ± 0.6 |
| C | TNP-C | – | 1.5 ± 0.5 | 7.6 ± 1.2 |
| Fresh responders | TNP-A | 19.6 ± 1.6 | – | – |
| C | TNP-A | 9.0 ± 0.9 | – | – |

[a]$n = 4$.

### 2. *I*-Region Restriction of Proliferating and Helper T Cells

A variety of different T-cell responses to various antigens are restricted by *I*-region structures. Initially this phenomenon was pointed out by Shevach and Rosenthal (1973) for proliferating T cells, by Katz and co-workers (1973) for helper T cells interacting with B cells, and by Vadas *et al.* (1977) in delayed-type hypersensitivity to a protein antigen. These studies have been extended to show that the restriction is related to *Ir*-gene control of immune responses, since in each case $F_1$ animals, primed to an antigen to which one parent is a responder and one a nonresponder, have T cells that behave as responder cells when presented with antigen on responder parental or $F_1$ cells, but as nonresponder T cells when presented with antigen on nonresponder parental cells. Again, in this instance von Boehmer *et al.* (1975) formed chimeras by transferring bone marrow from two different strains to a lethally irradiated $F_1$ recipient. Those T cells in the chimera that were derived from one of the parents would now cooperate with B cells from the other parent, suggesting that, as with killer cells, the restriction is not fixed in the genome of the T cell but rather is "learned" in the thymus of the recipient animal. This strongly suggests, but does not prove, that recognition of the *I* region by the T cell is mediated not by the T cell's own *I*-region structures, but by some highly variable set of receptors that becomes fixed during differentiation in the thymus.

**Table V. Inhibition of the Response of T Cells to *Mls* Locus with Anti-Ia Antibody**

| | | | | Responders: $(C_H3 \times BALB/c)F_1$ spleen T cells | | |
|---|---|---|---|---|---|---|
| | | | | Residual response in anti-$Ia^k$ (as % of control response) | | |
| Stimulators (2000 R) | H-2 | Mls | Response in PBS (cpm, E-C) | IgM | IgG | IgG 1:5 |
| $(C_H3 \times BALB/c)F_1$ | k × d | b × c | (1007) | (677) | (1932) | (1120) |
| AKR | k | a | 43332 | 23 | 8 | 37 |
| C57BL/6 | b | b | 78229 | 247 | 274 | 141 |
| CBA/J | k | d | 159964 | 15 | 13 | 54 |
| DBA/2J | d | a | 187661 | 93 | 111 | 105 |
| $(AKR \times DBA/2)F_1$ | k × d | a | 183345 | 96 | 40 | 127 |

Antiserum: A.TH anti-A.TL, ammonium sulfate precipitate passed on Sephadex G-200, 19 S and 7 S peaks taken, dialysed v. PBS, concentrated by Amicon, sterile filtered, and absorbed with BALB/c spleen cells. One ml serum gave rise to 5 ml of each peak, and 20 μl of each peak was used in 200 μl of culture fluid. Absorption was with cells from one spleen per 0.3 ml of each peak.

MLC culture: Spleen cells were purified over Ig-anti-Ig columns, and cultured at $1.5 \times 10^5$ per well in flat bottom plates with $5 \times 10^5$ irradiated spleen cells as stimulators. Stimulators were incubated 1 h with anti-Ia before the addition of responders. Medium was EHAA with 5% heat-inactivated fetal calf serum.

The mouse contains a single autosomal, non-MHC mixed-lymphocyte-stimulating antigenic locus, called the *M1s* locus. This has been shown by Peck *et al.* (1977) to be recognized by primed T cells only when presented on a stimulating cell bearing *I*-region determinants of the immunizing strain. Recent experiments in my laboratory using either BUdR and light suicide or specific blocking with purified anti-Ia antibody have shown that unprimed T cells also recognize *Mls*-locus antigens in association with *I*-region structures, and that in $F_1$ animals, different cells recognize the same *Mls*-locus antigen depending upon the *I* region with which the antigen is associated (Table V).

Thus, findings for *I*-region restriction are analogous to those for *K*/*D* restriction. However, in this instance there are a number of apparent exceptions to the general rule that recognition of nominal antigen involves coincident recognition of MHC antigens (Swain *et al.*, 1976; Pierce *et al.*, 1976). The reason for these exceptions is not yet known, but their existence suggests that further complexity awaits us in the future.

In summary, the following points have emerged from studies of T-cell antigen recognition:

1. Mature peripheral T cells are committed to recognize antigen in association with a particular self-MHC gene product.
2. This commitment is acquired during the cell's differentiation in the thymus. In chimeras, restriction is dictated by the MHC of the thymus, rather

than the MHC genes of the T-cell, although the MHC antigens carried by that T cell are not detectably different from those of donor T cells.
3. This recognition of self-MHC antigens is in general very precise, since it can discriminate apparent point mutations in MHC antigens absolutely.
4. The recognition of the nominal antigen is equally precise.

## V. SUBPOPULATIONS OF T CELLS

In the past few years, a great deal has been learned about T-cell function and specificity through the use of surface-antigenic markers known as Ly, or Lyt, antigens. These are alloantigens that fall under the heading of differentiation antigens, since they are selectively expressed on different populations of cells. By definition, Lyt antigens are found only on cells of the T-lymphocyte lineage. Thus far, the antigens known as Ly-1, Ly-2, and Ly-3 have been most extensively studied, and have led to the discrimination of three distinct subpopulations of mature T cells (Cantor and Boyse, 1975). These subpopulations are: Ly-$1^+$, Ly-$2,3^-$ (Ly1 cells), Ly-$1^-$, Ly-$2,3^+$ (Ly23 cells), and Ly-$1^+$, and Ly-$2,3^+$ (Ly123 cells). These are present in varying proportions in peripheral lymphoid organs (Table VI). Largely through the work of Cantor and Boyse (1976), each of these cell types has been assigned distinct functions. Not only do these different cell populations have unique functions, they also appear to respond to unique portions of the MHC, either in allogeneic responses, or in responses to nominal antigen in association with self-MHC antigens. The functions of these different cells will now be described.

### A. Ly1 Cells

Ly1 cells respond to *I*-region differences in responses to allogeneic cells (Cantor and Boyse, 1975). Furthermore, Nagy *et al.* (1976) have shown that after activation with allogeneic cells, foreign Ia molecules are specifically bound by responding Ly1 T cells; such cells do not bind foreign *K*/*D* molecules. Cantor and Boyse (1975) also showed that Ly1 cells responding to *I*-region differences synergize with Ly23 precursors of cytotoxic effector cells in the generation of cytotoxic activity.

When one examines the activity of Lyl cells in syngeneic systems, they can be seen to be responsible for helper effects in antibody responses (Cantor and Boyse, 1975), delayed-type hypersensitivity responses (Huber *et al.*, 1976*b*), and *in vitro* proliferative responses to protein antigens (R. H. Schwartz, personal communication). Since all of these responses involve recognition of antigen in association with self *I*-region structures, one could as well associate the activity of

**Table VI. Proportions of T-Lymphocyte Subpopulations in C57BL/6J Spleen T Cells[a]**

| Cell type | Ly antigen phenotype | As % of spleen T cells |
|---|---|---|
| Ly1 | Lyt-1.2$^+$, Lyt-2.2$^-$, Lyt-3.2$^-$ | 45% |
| Ly23 | Lyt-1.2$^-$, Lyt-2.2$^+$, Lyt-3.2$^+$ | 14% |
| Ly123 | Lyt-1.2$^+$, Lyt-2.2$^+$, Lyt-3.2$^+$ | 35% |

[a] Data obtained by preparing spleen T cells on anti-Ig columns, incubating cells with antisera specific for different Ly alleles, and counterstaining with fluoresceinated anti-mouse Ig. Antisera a kind gift of F.-W. Shen.

Ly1 cells with the MHC structures to which they respond as with their function. It is an open question as to which of these distinctions (function or specificity) is most directly correlated with Ly phenotype. This is important, because if Lyt-antigen phenotype determines which type of MHC structure the T cell will respond to, then it seems likely that the Lyt antigens will be involved either directly or indirectly in T-cell-receptor formation (Janeway *et al.*, 1976), while if the correct correlation is with function, then Lyt antigens are probably not involved in antigen-binding-receptor formation.

## B. Ly23 Cells

Ly23 cells responding to allogeneic cells recognize *K* and *D* differences (Cantor and Boyse, 1975). This response leads to both proliferation and the production of cytotoxic effector cells, which are also Ly23 cells. Furthermore, Nagy *et al.* (1976) have shown that after activation with allogeneic stimulators, Ly23 cells specifically bind allogeneic *K*/*D* molecules and do not bind allogeneic Ia antigens.

Responses of Ly23 cells in syngeneic systems are more complex. While cytotoxic effector cells for a variety of modified autologous target cells are clearly Ly23 cells—as one would expect from the *K*/*D* restriction of such responses—it is not clear whether the precursors of such cells are also Ly23 cells, or whether they are Ly123 cells (Cantor and Boyse, 1976). Although it has been shown that a mixture of Ly1 and Ly23 cells responds well to alloantigen but does not produce cytotoxic effector cells specific for TNP-modified syngeneic cells, this only demonstrates that Ly123 cells are required for the latter response, and not that they are precursors of the effector cells.

Ly23 cells also suppress antibody responses in a variety of different systems. The question of MHC restriction of suppressor-cell activity has not been examined in detail in syngeneic systems. However, in an allogeneic system it has been shown that Ly23 cells responding to H-2D antigens lead to suppression, while in situations in which the only differences were in the *I* region, no suppression occurred. These findings again imply that there is as good a correlation between Ly-antigen phenotype of a T cell and the type of MHC antigen it recognizes as there is with function.

### C. Ly123 Cells

Ly123 cells have been much more difficult to study, since there is at present no good way to isolate them in relatively pure form. Since they carry both Ly-1 and Ly-23 antigens, they are killed by antisera directed at either antigen. Instead, their activity is usually detected by differences in behavior between unselected T-cell populations and mixtures of Ly1 and Ly23 cells. Thus, their precise role in responses to allogeneic cells has not been determined, although from studies of Huber *et al.* (1976*a*) it has been shown that they do play a role in such responses.

As mentioned above, it has been proposed that Ly123 cells are the precursors of Ly23 killer cells in responses to TNP-modified syngeneic cells. Further studies on this point seem warranted, since there is only indirect evidence of the maturation of Ly123 cells into either Ly1 cells or Ly23 cells. In several other systems, Ly123 cells have been shown to play an amplifying role in the responses of Ly1 or Ly23 cells, but not to be converted from one to the other (Feldmann *et al.*, 1976). A more extensive examination of the regulatory functions of these fascinating cells will be undertaken later in this chapter.

Thus we have at least three distinct subpopulations of T cells, and there is strong evidence that further subdivisions of these cells on the combined bases of function and surface-antigenic phenotype will be forthcoming. For the present, it is important to note that Ly-antigen phenotype appears to correlate well with certain functional activities, and also that it correlates equally well (and, in this author's opinion, more simply) with the type of MHC antigen to which the cell responds, and which it will bind to its surface. This is true both when responses to allogeneic MHC are examined and when one looks at the responses of these cells in syngeneic systems. Their responses to allogeneic MHC involve the same class of MHC structure as do their MHC-restricted responses to a variety of different nominal antigens.

## VI. THE HIGH FREQUENCY OF ALLOREACTIVE T CELLS AND THEIR RESPONSIVENESS TO NOMINAL ANTIGEN

Simonsen (1968) and Wilson *et al.* (1967) have pointed out the surprisingly high frequency of T cells reactive to foreign MHC antigens. These studies were initially carried out either by limiting dilution analysis of cells inducing graft-versus-host reactions (Simonsen, 1968) or by studying the number of T cells activated by a given allogeneic stimulator cell (Ford *et al.*, 1975; Wilson *et al.*, 1967). These approaches gave numbers of the order of 2–10% of T cells specific for a given antigen. There have been at least two objections raised to these experiments. One is that only a few of the responding cells are actually specific for the activating antigen, and the rest are recruited by factors secreted by the responding cells. This seems unlikely in view of the way in which the Simonsen experiments were performed, in which single cells gave rise to measurable effects, and particularly in light of recent studies using antiidiotypic antibodies. Thus, Binz and Wigzell (1977) showed that about 6% of Lewis rat T cells bear an idiotype specific for responses to DA rat alloantigens, and that the cells bearing this idiotype account for responses to these alloantigens, and do not respond to other alloantigens following positive selection of such cells. More recently, Krammer (1978) has confirmed these findings by showing a similar idiotype on about half of the blasts (enlarged, responding lymphocytes) in a specific mixed-lymphocyte reaction. These findings cannot be accounted for by recruitment phenomena. The second objection is that alloantigenic differences are actually highly complex, and while many cells respond to allogeneic stimulation, in fact these responding cells represent a variety of T cells specific for a large number of different antigenic determinants. This argument is more difficult to overcome. It cannot be answered with the use of antiidiotypic antisera, which may contain many specificities, but it might be possible to do so with monoclonal antiidiotypic immunoglobulin produced by a somatic-cell hybrid. However, the fact that apparent point mutations in MHC antigens lead to typical MHC responses—involving graft rejection, cell proliferation, and cell-mediated lympholysis—would tend to suggest that the high frequency of alloreactive T cells is a real phenomenon directly related to the nature of MHC antigens and the T-cell receptor, and is not due to the presence of very large numbers of antigenic differences between different MHC gene products.

Wilson (1974) and his colleagues then went on to enrich for alloreactive T cells specific for a given alloantigen. This was done in different ways and led to T-cell populations that responded well to a particular alloantigen, but did not respond to other alloantigens at all, even after extensive sojourns in T-cell-depleted syngeneic rats. These cells were then tested for their ability to help B cells respond to sheep red blood cells in a quantitative helper-T-cell assay (Heber-Katz and Wilson, 1976). It was found that these T cells helped as well as unselected T cells in B-cell responses to sheep red blood cells. Thus, while these T cells did not respond to alloantigens other than the initial selecting alloantigen (i.e., they were *depleted* of alloreactive cells to all other MHC antigens), they contained normal numbers of helper T cells specific for the nominal antigen, sheep red blood cells.

If one accepts that this experiment demonstrates that the same T cell can respond specifically to allogeneic MHC antigens and to the nominal antigen, sheep red blood cells, and that this finding is generalizable, then a number of different models for antigen recognition by T cells are possible. It must be remembered that helper T cells recognize the nominal antigen sheep red blood cells in association with self-MHC antigens, in this case *I*-region structures (Sprent, 1978). Thus, the following models are all possible:

One receptor, recognizing either alloantigen or the complex of self-MHC antigen with sheep red blood cells resembling alloantigen.

Two receptors, one recognizing alloantigen, the other the complex of sheep red blood cells and self-MHC.

Two receptors, one recognizing either alloantigen or self-MHC antigens, the other specific for sheep red blood cells.

Three receptors, one each for self- and allo-MHC antigens, and the third specific for sheep red blood cells.

At present, it is not possible to choose between these alternatives. Furthermore, there are potential problems in interpreting the experiments of Heber-Katz and Wilson (1976). Thus, the failure to respond to alloantigen could be due to specific suppression rather than positive selection of responding clones of cells. Secondly, it has not been determined if MHC restriction exists in the quantitative helper-cell assay used by these authors, and while their own evidence (Heber-Katz and Wilson, 1975) suggests that it does not, other work in the same laboratory suggests that such responses are MHC-restricted (Sprent, 1978). Thus, the findings of Heber-Katz and Wilson (1976), although highly suggestive, need confirmation in other systems before they can be used in detailed model building. It is this author's opinion that in fact alloreactive T cells *can* also respond in an MHC-restricted fashion to nominal antigens, in a perfectly conventional way, and that the experiment of Heber-Katz and Wilson (1976) leads one to a unique and correct understanding of the specificity of T-cell responses to both types of antigen (Janeway *et al.*, 1976).

## VII. T-CELL RECEPTORS FOR ANTIGEN ARE ENCODED IN CONVENTIONAL $V_H$ GENES

John Humphrey (1967) was the first to suggest that T-cell receptors might consist of heavy chains without light chains. This strikingly accurate forecast has now been confirmed repeatedly in a variety of systems. The original studies of Ramseier and Lindenmann (1972) pioneered work in this field. More recent studies, particularly by Binz and Wigzell (1977) and Eichmann and Rajewsky (1975), have led to a more detailed understanding of the cellular, molecular, and genetic basis of T-cell idiotypy, and these studies will be discussed in detail in this section.

### A. T-Cell Receptors for Non-self MHC Antigens Carry Idiotypic Determinants

Ramseier and Lindenmann (1972) first proposed and tested the hypothesis that T cells carry idiotypic antigenic determinants. Their approach was based on the concept that $F_1$ hybrids derived from inbred parental strains should carry all the genes of both parents. Thus, the hybrids should express most, if not all, of the genetic information expressed in either parent. In particular, all MHC antigens should be expressed. However, one antigen they could not express would be an idiotypic determinant present on the receptor of one parent's T cells and directed at the MHC antigens of the other parent. This is so because T cells carrying such receptors would be anti-self-reactive and therefore "forbidden." To test this hypothesis, lymphoid cells from a parental-strain animal were injected into $F_1$ recipients, and the antisera were used to inhibit a modified mixed-lymphocyte reaction of the T cells of that parent against the other parent. Ramseier and Lindenmann found that such antisera inhibited mixed-lymphocyte reactivity, as detected by their assay in a highly specific fashion.

Binz and Wigzell (1977) subsequently produced antisera according to the techniques of Ramseier and Lindenmann (1972) by injecting Lewis rat T cells into (Lewis × DA) $F_1$ hybrid rats. These antisera used with complement would prevent mixed-lymphocyte reactivity of Lewis T cells for DA, but not for BN, stimulator cells. They would also kill cells required for a graft-versus-host reaction in the same strain combination. Furthermore, they could be used to fractionate Lewis T cells into idiotype-negative and idiotype-positive populations, which, when tested in graft-versus-host assays, showed the expected specificity: idiotype-positive T cells reacted only against DA and not against BN or other rat strains, while idiotype-negative T cells reacted to all alloantigens except those present on DA cells. As mentioned above, these sera were also used to stain and count the number of Lewis T cells with receptors specific for DA alloantigens. In normal Lewis rats, about 6% of T cells carry the idiotype. It is important to note that (Lewis × DA) $F_1$ hybrid rats did not have T cells bearing this idiotype, as expected. Nor were idiotypic T cells detected in the thymuses of Lewis rats.

The antisera were further characterized in terms of their reactions with serum antibody. Lewis anti-DA alloantibody could absorb the activity of the antiidiotypic antiserum when tested on T cells for inhibition of mixed-lymphocyte reactions, thus establishing a resemblance of the two structures. Furthermore, the heavy chains, but not the light chains, of Lewis anti-DA antibody would absorb the activity of antiidiotypic antisera, suggesting that the idiotype in question was carried by a $V_H$-like molecule. In order to demonstrate that the idiotypic receptor was indeed encoded in $V_H$ genes, a linkage analysis was performed in $F_2$ rats. In this study, only rats *not* carrying DA alloantigens were considered, since only such rats could express a Lewis anti-DA idiotype. These were then divided into those carrying the $C_H$ allotypes of Lewis and those not carrying this allotype. Only rats with Lewis $C_H$ allotype also had T cells bearing the Lewis anti-DA idiotypic determinant. This established that the genes encoding for the T-cell receptor were tightly linked to $C_H$, and these were surely the same $V_H$ genes encoding for Lewis anti-DA antibody.

In biochemical studies, molecules produced by purified normal Lewis T cells were characterized by Binz and Wigzell (1977). These had an approximate molecular mass of 140,000 daltons, and were probably present on the cells as a disulfide-linked dimer. Interestingly, isolated monomers would bind both to antiidiotypic antibody and to DA alloantigens, but not to Lewis antigens. These chains were tested with a large number of antisera directed against conventional Ig classes, light chains, and Lewis alloantigens, without reacting. Thus, the only known antigen found on these molecules is the $V_H$ idiotype.

From these studies one can conclude that the antigen-binding portion of the T-cell receptor is a $V_H$ region. It will bind alloantigen in the absence of light chain. It is part of a longer polypeptide chain that is quite susceptible to proteolysis, and which does not resemble any of the known immunoglobulin chains. Light chains are not involved in such receptors, the normal state of such receptors apparently being a dimer of similar or identical molecules.

### B. T-Cell Receptors for Conventional, Non-MHC Antigens Carry Idiotypic Determinants

Eichmann and Rajewsky (1975) have studied the effect of injecting guinea pig antimouse idiotypic antibody on the subsequent activity of T cells of the same specificity as the original immunizing antibody. This idiotype, carried on a molecule-binding streptococcal A polysaccharide called A5A, is found on 20–30% of antistreptococcal A polysaccharide antibodies in certain strains of mice.

In their studies it was observed that small doses of IgGl anti-A5A antibody would prime B cells and helper T cells to respond to strep A polysaccharide. Furthermore, the activity of such antiidiotype-primed T cells could be entirely inhibited with antiidiotype antibody. Subsequent studies showed that the ability to prime T cells with antiidiotype antibody was linked to the CH genes of the strains studies, and not to the MHC or to other genes tested for. Furthermore, antiidiotype antibody directed predominantly at $V_L$ would not prime T cells, while anti-$V_H$-idiotypic antibodies primed T cells well (Krawinkel *et al.*, 1976).

Biochemical studies have not been carried out in this system, but in a related system involving the isolation of antigen-binding receptors from T cells, such studies have been done (Krawinkel *et al.*, 1976). The mass of these antigen-binding, nonimmunoglobulin, T-cell derived molecules is approximately 150,000 daltons. They carry no known Ig determinants, but they do carry idiotypic determinants whose expression is linked to $C_H$. Interestingly, in one case analyzed by Krawinkel *et al.* (1976), the idiotype was associated with the presence of the unusual ($<5\%$ of total Ig) λ chains on serum antibody, but λ chains were not found in the T-cell-derived molecules. Nonetheless, such molecules bound antigen virtually identically with serum antibody, according to their analysis. Furthermore, these molecules did not carry any known MHC specificities. Thus, these molecules strongly resemble those isolated by Binz and Wigzell (1977), using antiidiotypic antibody in rats.

Finally, Krawinkel and his colleagues (1976) have isolated similar antigen-binding molecules from rabbits. These behave like those found in mice and carry rabbit $V_H$ allotypic markers, but lack the $C_H$ or $C_L$ allotypic markers of rabbits.

Thus, studies of idiotypic molecules derived from T cells tell us several very important things:

1. T cells use conventional $V_H$ genes to make antigen-binding sites. These sites strongly resemble those on antibody, since the same $V_H$ gene is used to make both T-cell receptors and antibody specific for a particular antigen.
2. Each T-cell receptor consists of two heavy chains, each of about 70,000 daltons, present on the cell as a dimer. It is not known what genes are used to make up the constant portion of the T-cell receptor, but available evidence suggests it is neither a conventional Ig heavy chain nor a known MHC gene product. Nor is it known whether both chains carry the same $V_H$ gene product, since single isolated chains will bind to MHC antigens.
3. $V_H$ gene products are used to make receptors to both allogeneic MHC antigens and to conventional, non-MHC antigens (nominal antigens). The nature of a postulated self-MHC-recognizing receptor has not been determined.

## VIII. SELF/NON-SELF DISCRIMINATION BY T CELLS

T cells are intimately involved in self/non-self discrimination. There is clear evidence that the genetic information needed to recognize self in a way identical to recognition of allogeneic MHC determinants is present in the precursors of T cells in all strains of a species. However, the experiments of Binz and Wigzell (1977) and Ramseier and Lindenmann (1972) show us that this potential is expressed in mature T cells only if those MHC antigens are not present in that animal. Thus, the Lewis $V_H$ gene that codes for the Lewis anti-DA receptor is present in (Lewis × DA) $F_1$ hybrid rats, since it can be detected in their offspring (see above), but it is not detectable as a T-cell idiotype in the $F_1$ hybrids themselves. There are several possible mechanisms by which this may occur, but experimental evidence currently suggests that self-reactive T cells are permanently inactivated in the thymus during their differentiation. This evidence comes primarily from studies of bone-marrow chimeras, such as those by von Boehmer *et al.* (1975).

However, there must be some kind of receptor for self-MHC antigens on T cells in order to explain the phenomenon of MHC restriction of T cells responding to a wide variety (perhaps all) of non-MHC or nominal antigens. This self-recognition is a property of T cells prior to their encounter with antigen, as discussed in Section IV.B. There is also strong evidence that this selection of T cells capable of recognizing self-MHC structures is a positive event, since only such cells are present, cells responsive to nominal antigen in the context of allogeneic MHC structures not being detected by most workers (for exceptions see Wilson *et al.*, 1977; Thomas and Shevach, 1977; also Section IV.B). The various chimera experiments also show that MHC antigens themselves do not serve as T-cell receptors accounting for self-MHC recognition. Indeed, as far as is known MHC-encoded structures are not highly variable in somatic cells, which makes them less likely candidates for self-recognizing structures capable of undergoing modulation by the environment in which they differentiate.

One final point is worth making. When chimeras are produced by transferring stem cells from $F_1$ animals into lethally irradiated parental recipients, the resulting T cells react only with nominal antigen presented on cells bearing the MHC antigens of the recipients. Thus, they behave like T cells of the recipient rather than like T cells of the donor. However, they differ from recipient T cells in one important respect, namely in lacking alloreactivity to the MHC antigens of the other parent. Thus, the negative selection against strongly anti-self-reactive T cells, presumed to occur in the thymus, must involve a significantly different process from that leading to the MHC-restricted behavior of T cells in responses to non-MHC antigens. This had been predicted to account for certain features of a model of T-cell receptor generation (Janeway *et al.*, 1976).

## IX. THE ASSOCIATION OF NOMINAL ANTIGENS WITH MHC STRUCTURES

Before trying to organize the above findings into a cohesive model for T-cell-receptor formation, one further problem should be discussed. It has been repeatedly stressed that nominal antigens are recognized in association with particular MHC-encoded structures. However, what does this mean at the level of the surface of the antigen-presenting cell? Does it mean that the nominal antigen complexes with a particular MHC product in a particular way, leading to activation of a T cell that recognizes the particular conjunction of antigen and MHC structure? It would appear that most T cells either do not bind antigen, or bind it very weakly. An example of this is the failure of either unmodified self cells or TNP-modified allogeneic cells to block the lysis of TNP-modified syngeneic cells by cytotoxic T cells, while TNP- modified synogeneic cells block this lysis very effectively. Thus, in this case at least, the presence of the nominal antigen on the same cell as the self-MHC antigen is required for inhibition to occur. What is not known is whether these molecules associate tightly on the cell surface, or whether simply being on the same cell is sufficient for binding to occur.

It is hard to believe that the large variety of different antigens that lead to MHC-restricted T-cell responses all bind avidly and specifically to one MHC antigen or another. Cohen and Eisen (1977) have proposed a novel solution to this paradox, which is satisfying at least for antigens that do adhere to cell surfaces in a nonspecific fashion. What they demonstrate is that when confined to a two-dimensional system, such as a cell membrane, the increase in the effective concentration of two molecules allows stable associations between them even when binding constants in solution would be too low to lead to detectable association of the molecules.

An example that would seem to require a particular association between a self-MHC antigen and a nominal antigen has already been discussed in Section IV.B.2. That is, $F_1$ T cells primed with antigen to which one parent is a responder while the other is a nonresponder behave as responder T cells. However, they will not respond to that antigen presented on nonresponder macrophages or B cells. This has suggested to many authors (Paul and Benacerraf, 1977; Janeway *et al.*, 1976; Schwartz, 1978) that nonresponder macrophages or B cells lack an *Ir*-gene product that can bind effectively to the genetically controlled antigen. This may be supported by the finding of numerous factors carrying Ia antigens and binding antigen in a specific fashion (Isac *et al.*, 1976). Perhaps the simplest explanation of these findings is that certain portions of antigens associate with relatively nonvariable *Ir*-gene products to give stable configurations, and it is these stable configurations that are recognized by T cells. Schwartz (1978) has recently proposed a hypothesis of *Ir*-gene action based on such a notion, in which particular, relatively nonpolymorphic self antigens associate with self *Ir*-gene products to give stable self structures that resemble the complex of genetically controlled antigen with *Ir*-gene product. T cells specific for these configurations would be eliminated during their differentiation, since they are self-reactive. This theory nicely explains *Ir*-gene function without having to postulate that there are *Ir*-gene products that are specific for each antigen in the sense in which antibodies are specific. Thus, in this model, *Ir*-gene products do not need to be variable as antibodies are variable. This model also leads to responsiveness being expressed in a dominant fashion, and to control primarily by MHC gene products.

There are also numerous instances of *K/D* specific associations with minor histocompatibility antigens, as described by Simpson and Gordon (1977). Thus, specific associations between cell-surface antigens and involving MHC gene products would appear to occur frequently. What is needed now is structural or biochemical evidence that these associations do indeed take place.

In concluding this section, the value of such a relatively complex mechanism of antigen recognition by T cells should be mentioned. If it is assumed that the major role of T cells is to deal with antigens on cell surfaces, such as tumor or viral antigens, while antibodies deal much more effectively with free antigen in solution, there must be some way to direct the attention of T cells to the cell-bound antigens. If T cells could bind soluble antigen such binding might prevent them from recognizing cell-bound antigen. Thus, the requirement that T cells recognize antigen in association with MHC antigens serves to direct T cells exclusively to cell-bound antigens.

## X. CELLULAR INTERACTIONS IN ANTIBODY RESPONSES

As was stated earlier, helper T cells are required in the production of antibody to most antigens. In this section, various cellular interactions involved in regulating antibody responses to antigen will be discussed.

### A. T-Cell–Macrophage Interaction in T-Cell Priming

When antigen is injected into an animal, most of it ends up in macrophages, where it is largely degraded by enzymes. However, some is retained for long periods of time, by mechanisms that are not well understood. It is probably this antigen that leads to T-cell priming. It makes sense for T cells to become primed to antigen on macrophage surfaces, not only because they retain antigen for long periods of time, but also because, unlike lymphocytes, macrophages carry passively acquired antibody of many specificities on their surfaces, allowing a single cell to bind avidly many different antigens. Thus, the macrophage carries on its surface three important classes of molecules: Ia antigens, nominal antigen, and antibody. It seems likely that T cells recognize antigen in this context during their primary immunization.

### B. T-Cell–B-Cell Interaction in Antibody Responses

It is difficult to prove definitively that macrophages are not intermediaries in T-B interaction, and there are many who argue that macrophages do play such a role. It is the opinion of this author that T cells and B cells must interact directly with one another. There are two reasons for this, which will be discussed is this and the subsequent section.

The first reason derives from the experiments of Katz *et al.* (1973), in which $F_1$ T cells transferred to $F_1$ recipients would help only responder parental B cells, and not nonresponder parental B cells. This type of finding has been independently confirmed recently by Swierkosz *et al.* (1978) and by Sprent (1978). It seems unlikely that such a finding could be based on any mechanism other than direct T-B interaction. This interaction would involve T cells' recognizing, on the B-cell surface, a complex of the nominal antigen, specifically bound to the B-cell Ig receptor (thus leading to specific activation of that B cell), and, in a way similar to its presentation by macrophages during T-cell priming, also bound to, or associated with, B-cell Ia antigens. These antigens have in fact been mapped to the *I-A* subregion (Katz *et al.*, 1975).

### C. Regulation of Immunoglobulin Quality by T Helper Cells

Initial studies on T helper cells focused on their regulation of the amount of antibody produced. However, subsequent studies have shown that T cells also affect the quality of the antibody response. Thus, helper T cells specifically involved in controlling antibody class, allotype, affinity, charge, or idiotype have been described. A general model to account for these findings grew out of studies on the kinetics of helper-T-cell–B-cell interactions in secondary antihapten antibody responses (Janeway *et al.*, 1977). These studies demonstrated that there are in fact two distinct helper T cells that can act synergistically in secondary antibody responses. One of these two helper T cells was absent in agammaglobulinemic mice, and was termed immunoglobulin-dependent. It is thought that one helper T cell recognizes antigen in association with Ia antigens on the B-cell surface, while the other recognizes both antibody (i.e., B-cell receptor) and antigen. In view of the apparently invariant requirement for MHC antigen in T-cell-antigen recognition, and the previously stated argument suggesting that T-cell responses are directed at cell-surface-bound antigen by this requirement, it may be that Ig and MHC are analogues in this instance. However, experimental evidence on this point is lacking, and thus the precise mechanism by which Ig-dependent T cells recognize the appropriate B cell is not known. One might argue that, in fact, antiidiotypic T cells may stimulate a non-antigen-binding B cell, and thus can give rise to idiotype-positive Ig that does not bind the appropriate antigen (Oudin and Cazenave, 1971). In any case, T helper cells do play a strong part in selecting which antigen-binding B-cell clones will be activated in any immune response, and thus they affect the various qualitative parameters outlined in Table VII. The helper T cells that perform this role are probably distinct from, and synergize with, those helper T cells that are specific for antigen in association with Ia antigens.

**Table VII. Evidence for an Ig-Recognizing T Helper Cell in Antibody Responses**

| Level of response affected | Treatment of T-cell donor | Addback synergy | Reference |
|---|---|---|---|
| Constant region | | | |
| Whole response | Anti-$\mu$ antibody from birth | + | Janeway *et al.*, 1977 |
| IgG/IgE ratio | Antigen dose and adjuvant | | Kishimoto and Ishizaka, 1973 |
| Allotype | Antiallotype antibody at birth | + | Herzenberg *et al.*, 1976 |
| Variable region | | | |
| Affinity | T-cell depletion | | Gershon and Paul, 1971 |
| Antibody charge | Charge of carrier | | Sela and Mozes, 1966<br>Karniely *et al.*, 1973 |
| Idiotype | Antiidiotype antibody | + | Ward *et al.*, 1977 |

### D. Suppressor T Cells in Antibody Responses

The immune system is highly regulated, giving carefully modulated responses to most antigens. There are numerous different mechanisms by which the magnitude and quality of immune responses are affected. Among the most prominent are suppressor T cells (Gershon, 1974). As stated previously, these cells are primarily of the Ly23 type. They are detected by reductions in total antibody response, or by a change in its quality, as in the instance of allotype suppression (Herzenberg *et al.*, 1976). Their mode of action probably varies, but one pathway is certain to affect the appropriate helper T cell. In the case of allotype suppressor cells, it is the T helper cell specific for allotype that is primarily affected, apparently leaving the carrier-specific helper T cell relatively unaffected. Other systems are antigen-specific and presumably affect the carrier-specific helper T cell preferentially (Tada, 1977). Yet other suppressor T cells may act directly on the B cell itself (Warren and Davie, 1977). Thus, for every cell involved in the induction of antibody production, there are counteracting suppressor T cells.

### E. Feedback Loops in Immunoregulation

If immune responses were regulated merely on the basis of competing helper and suppressor T cells, the system would function relatively well but would lack flexibility. However, regulation appears to be very flexible. This is owing to the functioning of Ly123 cells. These cells, while apparently not responding directly to antigen, do respond to signals produced by the immune system in response to antigenic challenge, and serve to amplify these signals in a variety of ways. Thus, Tada (1977) has described both helper and suppressor positive-feedback loops, in both of which Ly123 cells play a central, amplifying role. Eardley *et al.* (1978) have defined an opposite set of loops, in which helper cells communicate with Ly123 cells to produce Ly23 suppressor cells (feedback suppression), or Ly23 suppressor cells act via Ly123 cells to induce more helper cells (feedback help). Thus, virtually any result is possible, depending on the parameters of the response. The most important of these parameters appear to be the classes of cells present, the state of priming of each class, and the strength of the antigenic challenge. Thus, strong antigenic challenges tend to demonstrate suppressive activities, while weak challenges elicit optimal helper responses. Ly123 cells serve to modulate all of these responses. The simplest interpretation of these findings is to postulate that the Ly123 cells detect the intensity of the response itself and act on the response, rather than reacting directly with the antigen. In this they appear to be unique amongst lymphocytes. What structures they recognize on other cells is not known, but two possible ones are MHC antigens and idiotypes. This latter possibility leads to yet another aspect of immunoregulation.

### F. Idiotypic Networks and Immunoregulation

The role of idiotype-antiidiotype interactions in immunoregulation is covered in Chapter 8 of this book. Whether such networks are important in the cellular interactions discussed above is not known at present. What is known is that both T cells and B cells carry idiotypic receptors, and that both T cells and B cells with auto-antiidiotypic receptors have been described (Sakato *et al.*, 1976; Binz and Wigzell, 1976). Thus, the components for an idiotypic network of the type proposed by Jerne (1975) are certainly present.

## XI. DISCUSSION

The immune system is of great interest because of its central characteristics: specificity, inducibility, memory, and regulation. Each of these is also a characteristic of T cells. T cells play the central role in self/non-self discrimination for virtually all antigens. Thus, to understand the functioning of the immune system, and its evolutionary and biological significance, one must understand how T cells recognize antigen, and how they interact with other cells.

The T-cell receptor is still "elusive" (Crone *et al.* 1972), in that it has not yet been characterized sufficiently to explain functional T-cell specificity, but we do now know enough to begin to draw guidelines. These are:

1. The T-cell receptor is composed of two chains, each of about 70,000 daltons, carrying antigen-binding, $V_H$-gene-encoded sites. Single chains can bind

allogeneic-MHC antigens, but it is not known if single chains can bind self-MHC antigens or nominal antigen with sufficient affinity to be measurable. Light chains, although not found in many studies, have been found in some (see Marchalonis, this volume). If light chains are part of the T-cell receptor, they are not covalently linked nor are they essential for antigen binding of either MHC or conventional antigens.

2. T cells recognize antigen bound to cell surfaces, and do not bind soluble antigen in most cases. The apparent reason for this is that T cells can recognize antigen only when it is presented in association with self-MHC antigens. This so-called MHC restriction is not a function of the MHC type of the T cell, in that T cells differentiating in a semiallogeneic thymus can respond to antigen presented on the other parent's (allogeneic) cells. This ability to recognize antigen in association with non-self cells is independent of tolerance to the other parent's cells, as shown by $F_1$ into parental chimeras, where the T cells are tolerant of both parental MHC types but will recognize antigen only in association with the recipient parental MHC antigens. Furthermore, these represent two quite different processes, tolerance being a negative selection *against* responsiveness to self-MHC antigens, while MHC restriction results from a positive selection for those T cells that will recognize antigen associated with self MHC. The cell that is responsible for tolerance induction must be the thymocyte itself, whereas it has been clearly shown that the thymic epithelial cells are responsible for self-MHC recognition.

3. A very high proportion of T cells are reactive to allogeneic-MHC antigens. Whether this is true of all T cells is not known. However, in experiments in which T cells of selected alloreactivity were tested for recognition of a nominal antigen, this activity was found to be normal. The implication of this finding is that reactivity to nominal antigen is independently expressed on alloreactive T cells. If this is true, then it seems likely that the T cell displays at least two receptor sites, one of which is specific for allogeneic-MHC antigens. It has been proposed (Janeway *et al.*, 1976) that this same receptor recognizes self-MHC antigens of the same type (e.g., self *K*/*D* in cells reactive to allogeneic *K*/*D* molecules), and accounts for MHC restriction. If this were so, it would have somehow to act in concert with a receptor for the nominal antigen. These two different kinds of binding would have to convey a unique signal, since if this were not so a T cell with multiple self-MHC-reactive receptors would be perpetually activated by self cells. Likewise, allogeneic-MHC antigens must bind to give a unique signal, perhaps on the basis of the stability of the antigen–receptor interaction, as outlined previously (Janeway *et al.*, 1976).

4. To talk about T cells as a single entity is obviously erroneous. There are at least three subpopulations, distinguished solely by Ly-antigen phenotype. Each of these classes can be further subdivided, and will be. There is no reason to believe that all T cells will have identical receptors, although it may be true

that all receptors in the immune system utilize the immunoglobulin-V genes for their antigen-combining sites. However, numerous other structures may get involved in receptor formation. These include: Ly antigens, which are associated with cells of particular MHC-recognizing types; I-region-gene products, which are found on a large number of T-cell-derived factors, although they have not been conclusively shown to be synthesized by the T cell itself; and the unknown structural genes for the constant region of the T-cell receptors thus far characterized. What is needed now are techniques for isolating different subpopulations of T cells, and then a characterization of the antigen-binding or idiotypic molecules on such subpopulations.

5. As mentioned above, one function of Ir genes may be to form portions of the T-cell receptor for antigen, or else to be a part of secreted T-cell factors. A distinct and different role of these molecules appears to be in antigen presentation. Thus, the conjunction of *Ir*-gene product with nominal antigen appears to present the T cell with a unique antigenic complex. Nonresponder animals either lack the appropriate binding *Ir*-gene product, or have been tolerized to the complex, which resembles a complex of self cell-surface molecules and *Ir*-gene product. Neither of these models requires that *Ir*-gene products be highly variable in the sense that antibody molecules are variable, since the orientation of the complex may be as essential in its recognition by T cells as the fact that it is present on the cell surface. The *Ir*-gene product could bind different antigens in different ways, thus behaving in a selective fashion, even though it is not antigen-specific in the sense that antibody is specific. Furthermore, the *Ir*-gene system is heavily tilted in the direction of responsiveness, since only relatively simple antigens are under absolute *Ir*-gene control.

6. Different T-cell subpopulations play different roles in cellular interactions, as exemplified by T-B cooperation in antibody formation. There appear to be at least two types of antigen-specific T helper cells, one responsive to carrier in association with self *I*-region gene products, the other responsive to autologous immunoglobulin. Both of these cells are Lyl cells. However, the interplay of Lyl and Ly23 cells would lead to a very inflexible system were there no way for T cells to perceive their own activity. This is the role of the Ly123 cell, about which little else is known. Questions still to be answered about such cells are: Do they differentiate into Ly1 and Ly23 cells, or are they a distinct line of mature T cell? Are there two types of Ly123 cell, one a precursor of all three mature forms? Do Ly123 cells have receptors for antigen? Can they be primed? Are they antiidiotypic in nature, responding not to antigen but to immune-system signals in the form of idiotypic determinants? The great need in this area is a pure population of Ly123 cells from mature peripheral lymphoid tissue. Thus far, this has not been possible to obtain.

7. The carrier specificity of T-cell responses to hapten-carrier conjugates can also be regarded in a new light. Since the unit recognized by the T cell would ap-

pear to be antigen plus self *I*-region structures, the failure of haptens to serve as carriers may relate to a failure to form appropriate complexes with self *I*-region structures. Another way to look at this is to say that the association of a hapten–carrier conjugate on a cell surface with self *I*-region structures is dictated by the carrier rather than by the hapten; thus, the dominant T-cell response is to carrier plus self *I*-region structures. It is interesting to note that, while azobenzenearsonyl-tyrosine in adjuvant induces T-cell responses to the hapten on many carriers, the same hapten on a protein carrier induces carrier-specific T-cell responses. This mechanism may also explain the exceptions to carrier specificity mentioned previously. Lipid-containing antigens appear to bind very tightly to cell surfaces, and behave as though they associate with self *I*-region structures in such a way as to mimic any hapten–protein conjugate (Janeway *et al.*, 1979). Thus, a great variety of hapten-reactive, but not strictly hapten-specific, T cells become activated to such compounds. Likewise, with hapten presented on autologous Ig there may be a nonspecific association with self *I*-region structures, perhaps related to the association between receptors for the Fc piece of Ig and *I*-region structures. An alternative explanation in this case would be that it is the Ig-recognizing T cell that responds to hapten-autologous Ig in a hapten-reactive fashion. Finally, even in these instances T cells have not been shown to be hapten-specific in the sense that B cells are hapten-specific, probably because, unlike B cells, they must see not only the hapten but also self MHC structures in order to respond.

## XII. SUMMARY

T cells are responsible for virtually all the characteristics of the mammalian immune system except the production of serum antibody, in which they play a vital regulatory role. As such, they are central to our understanding of the immune system. T cells recognize cell-bound antigens with great precision, in association with self MHC antigens. They do this by means of antigen-specific receptors, whose antigen-combining sites are encoded in conventional $V_H$ genes. There is evidence that T cells carry at least two kinds of specific receptors, one for MHC antigens and one for non-MHC antigens. Both of these would bear $V_H$-encoded and distinct idiotypic determinants. The process by which antigens associate with MHC-gene products on cell surfaces is poorly understood at present, and so is the process by which the two types of receptors communicate with each other. T cells are divisible into a number of subpopulations playing unique functional roles in the regulation of antibody responses. If one examines them further for other functions, even greater complexity emerges. Thus, all T cells may not have the same kind of receptor, which would not be surprising given the wide variety of functions they perform. Future work will undoubtedly focus on these important questions.

## XIII. REFERENCES


Barcinsky, M. A., and Rosenthal, A. S., 1977, Immune response gene control over determinant selection. I. Intramolecular mapping of the immunogenic sites on insulin recognized by guinea pig T and B cells, *J. Exp. Med.* **145**:726.

Bevan, M. J., 1978, In radiation chimeras host H-2 antigens determine the immune responsiveness of donor cytotoxic cells, *Nature* **269**:417.

Binz, H., and Wigzell, H., 1976, Successful induction of specific tolerance to transplantation antigens using autoimmunization against the recipient's own, natural antibodies, *Nature* **262**:294.

Binz, H., and Wigzell, H., 1977, Antigen-binding idiotypic T lymphocyte receptors, in: *Contemporary Topics in Immunobiology,* Vol. 7: T Cells (O. Stutman, ed.), pp. 113–117, Plenum Press, New York.

Boehmer, H. von, and Haas, W., 1976, Cytotoxic T lymphocytes recognize allogeneic tolerated TNP-conjugated cells, *Nature* **261**:141.

Bohmer, H. von, and Sprent, J., 1976, T cell function in bone marrow chimeras: absence of host-reactive T cells and cooperation of helper T cells across allogeneic barriers, *Transpl. Rev.* **29**:3.

Boehmer, H. von, Hudson, L., and Sprent, J., 1975, Collaboration of histoincompatible T and B lymphocytes using cells from tetraparental bone marrow chimeras, *J. Exp. Med.* **142**:989.

Cantor, H., and Boyse, E. A., 1975, Functional subclasses of T lymphocytes bearing different Ly antigens. I. The generation of functionally distinct T cell subclasses is a differentiation process independent of antigen, *J. Exp. Med.* **141**:1376.

Cantor, H., and Boyse, E. A., 1976, Regulation of cellular and humoral immune responses by T cell subclasses, *Cold Spring Harbor Symp. Quant. Biol.* **41**:23.

Cohen, R. J., and Eisen, H. N., 1977, Hypothesis: Interactions of macromolecules on cell membranes and restrictions of T-cell specificity by products of the major histocompatibility complex, *Cell. Immunol.* **32**:1.

Crone, M. M., Koch, C., and Simonsen, M., 1972, The elusive T cell receptor, *Transpl. Rev.* **10**:36.

Eardley, D. D., Hugenberger, J., McVay-Boudreau, L., Shen, F. W., Gershon, R. K., and Cantor, H., 1978, Immunoregulatory circuits among T cell sets. I. T helper cells induce other T cell sets to exert feedback inhibition, *J. Exp. Med.* **147**:1106.

Eichmann, K., and Rajewsky, K., 1975, Induction of T and B cell immunity by anti-idiotypic antibody, *Eur. J. Immunol.* **5**:661.

Erb, P., Feldmann, M., and Hogg, N., 1976, Role of macrophages in the generation of T helper cells. IV. Nature of genetically related factor derived from macrophages incubated with soluble antigens, *Eur. J. Immunol.* **6**:365.

Feldmann, M., Beverley, P., Erb, P., Howie, S., Kontiainen, S., Maoz, A., Mathies, M., McKenzie, I., and Woody, J., 1976, Current concepts of the antibody response: Heterogeneity of lymphoid cells, interactions, and factors, *Cold Spring Harbor Symp. Quant. Biol.* **41**:113.

Ford, W. L., Simmonds, S. J., and Atkins, R. C., 1975, Early events in a systemic graft-versus-host reaction. II. Autoradiographic estimation of the frequency of donor lymphocytes which respond to each Ag-B determined antigenic complex, *J. Exp. Med.* **141**:681.

Gershon, R. K., 1974, T cell control of antibody production, in: *Contemporary Topics in Immunobiology*, Vol. 3 (M. D. Cooper and N. L. Warner, eds.), pp. 1–40, Plenum Press, New York.

Gershon, R. K., and Paul, W. E., 1971, Effect of thymus derived lymphocytes on amount and affinity of anti-hapten antibody, *J. Immunol.* **106**:872.

Gowans, J., 1970, Lymphocytes, in: *The Harvey Lectures*, Series 64, pp. 87–119, Academic Press, New York.

Hansen, T. H., Cullen, S. E., Melvold, R., Kohn, H., Flaherty, L., and Sachs, D. H., 1977, Mutation in a new *H-2*-associated histocompatibility gene closely linked to H-2D, *J. Exp. Med.* **145**:1550.

Heber-Katz, E., and Wilson, D. B., 1975, Collaboration of allogeneic T and B lymphocytes in the primary antibody response to sheep erythrocytes *in vitro*, *J. Exp. Med.* **142**:928.

Heber-Kratz, E., and Wilson, D. B., 1976, Sheep red blood cell-specific helper activity in rat thoracic duct lymphocyte population positively selected for reactivity to strong specific histocompatibility alloantigen, *J. Exp. Med.* **143**:701.

Herzenberg, L. A., Okumura, K., Cantor, H., Sato, V. L., Shen, F. W., Boyse, E. A., and Herzenberg, L A., 1976, T cell regulation of antibody responses: demonstration of allotype-specific helper T cells and their specific removal by suppressor T cells, *J. Exp. Med.* **144**:330.

Huber, B., Cantor, H., Shen, F. W., and Boyse, E. A., 1976*a*, Independent differentiative pathways of Ly1 and Ly23 subclasses of T cells: Experimental production of mice deprived of selected T cell subclasses, *J. Exp. Med.* **144**:1128.

Huber, B., Devinsky, O., Gershon, R. K., and Cantor, H., 1976*b*, Cell-mediated immunity: delayed-type hypersensitivity and cytotoxic responses are mediated by different T cell subclasses, *J. Exp. Med.* **143**:1424.

Humphrey, J. H., 1967, Cell mediated immunity–General perspectives, *Br. Med. Bull.* **23**: 93.

Isac, R., Mozes, E., and Taussig, M., 1976, Antigen-specific T cell factors in the immune response to poly(Tyr, Glu)-poly(Pro)-poly(Lys), *Immunogenetics* **3**:409.

Janeway, C. A., 1975, Cellular cooperation during *in vivo* anti-hapten antibody responses. I. The effect of cell number on the response, *J. Immunol.* **114**:1394.

Janeway, C. A., 1976, The specificity of T lymphocyte responses to chemically defined antigen, *Transpl. Rev.* **29**:164.

Janeway, C. A., and Paul, W. E., 1976, The specificity of cellular immune responses in guinea pigs. III. The precision of antigen recognition by T lymphocytes, *J. Exp. Med.* **144**:1641.

Janeway, C. A., Wigzell, H., and Binz, H., 1976, Hypothesis: Two different VH genes products make up the T cell receptors, *Scand. J. Immunol.* **5**:993.

Janeway, C. A., Murgita, R. A., Weinbaum, F. I., Asofsky, R., and Wigzell, H., 1977, Evidence for an immunoglobulin-dependent antigen-specific helper T cell, *Proc. Natl. Acad. Sci. USA* **74**:4582.

Janeway, C. A., Murphy, P. D., Kemp, J., and Wigzell, H., 1978, T cells specific for hapten-modified self are precommitted for self major histocompatibility antigens before encounter with the hapten, *J. Exp. Med.* **147**:1065.

Janeway, C. A., Horowitz, M., Dailey, M. O., Hunter, R. A., and Wigzell, H., 1979, Lipid-modified hapten–carrier conjugates. I. Evidence for association with cell surface I region determinants, *J. Immunol.* **122**:1482.

Jerne, N. K., 1975, The immune system: a web of V domains, in: *The Harvey Lecture Series*, pp. 93–110, Academic Press, New York.

Jones, P. P., Cebra, J. J., and Herzenberg, L. A., 1974, Restriction of the gene expression in

B lymphocytes and their progeny. I. Commitment to immunoglobulin allotype, *J. Exp. Med.* **139**:581.

Julius, M. H., Janeway, C. A., Jr., and Herzenberg, L. A., 1976, Isolation of antigen binding cells from unprimed mice. II. Evidence for monospecificity of unprimed cells, *Eur. J. Immunol.* **6**:288.

Karniely, Y., Mozes, E., Shearer, G. M., and Sela, M., 1973, The role of thymocytes and bone marrow cells in defining the response to the dinitrophenyl hapten attached to positively and negatively charged synthetic polypeptide carriers, *J. Exp. Med.* **137**:183.

Katz, D. H., 1977, *Lymphocyte Differentiation, Recognition, and Regulation*, Academic Press, New York.

Katz, D. H., Hamaoka, T., Dorf, M. E., Maurer, P. H., and Benacerraf, B., 1973, Cell interactions between histoincompatible T and B lymphocytes. IV. Involvement of the immune response (Ir) gene in the control of lymphocyte interactions in responses controlled by the gene, *J. Exp. Med.* **138**:734.

Katz, D. H., Graves, M., Dorf, M. E., DiMuzio, H., and Benacerraf, B., 1975, Cell interactions between histoincompatible T and B lymphocytes. VII. Cooperative responses between lymphocytes are controlled by genes in the I region of the *H-2* complex, *J. Exp. Med.* **141**:263.

Kishimoto, T., and Ishizaka, K., 1973, Regulation of the antibody response *in vitro*. VI. Carrier-specific helper cells for IgG and IgE antibody response, *J. Immunol.* **111**:720.

Klein, J., 1975, *Biology of the Mouse Histocompatibility-2 System*, Springer-Verlag, New York.

Krammer, P. H., 1978, Alloantigen receptors on activated T cells in mice. I. Binding of alloantigens and anti-idiotypic antibodies to the same receptor, *J. Exp. Med.* **147**:25.

Krawinkel, U., Cramer, M., Berek, C., Hämmerling, G., Black, S. J., Rajewsky, K., and Eichmann, K., 1976, On the structure of the T cell receptor for antigen, *Cold Spring Habor Symp. Quant. Biol.* **41**:285.

Kuhn, T. S., 1962, *The Structure of Scientific Revolutions*, University of Chicago Press, Chicago.

Laskin, J. A., Gray A., Nisonoff, A., Klinman, N. R., Gottlieb, P. D., 1977, Segregation at a locus determining an immunoglobulin $V_L$-region genetic marker affects inheritance of expression of an idiotype, *Proc. Natl. Acad. Sci. USA* **74**:4600.

Miller, J. F. A. P., and Vadas, M. A., 1976, Antigen activation of T lymphocytes: Influence of major histocompatibility complex, *Cold Spring Harbor Symp. Quant. Biol.* **41**:579.

Mitchison, N. A., 1971, The carrier effect in the secondary response to hapten–protein conjugates. II. Cellular cooperation, *Eur. J. Immunol.* **1**:18.

Nagy, Z., Elliott, B. E., and Nabholz, N., 1976, Specific binding of K- and I-region products of the *H-2* complex to activated thymus-derived (T) cells belonging to different Ly subclasses, *J. Exp. Med.* **144**:1545.

Oudin, J., and Cazenave, P. A., 1971, Similar idiotypic specificities in immunoglobulin fractions with different antibody function or even without detectable antibody function, *Proc. Natl. Acad. Sci. USA* **68**:2616.

Ovary, Z., and Benacerraf, B., 1963, Immunological specificity of the secondary response with dinitrophenylated proteins, *Proc. Soc. Exp. Biol. Med.* **114**:72.

Paul, W. E., and Benacerraf, B., 1977, Functional specificity of thymus-dependent lymphocytes, *Science* **195**:1293.

Peck, A. B., Janeway, C. A., and Wigzell, H., 1977, T lymphocyte responses to Mls-locus antigens involve recognition of *H-2* I region products, *Nature* **266**:840.

Pfizenmaier, D., Starzinki-Powitz, A., Rodt, H., Rollinghoff, M., and Wagner, H., 1976, Virus and trinitrophenyl hapten-specific T-cell-mediated cytotoxicity against *H-2* incompatible target cells, *J. Exp. Med.* **143**:999.

Pierce, C. W., Kapp, J. A., and Benacerraf, B., 1976, Genetic restriction of macrophage–

lymphocyte interactions in secondary antibody responses *in vitro, Cold Spring Harbor Symp. Quant. Biol.* **41**:563.

Poljak, R. J., Amzel, L. M., Chen, B. L., Phizackerley, R. P., and Saul, F., 1974, The three dimensional structure of the Fab′ fragment of a human myeloma immunoglobulin at 2.0–Å resolution, *Proc. Natl. Acad. Sci. USA* **71**:3440.

Raff, M. C., Feldmann, M., and dePetris, S., 1973, Monospecificity of bone marrow–derived lymphocytes, *J. Exp. Med.* **137**:1074.

Ramseier, H. R., and Lindenmann, J., 1972, Alliotypic antibodies, *Transpl. Rev.* **10**:57.

Sakato, N., Janeway, C. A., and Eisen, H. N., 1976, Immune responses of BALB/c mice to the idiotype of T15 and other myeloma proteins of BALB/c origin: implications for an immune network and antibody multispecificity, *Cold Spring Harbor Symp. Quant. Biol.* **41**:719.

Schwartz, R. H., 1978, A clonal deletion model for Ir gene control of the immune response, *Scand. J. Immunol.* **7**:3.

Segal, D. M., Paddlan, E. A., Cohen, G. H., Rudikoff, S., Potter, M., and Davies, D. R., 1974, The three-dimensional structure of a phosphorylcholine-binding mouse immunoglobulin Fab and the nature of the antigen binding site, *Proc. Natl. Acad. Sci. USA* **71**:4298.

Sela, M., and Mozes, E., 1966, Dependence of the chemical nature of antibodies on the net electrical charge of antigens, *Proc. Natl. Acad. Sci. USA* **55**:445.

Shevach, E. M., and Rosenthal, A. S., 1973, The function of macrophages in antigen recognition by guinea pig T lymphocytes. II. The role of macrophages in the regulation of genetic control of the immune response, *J. Exp. Med.* **138**:1213.

Simonsen, M., 1968, The clonal selection hypothesis evaluated by grafted cells reacting against their hosts, *Cold Spring Harbor Symp. Quant. Biol.* **32**:517.

Simonsen, M., 1974, The heterogeneity of lymphocytes: Return to square one, in: *Allergology*, International Congress Series No. 323, pp. 146–154, Excerpta Medica, Amsterdam.

Simpson, E., and Gordon, R. D., 1977, Responsiveness to H-Y antigen: Ir gene complementation and target cell specificity, *Immunol. Rev.* **35**:59.

Sprent, J., 1978, Restricted helper function of F1 hybrid T cells positively selected to heterologous erythrocytes in parental strain mice. II. Evidence for restrictions affecting helper cell induction and T–B collaboration, both mapping to the *K* end of the *H-2* complex, *J. Exp. Med.* **147**:1159.

Swain, S. L., Trefts, P. E., Tse, H. Y.-S., and Dutton, R. W., 1976, The significance of T-B collaboration across haplotype barriers, *Cold Spring Harbor Symp. Quant. Biol.* **41**:597.

Swierkosz, J. G., Rock, K., Marrack, P., and Kappler, J. W., 1978, The role of *H-2*-linked genes in helper T-cell function. II. Isolation on antigen pulsed macrophages of two separate populations of F1 helper T cells each specific for antigen and one set of parental *H-2* products, *J. Exp. Med.* **147**:554.

Tada, T., 1977, Regulation of the antibody response by T cell products determined by different I subregions, in: *Immune System: Genetics and Regulation* (L. A. Herzenberg, E. E. Sercarz, and C. F. Fox, eds.), pp. 345–361, Academic Press, New York.

Tada, T., Taniguchi, M., and David, C. S., 1977, Suppressive and enhancing T cell factors as I region products: properties and subregion assignment, *Cold Spring Harbor Symp. Quant. Biol.* **41**:119.

Thomas, D. W., and Shevach, E. M., 1977, Nature of the antigenic complex recognized by T lymphocytes. III. Specific sensitization by antigens associated with allogeneic macrophages, *Proc. Natl. Acad. Sci. USA* **74**:2104.

Thomas, D. W., Yamashita, U., and Shevach, E. M., 1977, The role of Ia antigens in T cell activation, *Immunol. Rev.* **35**:97.

Tonegawa, C., Brock, C., Hozumi, N., Matthyssens, G., and Schuller, R., 1977, Dynamics of immunoglobulin genes, *Immunol. Rev.* **36**:73.

Vadas, M., Miller, J. F. A. P., Whitelaw, A. M., and Gamble, J. R., 1977, Regulation by the *H-2* gene complex of delayed type hypersensitivity, *Immunogenetics* **4**:137.

Ward, K., Cantor, H., and Boyse, E. A., 1977, Clonally restricted interactions among T and B cell subclasses, in: *Immune System: Genetics and Regulation* (L. A. Herzenberg, E. E. Sercarz, and C. F. Fox, eds.), pp. 363–410, Academic Press, New York.

Warren, P. W., and Davie, J. M., 1977, Antigen mediation of a late-acting suppressor T cell activity, *J. Exp. Med.* **146**:1627.

Weigert, M., and Potter, M., 1977, Antibody variable region genetics: Summary and abstracts of the homogeneous antibody workshop VII, *Immunogenetics* **5**:491.

Wilson, D. B., 1974, Immunologic reactivity to major histocompatibility alloantigens: HARC, effector cells, and the problem of memory, *Prog. Immunol.* **2**:145.

Wilson, D. B., Silvers, W. K., and Nowell, P. C., 1967, Quantitative studies on the mixed lymphocyte culture interaction in rats. II. Relationship of the proliferative response to the immunological status of the donors, *J. Exp. Med.* **126**:655.

Wilson, D. B., Lindahl, K. F., Wilson, D. H., and Sprent, J., 1977, The generation of killer cells to trinitrophenyl-modified allogeneic targets by lymphocyte populations negatively selected to strong alloantigens, *J. Exp. Med.* **146**:361.

Zinkernagel, R. M., 1976, Virus-specific T-cell mediated cytotoxicity across the *H-2* barrier to virus altered alloantigen, *Nature* **261**:139.

Zinkernagel, R. M., Callahan, G. N., Althage, A., Cooper, S., Klein, P., and Klein, J., 1978*a*, On the thymus in the differentiation of *H-2* self-recognition by T cells: evidence for dual recognition, *J. Exp. Med.* **147**:882.

Zinkernagel, R. M., Callahan, G. N., Althage, A., Cooper, S., Streilein, J. W., and Klein, J., 1978*b*, The lymphoreticular system in triggering virus-plus-self-specific cytotoxic T cells: evidence for T help, *J. Exp. Med.* **147**:897.

*Chapter 8*

# *An Immunologic Network*

**Donald A. Rowley**

*La Rabida–University of Chicago Institute*
*Chicago, Illinois 60649*
and
*Departments of Pathology and Pediatrics*
*University of Chicago*
*Chicago, Illinois 60637*

**Heinz Köhler**

*La Rabida–University of Chicago Institute*
*Chicago, Illinois 60649*
and
*Departments of Pathology and Biochemistry*
*University of Chicago*
*Chicago, Illinois 60637*

**and**

**Jack D. Cowan**

*Department of Biophysics and Theoretical Biology and the College*
*University of Chicago*
*Chicago, Illinois 60637*

## I. INTRODUCTION

A description of complex networks paraphrased and abbreviated from Waddington (1977) seems to apply nicely to the immune system:

> Input signals are parcelled into different circuits which branch and rebranch to give different output signals or products which need not be independent. Within the network positive feedback circuits tend to destabilize while negative feedback circuits tend to stabilize the system. Networks are difficult to model and often behave in unexpected ways because of difficulties in estimating rates of reactions, because of the absence or failure of components, or because the system is oscillating to a new equilibrium.

The immune system is capable of responding to a very large number of different antigens by producing an even greater number of different kinds of antibodies and cells that are specifically reactive with the antigen. The process involves multiple types of circulating and fixed cells and amplifier circuits conditioned by prior experience with the antigens. And probably most immunologists have been surprised one time or another by results contrary to those expected from perturbing the system in an exceptionally controlled way.

Niels Jerne used the term *network* to describe the immune system as a web of idiotypes, and by now the term is used frequently in this context (Jerne, 1974, 1976). We will broaden our discussion to include connectivity through antigen in order to construct a minimal network of reactants that might be involved in the response to any single antigen. While multiple factors permit or are necessary for connections to occur or to be effective, we will be concerned primarily with those aspects of connectivity in the network ultimately conferred by the recognition of antigen by variable (V) domains of receptors. Even so, a model of a simple or minimal network reveals great complexity of possible connections between reactants in the course of an immune response. While this complexity undoubtedly contributes to the usual reliability and stability of the system, it may also account for aberrant reactions observed as the cause or the result of some diseases.

## II. THE IMMUNE SYSTEM AND CONNECTIVITY THROUGH ANTIGEN

The immune system of an adult is capable of responding specifically to a large number (probably $>10^6$) of different epitopes. An epitope is a comparatively small "configuration" specified, for example, by short peptides (as few as 3 to 5 amino acids) or equally short oligosaccharides. Complex materials such as proteins, cell membranes, or microorganisms may contain many of the same or different epitopes. These materials, ranging from large molecules to complex unicellular organisms, are referred to as antigens. An epitope is recognized by noncovalent binding with the V domain of a receptor on a lymphocyte or of an antibody molecule produced by the lymphocyte. The specificity of the V domain is determined by the amino-acid sequence of 3 to 4 or fewer hypervariable regions of a heavy chain and 3 or fewer hypervariable regions of a light chain. Each hypervariable region consists of 3 to 5 amino-acid residues. The chains are folded so that one or more of the amino-acid residues from several hypervariable regions form a configuration, or "recognition patch," which is complementary to the epitope and binds to it by the "closeness of the fit."

Antibody is produced by bone-marrow-derived (B) lymphocytes that are unispecific; i.e., the antigen receptors and the antibody produced by a B lymphocyte share the same V domain. On immunization, stimulated B lymphocytes give rise to cells that sustain the capability of the response and to cells that divide rapidly, synthesize, and release antibody. The B-lymphocyte population includes recirculating cells and cells that are at least temporarily immobilized in lymphoid tissues; the antibodies produced by B lymphocytes have half-lives of 1 to many days, depending on the class of antibody and animal species.

Thymus-derived (T) lymphocytes comprise at least three broad classes that differ in function and surface molecules other than antigen receptors. One class, T helper ($T_H$) cells, collaborates with B or T lymphocytes to cause proliferation and differentiation of these cells. A second class, T suppressor cells, ($T_S$) suppresses immune reactions by interaction with $T_H$ cells, with B cells, or possibly with antigen in association with these or accessory cells. A third class, T effector cells, ($T_E$) consists of cells that interact with target antigens to initiate cytotoxic or other effects. Insofar as is known, T lymphocytes are also unispecific and the V domain of their receptors is shared by receptors and antibodies produced by B lymphocytes, except that the light and heavy chains of T-cell receptors are not covalently linked. Upon immunization T lymphocytes proliferate; progeny recirculate and mediate help or suppression of other B or T cells by direct cell–cell interaction or cytotoxicity against foreign cells or organisms through cell-target contact (Golub, 1977; Cantor and Boyse, 1976; Feldmann *et al.*, 1975, 1977; Evans *et al.*, 1977; Phillips and Waldman, 1977; Eardley *et al.*, 1978; Sigal and Klinman, 1978; McKearn, 1974; Eichmann and Rajewsky, 1975; Binz *et al.*, 1976; Binz and Wigzell, 1976*a*; Marchalonis *et al.*, 1976; Szenberg *et al.*, 1977; Owen *et al.*, 1977). Various factors isolated from cells *in vitro* or culture media substitute or replace activity provided by intact lymphocytes, but it is not known whether such factors are released *in vivo* and are active at a distance from the cells producing them (Munro and Taussig, 1975; Taniguchi *et al.*, 1976; Kapp *et al.*, 1976; Harwell *et al.*, 1977; Kindred and Corley, 1977; Diamanstein and Naher, 1978).

The hypervariable sequences responsible for the unique combining specificity of a V domain may in turn specify one or more unique epitopes. These epitopes are referred to as idiotypes (Oudin and Michel, 1963; Kunkel *et al.*, 1963). For convenience of discussion we will assume that the commitment of a stem cell to the expression of a given set of idiotypic epitopes marks the appearance of a clone of lymphocytes. By this definition a clone includes the multiple subpopulations of B lymphocytes that differ in their responses to various forms of antigen and/or differ in their production of different classes of antibody, and the different subpopulations of $T_H$, $T_S$, and $T_E$ lymphocytes, all of which have the same idiotypes and specificity for an epitope.

We emphasize that binding of epitopes to lymphocyte receptors is required for the specificity of interactions, but binding by itself is not sufficient to trigger the entire sequence of events leading to activation (or suppression) of an immune response. The different factors responsible for triggering the various kinds of responses are usually not known, though empirically different kinds of responses to the same epitope may be obtained depending on the form, amount, and route of exposure to the antigen; previous experience with the antigen; the size of the responding clones, etc.

## III. CONNECTIVITY THROUGH ANTIGEN AND A CELLS

Complex antigens such as bacteria and viruses containing multiple epitopes connect otherwise unrelated clones so that the separate responses become strongly interdependent. This occurs because many clones of B cells require $T_H$ cells either to respond at all or for maximal proliferation and antibody synthesis. In most experimental systems, $T_H$ cells specific for one epitope collaborate with B cells responding to a different epitope; thus, for a response to occur, one clone of B lymphocytes is usually linked through antigen to another clone of $T_H$ lymphocytes, as depicted in Fig. 1. The antibodies depicted in Fig. 1 are produced in large numbers and are active at a distance from the cells producing them; but if collaboration between B and $T_H$ cells requires cell–cell interaction, then a critical question arises: How are a relatively few lymphocytes specific for one epitope ($<0.1\%$ of lymphocytes) brought together or connected with an equally small number of lymphocytes specific for a different epitope on an antigen, particularly when these cells are recirculating in a large volume of blood and lymph? A relatively few, possibly antigen-specific, accessory or adherent cells (A cells) that, after interaction with antigen, display epitopes of the antigen on their surface may serve this function. Several findings support this possibility.

Upon immunization, antigens are localized in macrophages in the spleen and/or lymph nodes. Most phagocytized antigens are rapidly degraded, though demonstrable immunogenic material is retained (Franzl, 1962, 1972; Unanue and Askonsas, 1968; Pike and Nossal, 1976). Lymphocytes specific for the immunizing antigen are selectively recruited from the blood and lymph so that by 24 hours after immunization the lymph and blood are depleted and the spleen and lymph nodes are enriched with lymphocytes specific for the immunizing antigen. Antibody to antigen given passively markedly suppresses immunization, presumably by combining with antigen, but with passive immunization lymphocytes specific for the antigen remain in the lymph and blood and are normally responsive when transferred to another animal (Sprent *et al.*, 1971; Rowley *et al.*, 1972; Ford, 1975). Together these findings indicate that a small amount of antigenic material localized in critical fixed sites is responsible for the selective recruitment and connection of specific lymphocytes.

A model of the immune response *in vitro* permits additional analysis. Cells that phagocytize antigens can be separated from lymphocytes because they tend to adhere to plastic or other surfaces. Almost all of these cells ($>95\%$) can phagocytize a wide variety of foreign particles (e.g., carbon particles, foreign

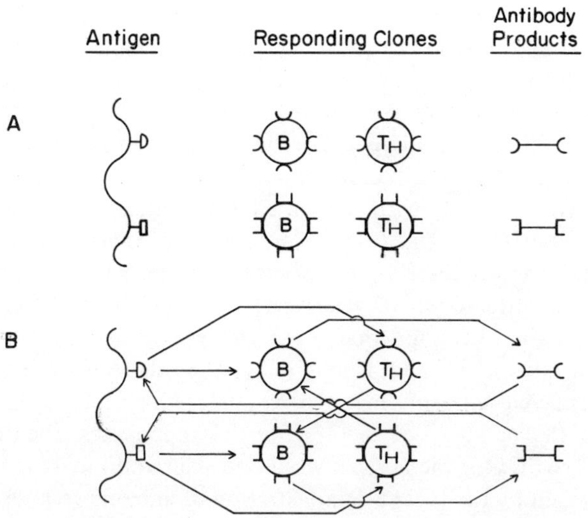


Figure 1. A network of clones connected through antigen. (A) Antigen is drawn as a carrier with 2 different epitopes, —∋ and —□. The combining sites of antibody and receptors on lymphocytes are represented as complementary to the epitopes, —∋ ⊃— and —□ ]—. Only a single B and a single T lymphocyte in each clone are drawn. Upon immunization, responding B lymphocytes proliferate and produce antibodies, ⊃—⊂ and ]—[. Similarly, $T_H$, $T_S$, and $T_E$ lymphocytes give rise to active cells having specificity for the epitopes. (B) The responses are interdependent because $T_H$ lymphocytes specific for —∋ collaborate for amplification of B lymphocytes specific for —□, and $T_H$ lymphocytes specific for —□ collaborate for amplificant B lymphocytes specific for —∋. Also, the antibody products of either response may interact with antigen to alter the original stimulus. The complexity of the interconnections can be appropriately increased by adding the multiple additional responding $T_S$, $T_H$, and $T_E$ lymphocytes and the cellular products of these cells. In the more complete scheme, $T_E$ lymphocytes may also interact with antigen to alter the original stimulus, and $T_S$ and $T_H$ lymphocytes specific for one epitope may affect the response to the other epitope by interacting with B and/or T lymphocytes responding to the other epitope. Though only 2 epitopes are depicted, most complex antigens contain multiple epitopes. Probably within limits, $T_H$ activity is cumulative, i.e., the sum of $T_H$ lymphocytes specific for multiple different epitopes on an antigen causes greater amplification of the B-lymphocyte response to an epitope than do $T_H$ lymphocytes specific for only a single epitope.

erythrocytes, etc.). These A cells obtained from mice recently injected with antigen (or alternatively, A cells from normal mice "fed" antigen *in vitro* and then washed throughly) stimulate a high antibody response when normal B and T lymphocytes are added to them. A cells exposed to antigen *in vitro* or *in vivo* and then treated with antibody to the antigen and washed did not stimulate a response of normal B and T lymphocytes; similarly, A cells fed antigen and treated chemically to inactivate the antigen did not stimulate normal lymphocytes, though the A cells that were re-fed the antigen were effective. Both the phagocytic and immunologic functions of A cells are quite resistant to X irradiation, and the number and function of these cells does not change measurably after immunization, which indicates that the A cells do not (or need not) proliferate in an immune response (Rowley *et al.*, 1975; Lee *et al.*, 1976; Landahl, 1976).

Both the kinetics of responses *in vitro* and *in vivo* and the physical conditions necessary for responses in culture indicate that only a very few of all of the A cells that have interacted with antigen are required, and too many A cells may prevent responses (Mosier and Coppleson, 1968; Weiss and Fitch, 1978). These findings are expected if the function of cells that have interacted with antigen is to focus cell–cell interaction of relatively few lymphocytes. Too many A cells should decrease the likelihood that 2 lymphocytes would be connected by the same A cell. On the other hand, if only a few of all the A cells that phagocytized an antigen displayed antigenic material on surface membranes, and if these cells were fixed in the pathway of the traffic of lymphocytes, then connection of lymphocytes specific for the antigen would be assured. In making this suggestion we are encouraged by the recent demonstration of immune-response-gene control of antigen recognition that operates at the level of the macrophage (Rosenthal *et al.*, 1977). In suggesting the existence of a subpopulation of antigen-specific A cells we mean to imply that each subpopulation is specific for one epitope, as are B and T cells, but on interaction with the antigen the other epitopes of the antigen may be displayed. Thus, the total number of A cells involved in a response to an antigen should approximate the number of A cells specific for all of the epitopes on the antigen. Early studies demonstrating that A cells and 2 different populations of lymphocytes were required for an antibody response *in vitro* also demonstrated that the subpopulation of A cells required for the response approximated in number the interacting lymphocytes. Alternatively, A cells may be nonspecific in both ingestion and display of antigen, but only the combination of A cells and antigen that has recruited B lymphocytes may be effective in recruiting $T_H$ lymphocytes specific for carrier determinants (or vice versa). Also, A cells are required for antigen-specific T-cell as well as B-cell proliferation *in vitro* (Rosenthal *et al.*, 1978; Pierce and Kapp, 1978; Beller *et al.*, 1978; Erb *et al.*, 1978; Möller, 1978). It is not known whether the different subpopulations of B and T lymphocytes responding to antigenic stimulation are triggered by the same or different populations of A cells that have interacted with antigen. Thus, A cells that have interacted with antigen are probably crucial sites for connections in the immune system and therefore potential targets for suppression by appropriate classes of specific antibody and subpopulations of $T_S$ lymphocytes.

The specificity of the interactions discussed so far is determined by exogenous antigens and the V domains that recognize the epitopes of the antigen; but if V domains themselves specify epitopes, then an additional level of connectivity must be considered.

## IV. COMPLEMENTARY IDIOTYPES

If a combining site of one antibody is directed against a combining-site structure of another antibody, then the two antibodies can be considered at least partially complementary; each antibody is an antiidiotypic antibody to the other (so it is arbitrary as to which is referred to as idiotype and which is referred to as antiidiotype). The concept of complementary idiotypes, in Fig. 2, includes two essential ideas: (1) complementary responses may be stimulated by a single epitope, since the antibody product is potentially immunogenic, and (2) the products of either complementary response can suppress the other response.

The evidence for idiotypy and antiidiotypy obtained by Oudin, Kunkel, Nisonoff, and others (Oudin and Michel, 1969; Kelus and Gell, 1968; Daugharty *et al.*, 1969; Braun and Krause, 1968) was derived from experiments using anti-

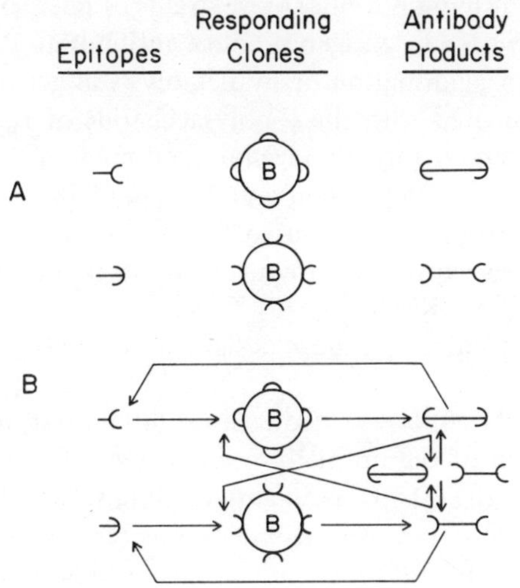


Figure 2. Complementary idiotypes. (A) The epitopes can be components of complex exogenous antigens or of autogenous idiotypes (V domains of receptors or antibodies). Epitopes, regardless of origin, that combine with and stimulate or inhibit the same lymphocytes are assumed to have similar 3-dimensional configurations of charge and shape, though they may be chemically different. The pairs of epitopes on B lymphocytes and antibodies are complementary. (B) Since the combining site structures of receptors for epitopes on B cells are identical with the combining site structures of the antibody the cells produce, the complementary antibody can be considered an "antireceptor" antibody. Thus, the antibody product of an response to an epitope may: (1) combine with the original epitope, (2) act as antigen to stimulate a complementary response, or (3) act as "antireceptor antibody" to inhibit the complementary response. Also, the products of simultaneous or coexisting complementary responses may combine to form complexes. Of course, the possible interacting clones and products include $T_H$, $T_S$, and $T_E$ lymphocytes, as well as the B lymphocytes and antibody drawn, so that the complexity of interconnections is much greater than depicted.

body as putative antigen. The antisera raised against antibody were absorbed with control sera or purified immunoglobulin (Ig), and the remaining antibody that combined with the original antibody was presumably directed against V-domain structures. Much of the evidence supporting a concept of a "network of idiotypes" can be deduced or inferred from these studies, but probably the broadest base of experimental data on complementary idiotypes has been obtained from a model using antigens containing phosphorylcholine (Pc) as a major epitope. For this reason the model will be described in some detail.

The model depended on the identification of plasmacytomas that produce Ig with combining activity to Pc. These tumors, which occur spontaneously in BALB/c mice and are serially transplantable in this strain, provide a source for large quantities of homogenous Ig that can be used as a putative antigen or idiotype. Pc, a constituent of the C-polysaccharide from the rough strain of pneumococcus R36A, or Pc coupled as a diazonium derivative with any of a large number of carrier molecules is immunogenic. Most strains of mice, or their spleen cells in culture immunized with a Pc antigen produce antibody to Pc, which can be measured by passive hemagglutination or by hemolysis in gel (plaque formation) of sheep erythrocytes coated with the C-polysaccharide of R36A or coupled with Pc. The antibody is remarkably homogenous and predominantly IgM (Potter and Leon, 1968; Cohn *et al.*, 1969; Leon and Young, 1971; Potter and Lieberman, 1970; Claflin and Davie, 1975; Rudikoff and Claflin, 1976; Gearheart *et al.*, 1977). Earlier findings supporting a concept of an immunologic network in the Pc system were reviewed (Köhler, 1975).

Several plasmacytomas, e.g., those designated as TEPC-15 and HOPC-8 (which we will refer to collectively as T15), produce Pc-binding IgA having a V domain identical with the IgM antibody produced on immunization with Pc. The identity of the V domain of the normally occurring anti-Pc antibody and T15 was shown by the use of the T15 Ig as an antigen to raise antiidiotypic antisera. The antisera were absorbed to remove antibodies directed against epitopes not associated with the V domain. Antisera raised against T15 inhibited plaque formation by cells from BALB/c mice immunized to Pc. Other plasmacytomas, e.g., MOPC-167, produce a different Pc-binding IgA; antisera raised against the Ig produced by MOPC-167, or against non-Pc-binding myeloma proteins, did not have this activity. Thus, by serologic analysis, the V-region structure of the predominant antibody produced on immunization with Pc is identical with the V-region structures of the Ig produced by the T15 tumor, a conclusion that has been validated by comparing the structures of the immunoglobulins.

The antisera to T15 also suppressed immunization to Pc. This was shown by giving homologous, heterologous, or syngeneic antisera to T15 to mice, or by adding the antisera to cultures at the time of immunization with Pc. Peak responses at 4 to 5 days were suppressed >90% by high dilutions of antisera. Antibody to T15 undoubtedly suppresses by combining with the receptors for Pc on B lymphocytes specific for Pc. Indeed, such receptor-bearing cells were identified in the spleens of normal mice, but not after passive immunization with antibody to T15; the receptor-bearing cells reappeared when the passively immunized cells were washed and incubated briefly (Cosenza and Köhler, 1972; Köhler *et al.*, 1974).

The existence of $T_S$ cells for the Pc idiotype was inferred from the fact that the response of mice to forms of Pc antigens that do not require T-cell help was remarkably enhanced in mice treated to eliminate T cells or in nude mice with congenital absence of the thymus. In both instances the response to Pc was reduced to normal levels by a normal thymus graft (Hopkins, 1975, 1978). It was not known whether suppression was due to a subpopulation of specific $T_S$ cells. However, in subsequent experiments spleen cells from mice made neonatally tolerant to Pc were enriched to contain predominantly T cells; these cells suppressed immunization of normal syngeneic spleen cells to Pc but not to other epitopes. Subsequent studies indicated that the specificity of the cells was for the T15 idiotype (DuClos and Kim, 1977; Schreiber *et al.*, 1977). $T_H$ cells for idiotypic determinants on DNP-binding myeloma proteins and $T_H$ cells for Pc used as a carrier determinant have been demonstrated (Janeway *et al.*, 1975; Eichmann, 1975; Julius *et al.*, 1977), but to our knowledge $T_E$ cells specific for Pc have not been reported.

In other models considerable evidence indicates that antibodies raised against idiotypes of antibodies directed against alloantigens will suppress various T-cell reactions and are therefore probably directed against antigen receptors or idiotypes of alloreactive T lymphocytes. The essential findings are that antiidiotypic antibodies can be raised in inbred Lewis (L) rats with the use as antigen of partially purified L antibody directed against inbred Brown Norway (BN) alloantigens. The antiidiotypic antibody given passively can suppress graft-versus-host disease and mixed-lymphocyte reactions *in vitro* which are T-cell mediated (McKearn *et al.*, 1974*b*; Stuart *et al.*, 1974; Binz and Wigzell, 1976*b*, 1978; Andersson *et al.*, 1976; Bellgrave and Wilson, 1978; Woodland and Wilson, 1977).

In other studies complementary idiotypes have been demonstrated in individual rabbits, guinea pigs, rats, and multiple stains of mice (Hart *et al.*, 1972; Trenkner and Riblet, 1975; Yakulis *et al.*, 1972; Rodkey, 1974; Geczy, 1977; Frischknecht *et al.*, 1978). The evidence, though fragmentary, is sufficient to suggest that complementary idiotypes can be found wherever they are sought, which merely states in another way the idea that a very large repertoire of V domains will probably include at least one V domain that will be complementary to any selected idiotype.

## V. A MINIMAL NETWORK

If unrelated clones are usually linked through antigens, and if each clone is usually linked with a complementary clone, then an idealized minimal network can be constructed involving 4 clones, the smallest number potentially involved in response to an antigen having only two different epitopes, Fig. 3. The essential features of the minimal network are: (1) The products of any one clone may cause reciprocal regulation of the complementary clone or combine to form complexes with products of the complementary clone, and (2) the products of a clone responding to one epitope potentially can regulate either of the complementary responses to the other epitope through connection by antigen.

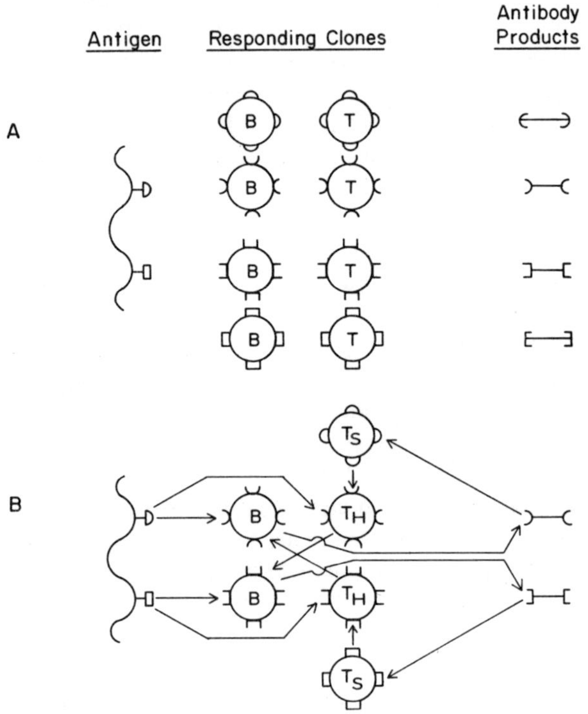


Figure 3. A network of clones connected through antigen and complementary idiotypes. (A) Antigen is drawn as a carrier with 2 different epitopes. The possible reactants include B and T lymphocytes from 4 different clones. (B) The products of one responding clone may cause reciprocal regulation of the complementary clone or else combine to form complexes with the products of the complementary clone; also, the complementary responses to either epitope are interdependent, as described in Fig. 2. The products of clones specific for one epitope can potentially regulate either of the complementary responses to the other epitope because of the connection of T lymphocytes through antigen; see Fig. 1. Thus, the responses of all 4 clones are potentially linked to one another. The interconnections between reactants can be drawn as in Figs. 1 and 2, but the meaning of the drawing (particularly if the responding clones of $T_H$, $T_S$, $T_E$ and the cellular products of these clones are included) tends to be lost, except to demonstrate the great complexity of possible connections. However, one possible set of linkages that connect 4 clones having different idiotypes is depicted.

The network is considered as though there were for each epitope a single specific V domain and a single complementary V domain. If fidelity were this absolute, the system might be considered a repertoire of pairs of complementary clones connected to one another through antigen. But even with such a limited construction, cross-connectivity between complementary pairs through antigen could be great. For example, immunization with relatively simple molecules such as dinitrophenol (DNP) coupled with complex carriers stimulates production of antibodies having different V domains but all capable of combining with DNP, or DNP coupled with other carriers. This "degeneracy" can be accounted for in two ways, which are not exclusive: (1) DNP may specify separate epitopes, the fidelity of each clone for each epitope of DNP may be high but the collective response is observed as heterogeneous. (2) Multiple clones having receptors with different V domains that combine more or less well with the same epitopes of DNP respond so that the antibody produced is heterogeneous. But for our purposes the conclusion is the same: The web of connectivity of clones through antigens must be at least as intricate as that depicted in Figs. 1 and 3.

Similarly, cross-connectivity through complementary V domains may be extensive. Certainly homogeneous antibodies can have multiple idiotypes, some of which are specified by both heavy and light chains and others of which are specified by the heavy chain only. Also, a large number of different antiidiotypic antibodies were obtained in different mice immunized with one dinitrophenylated syngeneic myeloma protein (Claflin and Davie, 1975; Schuler *et al.*, 1977). The validity of the interpretations of the latter study—i.e., that there is a large repertoire of BALB/c antiidiotypic antibodies to the idiotype of a mouse myeloma protein produced by the J558 tumor—may depend on the investigators use of dinitrophenylated myeloma protein to raise antiidiotypic responses. Because an idiotype potentially has several idiotypic epitopes, a complex network of complementary determinants can develop. However, we believe the weight of evidence supports the likelihood of relatively high fidelity of connectivity at the level of individual idiotypes. For example, homologous or syngeneic antiidiotypic antibodies bind to the idiotype that was used to induce them in an exquisitely specific manner. In the Pc system, antibody to T15 raised in BALB/c or A/He mice can distinguish between the T15 idiotype and the idiotypes of other Pc-binding myelomas produced by BALB/c lines: McPC-603, MOPC-167, or MOPC-511; also, antibody to T15 selectively suppresses immunization to Pc *in vivo* or *in vitro* of antibody of T15 idiotype but not responses of the other idiotypes. In keeping with these findings, the spectrotypes of antibodies in sera raised against MOPC-167 and T15 are very limited (Sakato *et al.*, 1977; Köhler and Smyk, 1978). It is conceivable that in the evolution of the immune system, V domain variants may have been positively selected for because of existing idiotypes that were complementary. In this way the repertoire may have expanded as a hierarchy of complementary pairs of V domains (Köhler *et al.*, 1977).

The question of fidelity in complementary interactions has been approached in another way, by asking what kinds of responding clones can be detected when antiidiotypic antibody is used as antigen. This experiment was first done by Urbain *et al.* and Cazenave, using outbred rabbits according to the scheme $AB_1$ (from rabbit 1) → $AB_2$ (from rabbit 2) → $AB_3$ in rabbit 3. Rabbit 3 either had AB very similar to $AB_1$ or was primed to produce $AB_1$. We have used a similar protocol for BALB/c mice and the Pc system. Using anti-T15 as ≅ to $AB_2$, we could induce in mouse 3 an antibody that reacted with the T15 idiotype (≅ $AB_1$ in the scheme) (Cazenave, 1977; Urbain *et al.*, 1977; Köhler, 1979). So far, attempts to forcibly induce an $AB_3$ idiotype that would represent an antibody outside the pair have not succeeded, though this may only reflect the limitation of observations in the present experimental systems. Even if the fidelity of complementary responses is not high, we suspect that responses are dampened quickly either because autogenous idiotypes are poorly immunogenic or because regulatory mechanisms may function rapidly enough to prevent a cascade of complementary responses. For example, if non-binding-site idiotypic determinants (paratopes) are shared by antibodies of differing specificity, then such an additional level of "antiidiotypic" regulation may prevent extensive excitation of complementary idiotypes so that only high-affinity complementary interactions dominate and are therefore observable. The evidence for combining site-specific and noncombining site-specific antiidiotypes has been recently reviewed (Eichmann, 1978; Richter, 1975; Hoffmann, 1975). Both models based on simplified assumptions about the nature of the system account for many aspects of its function, but in the Richter model idiotypic epitopes are considered to be specified by nonbinding site structures (paratopes) of antibodies or antigen receptors, while in the Hoffmann model idiotypes are assumed to be complementary or nearly complementary binding site structures, an assumption we favor, according to experimental findings discussed in this paper.

In the Hoffmann model, there exist both B and T cells specific for antigen, $B_+$ and $T_+$, and $B_-$ and $T_-$, specific for the complementary idiotype. The ($B_+$, $B_-$) and ($T_+$, $T_-$) pairs act in an autocatalytic fashion when triggered by antigen. Regulation is presumed to occur by T-cell suppression of complementary T and B cells. In such a network a number of differing stable or quasi-stable states can exist in response to external antigen: the zero, or "virgin," state (0,0;0,0), in which both pairs of B and T cells are below threshold concentration for the triggering of autocatalytic activity; the "suppressed" state (0,0;$T_+$,$T_-$), in which the T cells predominate, releasing factors that inhibit B-cell activity; the "immune" state ($B_+$,0;$T_+$,0), in which the positive-cell populations dominate and suppress the negative ones; and the "antiimmune" state (0,$B_-$,0,$T_-$), in which the negative-cell populations dominate. In all cases T cells are presumed to be more sensitive than B cells, so that regulation is primarily a T-cell property. Tolerance would then be equivalent to the suppressed state (0,0;$T_+$,$T_-$).

A number of points are worth noting. Firstly, $T_+$ and $T_-$ cells function respectively as $T_H$ and $T_S$ cells for a given antigen, just as in Richter's model, since $T_+$ acts to suppress $T_-$. However, the targets of $T_H$ action in Hoffmann's model are $T_S$ and $T_-$ populations, and vice versa for $T_S$ action, whereas in the Richter model $T_S$ is the target of $T_H$ action, and $B_+$ that of $T_S$ action. There is as yet no direct evidence to support such proposals. Secondly, in the Hoffmann model T-cell specificity is presumed to be for the same antigenic determinants as B cells. This is apparently contrary to that $T_H$ specificity produced by hapten-carrier experiments in which $T_H$ binds to a carrier epitope distinct from that hapten epitope bound by $B_+$ cells. One way to resolve such a difference immediately suggests itself: antigenic determinants are polyepitypic, so that $B_+$ and $T_+$ responses, although not to the same epitope, would be triggered by the same antigen, as is suggested in this article. This in turn implies that in the normal, physiological case, T-cell specificity is neither identical to nor distinct from B-cell specificity, *but is a subset of it*, and that T-cell factors presumed to inhibit B- and T-cell responses are simple fragments of V regions that bind individual epitopes. Thus we begin to see some of the possible implications of connectivity through antigen in the T–B-cell interactions described above. A third point of interest concerns the response of the network to an antigen and its complementary idiotype, given simultaneously, e.g., to Pc and T15 in a BALB/c mouse. The normal immune responses to these antigens are respectively (using Hoffmann's notation) ($B_+$,0; $T_+$,0) and (0,$B_-$;0,$T_-$). Thus, if both responses obtain, there must be a quasi-steady state produced by mutual competition between the positive and negative T systems, each acting to suppress the other, so that the final state ($B_+$,$B_-$;0,0) emerges.

A fourth and final point relates to the question of complementary versus paratope–epitope responses. The experiments demonstrating in BALB/c mice neonatal suppression of the T15 idiotype of anti-Pc antibody by very small doses of anti-T15 Ab suggest that there is a noncomplementary as well as a complementary component to the normal immune response, since recovery from suppression leads to the expression of a spectrum of idiotypes different from T15. This suggests, once again, that antigens are polyepitypic, and that idiotypes comprise the complements of many differing subsets of the set epitopes. In such a hypothesis there will be many differing B- and T-cell populations with differing affinities with the antigen and its complements, all mutually inhibitory via T-cell factors, with the highest-affinity population dominant, and therefore suppressing all the rest, except possibly those with a very weak affinity with the antigen. In such a system Hoffmann's model corresponds to the high-affinity populations, and Richter's to all the other populations. Evidently a small dose of antiidiotypic Ab can counteract the suppressive effect of the complementary network by priming the T cells that act as suppressors of the dominant population, thus permitting an unrestricted clonal expansion of the other idiotypes to take place, subject only to mutual competition, as before, but not without a dominant idiotype to suppress them.

It will be seen, then, that there are many reasons to suppose that the immune system comprises a complex network of mutually interacting clones, each with a differing specificity, that may or may not have some overlap with another set of clones. Interactions may then be both complementary and noncomplementary in the sense defined earlier, and may be either excitatory or else suppressive. Such a system is capable of storing and retrieving a great many epitypic patterns in a stable yet sensitive fashion. The complementary network will act to provide high-fidelity recognition, and the noncomplementary networks could act to provide a redundant "buffer" against any potentially catastrophic failures and malfunctions, such as are manifest in autoimmune diseases.

## VI. REGULATION

The evidence for connectivity in the network depends in part on the demonstration of specific amplification or suppression using isolated antibody or cells as reagents. Thus, antibody to an epitope (or to a carrier epitope in some models) can be an extremely effective immunosuppressant when given as a reagent before or up to 24 hours after initial immunization. It is reasonable to assume that suppression is due to interference with interaction between epitopes and responding cells under these conditions, but suppression is probably not due to simple "masking" of antigen. Much less antibody is required to suppress than to mask all epitopes of an immunizing amount of antigen, and washed antigen-antibody complexes formed in antibody excess can suppress responses to free antigen. The Fc portion of the antibody molecule is important since some classes of Ig (e.g., IgA) suppress poorly or not at all, while other classes having the same idiotype (e.g., IgG) are effective. Also, $(FAB)_2$ fragments that retain full combining activity are ineffective immunosuppressants (Rowley *et al.*, 1973; Forni and Pernis, 1975; Fitch, 1975; Sidman and Unanue, 1976; Pierce and Klinman, 1977; Moretta *et al.*, 1978). In most previous reports antisera to complex antigens used to suppress immunization probably contained antibody to epitopes to which $T_H$ lymphocytes were directed, so that suppression observed may have resulted from the summation of inhibition of the interaction of both B and $T_H$ lymphocytes with antigenic epitopes. However, in recent studies homogenous antibody (antibody produced by hybridomas, which is then directed against a single epitope of alloantigens) can be effective in suppressing immunization *in vitro* and *in vivo* (McKearn *et al.*, 1979). Presumably, the antibody that suppresses links epitopes and Fc receptors on A and/or B lymphocytes, so that it is possible that immune complexes (specific or nonspecific) may interfere with this process.

During an infection or on reexposure to the agent, antibody should not turn off the immune response to the agent, and in fact, antibody is a very much less effective immunosuppressant when given more than 24 hours after a first immunization or before a second immunization, even if the second immunization is weeks or months after the first one. The changing mix of classes of antibody produced, the formation of antibody–antigen complexes, the generation of $T_H$ and $T_S$ cells, etc., probably account for this change; but at present it is impossible to assess the combined interactions of the reactants in the functioning of the network during the course of an immune response.

The potential for regulation through complementary antibody should be great. Antigen stimulates production of antibody; antibody stimulates production of complementary clones that regulate, directly or through their products, the interaction with cells having the idiotype of original responding cells. Several findings are consistent with this possibility. For example, mice immunized with Pc are subsequently specifically unresponsive to immunization with T15, and vice versa, and sera from the previously immunized mice specifically suppress the complementary response *in vivo* or *in vitro* (Rowley *et al.*, 1976). Clearly, regulation can be mediated by autogenous antiidiotypic antibody, though the experiments do not rule out a role for autogenous $T_S$ cells also. When adult mice are injected repeatedly at weekly or longer intervals with immunizing doses of Pc antigen, they have progressively lower responses to Pc with each immunization. This decline in responsivity correlates with the appearance of anti-T15 antibody in the serum and PFC in spleens. Similar observations have been made in mice immunized with Levan. The inference is that the anti-Pc and anti-Levan responses in these models are regulated by autoantiidiotypic antibody and/or cells (Kluskens and Köhler, 1974; Cosenza, 1976; Bona *et al.*, 1978). Analogous type observations have been made in L rats injected with allogeneic lymphocytes from BN rats. L rats injected repeatedly with BN antigen alone develop antiidiotypic antibody, i.e., antibody directed against a combining-site structure of antibody for BN antigen. Furthermore, L rats injected just once with BN antigen and L antibody to BN antigens also produce antiidiotypic antibody, which supports the idea that complexes are responsible for stimulating the complementary response. Interestingly, rats receiving LBN renal allografts at the peak of their antiidiotypic response do not reject the grafts, which suggests that autogenously produced antiidiotypic antibody may be essential for preventing sensitization to BN alloantigens (McKearn *et al.*, 1974; Stuart *et al.*, 1976).

The mechanisms of regulation by complementary idiotypes, however, must be more complex than simple binding of antibody to receptors. For example, $(FAB)_2$ fragments of antibody to T15 do not suppress immunization to Pc *in vitro*. Under these experimental conditions the fragments are not eliminated and retain full binding activity. The findings strongly suggest that cross-linking of antigen receptors with Fc receptors may be required for suppression (Köhler *et al.*, 1978). Also, when mice are intentionally immunized simultaneously with Pc and T15, reciprocal regulation does not occur; each response is undiminished, and circulating complexes of the complementary antibodies are formed. This absence of regulation cannot be accounted for by a shift in idiotypes of either of the complementary responses. Initially, the stimulated clones must proliferate and synthesize antibody in the absence of appreciable complementary idiotype. With progression of responses, released antibody, which can be considered shed antigen, may shield cells from being targets for complementary antibody. Alternatively, complexes of complementary antibodies may bind to Fc receptors that are required for regulation by complementary antibody and prevent regulation in this way (Rowley *et al.*, 1978). Certainly, other mechanisms can be suggested, but the point is to indicate that the role of autogenous complementary antibody in regulation is not simple or obvious.

A regulator role for autogenous $T_S$ and $T_H$ lymphocytes does rest on a strong base of experimental evidence. In the usual experimental model, $T_H$ or $T_S$ are stimulated by appropriate immunization with a complex antigen. The subsequent response to a new epitope coupled with that antigen is strongly modified by the previous immune experience, which correlates directly with demonstration of $T_S$ or $T_H$ cells in such animals. Presumably, the interdependence of responses of B and $T_H$ lymphocytes to different epitopes on the same antigen has advantage for providing greater specificity for anamnestic responses; i.e., only the same antigen with the same array of epitopes elicits maximum responses on subsequent exposure to the antigen; casual encounter with antigens that share only one or a few epitopes may elicit no or only low responses.

As for autogenous antibody, it is difficult to determine the regulatory role of $T_H$ or $T_S$ lymphocytes that are generated during the course of that response. $T_H$ cells for B lymphocytes are primarily involved in the triggering, or at least the early proliferation, of B lymphocytes, as is probably the case for $T_H$ cells that may be involved in the generation of $T_S$ or $T_E$ lymphocytes. The different populations of $T_S$ lymphocytes that are generated during the course of an immune response may be directed against sites that include epitopes of antigen in association with A cells or antigen in association with B lymphocytes, a possibility that may account for the remarkable capability of a population of T lymphocytes of shutting off secretion of antibody by B lymphocytes (Warren and Davie, 1977*a*,*b*). Targets may also include V domains of receptors of B or T lymphocytes, a possibility that may account for the self-limitation of an experimentally induced autoimmune hemolytic anemia (Cooke *et al.*, 1978) and other self-limiting responses where the existence of $T_S$ lymphocytes specific for the response but not for the antigen can be demonstrated.

Recent evidence indicates that the emergence of idiotypes is under specific regulation by complementary clones. In the Pc system, antibody to T15 given to neonatal mice produces tolerance to Pc lasting many months (Strayer *et al.*, 1974, 1975; Strayer and Köhler, 1976; Dorsch and Ross, 1977). When responsivity to Pc is regained, non-T15 clonotypes predominate, apparently because the reemergence of T15 clones is suppressed by complementary clones or their products. This is indicated by transferring neonatal lymphocytes to heavily irradiated adult mice. When the transfer is into irradiated normal adults, recovery of responsivity to Pc is with non-T15 clones, but when the transfer is into adult mice made neonatally tolerant to Pc, then the response to Pc is dominated by T15 clones (Kaplan *et al.*, 1978; Augustin and Cosenza, 1976; Augustin *et al.*, 1977, Ju *et al.*, 1977; Eig *et al.*, 1977; Ward *et al.*, 1978; Kaplan and Quintáns, 1979). Clearly, neonatal lymphocytes include precursors of the T15 clone and emergence is under idiotypic specific regulation, but the nature of the cellular or molecular regulation is not known.

## VII. IS THE NETWORK TOO COMPLEX?

The complexities of the network as presented in Figs. 1, 2, and 3 are sufficient so that almost any observed regulation of an immune reaction may be accounted for in any number of possible ways. We see no obvious escape from the apparent tyranny of this conclusion. Admittedly, the constructions depend on assumptions that may not or do not apply in all circumstances; for example, some clones of B lymphocytes do not require $T_H$ lymphocytes and therefore the regulation of these clones is presumably independent of clones' (or their products') responding to other epitopes on the same antigen; also, complementary idiotypes may not exist for all epitopes. In addition, many immunologists will argue vehemently that receptors on T cells recognize different epitopes from those on B lymphocytes or antibodies and that, therefore, T lymphocytes do not share extensively with B lymphocytes idiotypic determinants (Janeway and Paul, 1976; Krammer and Eichmann, 1977; Paul and Benacerraf, 1977; Benacerraf, 1978). If this is indeed the case, then the complexities of the network and the levels of regulation are even greater than we have indicated.

Earlier we emphasized the role of A cells that have reacted with antigen as sites for connecting reactants. We did this because we are convinced there must be a mechanism for assuring that very few circulating lymphocytes are focused for specific cell–cell interactions. But except for this constraint (which has not been depicted in the figures), we have considered all connections to be possible. Conceivably anatomical constraints may exclude some interactions. Quite likely some kinds of interactions are physically possible but ineffective. Certainly a large body of very important recent work demonstrates a fundamental role of regulatory genes of the major histocompatibility locus in controlling the interactions between B lymphocytes, T lymphocytes, and A cells and therefore in regulating immunity (Shreffler *et al.*, 1976; Katz and Benacerraf, 1976; Singer *et al.*, 1978; Tada *et al.*, 1978; Howie and Feldmann, 1978; Kappler and Marrack, 1978; Swerkosz *et al.*, 1978). Undoubtedly regulation at this level is extremely important in the programming and tuning of responses such as the determining of which of many clones that have identical or complementary idiotypes, but differ in other surface markers, are recruited to enter into an immune response. But we argue that regulation at this level is apparently superimposed on a network that already permits extensive connectivity of multiple components through both antigen and complementary idiotypes. When more of the uncertainties are resolved, an appropriate mathematical model can undoubtedly be constructed, which will generalize and simplify our understanding of the system.

## VIII. THE NETWORK AND DISEASE

Presumably the network evolved in complexity by addition of components and kinds of connectivity, so that regulated responses appropriate in type, magnitude, and duration were selected for that protected individuals against injurious agents; on the other hand, we strongly suspect that the system can fail in some situations, for reasons that are inherent in networks. Signals may be balanced or neutralized so that responses oscillate or are under- or overregulated. For example, the magnitude of antibody responses following immunization with some antigens does oscillate with slow dampening (Britton and Möller, 1968; Romball and Weigle, 1973; Gillespie and Barth, 1974; Mackey and Glass, 1977), so that some untoward effects of immunization may be only transitory while the system is coming to a new equilibrium. Also, as mentioned earlier, mice immunized simultaneously with Pc and T15 respond to both antigens without reciprocal regulation; in fact, responses may be enhanced and circulating complexes of the complementary antibodies are formed (Rowley *et al.*, 1976, 1978). An analogous type of balancing or neutralizing of inputs and outputs may account for the deregulation of immunity observed in some allergies and autoimmune or "immune-complex" diseases. Also, the capability for producing complementary antibodies may result in adverse effects through coupling with other systems. Antibodies specific for epitopes of hormones or neurotransmitters can be produced. These antibodies can neutralize hormonal activity or be used as antigen to raise complementary antibodies, some of which have hormonal acitivity. Both hormone-neutralizing and hormone-mimicking antibodies have been found in nature, which suggests that the products of immune responses can connect with the endocrine or neuronal systems to inhibit or stimulate these systems, probably in pathologic ways. Antiidiotypic antibodies raised against retinol-binding protein and to insulin have hormonal activity (Sege and Peterson, 1978*a*,*b*). Also, autoantibody produced *in vitro* by peripheral-blood lymphocytes from patients with Grave's disease has thyroid-stimulating properties (McLachlan *et al.*, 1977). Antibodies to the receptors for insulin or acetylcholine do not prevent binding of the respective agents to their receptors, though the antibodies have agonist or hormonal activity (Jacobs *et al.*, 1978; Heinemann *et al.*, 1977). Antibodies to the receptor for acetylcholine are present in the sera of patients with myasthenia gravis; such antibody may suppress acetylcholine activity by increasing the degradation of receptors for the agonist (Stanley and Drachman, 1978).

A complex network provides stability and redundancy, and such redundancy probably accounts for the fact that patients with some forms of immunodeficient diseases are protected by alternative immune responses, while patients with other immunodeficiencies may have point deletions of components essential for critical connectivity and therefore have diffuse abnormalities. In yet other conditions (e.g., aging, malnutrition, toxicity caused by some drugs and chemicals, irradiation, some viral infections, etc.) the function of multiple components may be altered to cause multiple breakdowns in the different regulatory loops controlling existing immunities. Because of differential effects on components and the differing states of existing immunities among individuals, the same condition or agent may cause quite different and bizarre abnormalities, e.g., altered absolute numbers or ratios of B and T lymphocytes, increased or decreased serum-Ig levels or ratios of Ig classes, increased or decreased numbers of $T_S$ or $T_H$ cells, autoimmune disorders, etc. (Talal, 1977; Cantor *et al.*, 1978).

## IX. SUMMARY

The immune system is a complex network of molecules and cells specifically connected by the complementarity of receptors for antigen and receptors for receptors. The network includes multiple positive- and negative-feedback loops, which modulate the type, magnitude, and duration of responses. The great challenge is to devise ways to manipulate the system specifically to induce effective autoimmunity to cancer, to prevent allograft rejection, and to turn off undesirable responses in allergies and autoimmune diseases. Recognition of the immune system as a network helps to explain why these objectives are so difficult and why manipulation of multiple components to achieve desired regulation may be required. But presumably manipulation must be focused on connectivity between receptor for epitope and receptor for receptor to achieve a high degree of specific regulation.

## X. REFERENCES

Andersson, L. C., Binz, H., and Wigzell, H., 1976, Specific unresponsiveness to transplantation antigens induced by auto-immunization with syngeneic, antigen-specific T lymphoblasts, *Nature* **264**:778.

Augustin, A., and Cosenza, H., 1976, Expression of new idiotypes following neonatal idiotypic suppression of a dominant clone, *Eur. J. Immunol.* **6**:497.

Augustin, A., Julius, M., and Cosenza, H., 1977, Changes in the idiotypic pattern of an immune response, following syngeneic haemopoietic reconstitution of lethally irradiated mice, in: *Immune Systems: Genetics and Regulation* (E. Sercarz, L. Herzenberg, and C. Fox, eds.), pp. 195–199, Academic Press, New York.

Beller, D. I., Farr, A. G., and Unanue, E. R., 1978, Regulation of lymphocyte proliferation and differentiation by macrophages, *Fed. Proc. Fed. Am. Soc. Exp. Biol.* **37**:91.

Bellgrave, D., and Wilson, D. B., 1978, Immunological studies of T-cell receptors. I. Specifically induced resistance to GVH disease in rats mediated by host T-cell immunity to autoreactive parental T cells, *J. Exp. Med.* **148**:103.

Benacerraf, B., 1978, A hypothesis to relate the specificity of T lymphocytes and the activity of I region specific Ir genes in macrophages and B lymphocytes, *J. Immunol.* **120**: 1809.

Binz, H., and Wigzell, H., 1976*a*, Antigen-binding, idiotypic receptors from T lymphocytes: An analysis of their biochemistry, genetics, and use as immunogens to produce specific immune tolerance, *Cold Spring Harbor Symp. Quant. Biol.* **61**:275.

Binz, H., and Wigzell, H., 1976*b*, Specific transplantation tolerance induced by autoimmunization against the individual's own, naturally occurring idiotype, antigen-binding receptors, *J. Exp. Med.* **144**: 1438.

Binz, H., and Wigzell, H., 1978, Induction of specific immune unresponsiveness with purified mixed leukocyte culture-activated T lymphoblasts as autoimmunogen. III. Proof for the existence of autoanti-idiotypic killer T cells and transfer of suppression to normal syngeneic recipients by T or B lymphocytes, *J. Exp. Med.* **147**:63.

Binz, H., Wigzell, H., and Bazin, H., 1976, T-cell idiotypes are linked to immunoglobulin heavy chain genes, *Nature* **264**:639.

Bona, C., Lieberman, R., Chien, C. C., Mond, J., House, S., Green, I., and Paul, W. E., 1978, Immune response to Levan. I. Kinetics and ontogeny of anti-Levan and anti-insulin antibody response and of expression of cross-reactive idiotype, *J. Immunol.* **120**:1436.

Braun, D. G., and Krause, R. M., 1968, The individual antigenic specificity of antibodies to streptococcal carbohydrates, *J. Exp. Med.* **128**:969.

Britton, S., and Möller, G., 1968, Regulation of antibody synthesis against *Eschericha coli* endotoxin. I. Suppressive effect of endogenously produced and passively transferred antibodies, *J. Immunol.* **100**:1326.

Cantor, H., and Boyse, E. A., 1976, Regulation of cellular and humoral immune responses by T cell subclasses, *Cold Spring Harbor Symposium on Origin of Lymphocyte Diversity* **41**:23.

Cantor, H., McVay-Boudreau, L., Hugenberger, J., Naidorf, K., Shen, F. W., and Gershon, R. K., 1978, Immunoregulatory circuits among T cell sets. II. Physiologic role of feedback inhibition *in vivo*: Absence in NZB mice, *J. Exp. Med.* **147**:1116.

Cazenave, P. A., 1977, Idiotypic–anti-idiotypic regulation of antibody synthesis in rabbits, *Proc. Natl. Acad. Sci. USA* **74**:5122.

Claflin, J. L., and Davie, J. M., 1975, Clonal nature of the immune response to phosphorylcholine (Pc). V. Cross-idiotypic specificity among heavy chains of murine anti-Pc antibodies and Pc-binding myeloma proteins, *J. Exp. Med.* **141**:1073.

Cohn, M., Notani, G., and Rice, S. A., 1969, Characterization of the anitbody to the C-carbohydrate produced by a transplantable mouse plasmycytoma, *Immunochemistry* **6**:111.

Cooke, A., Hutchings, P. R., and Playfair, J. H. L., 1978, Suppressor T cells in experimental autoimmune haemolytic anaemia, *Nature* **273**:154.

Cosenza, H., 1976, Detection of anti-idiotype reactive cells in the response to phosphorylcholine, *Eur. J. Immunol.* **6**:114.

Cosenza, H., and Köhler, H., 1972, Specific suppression of the antibody response by antibodies to receptors, *Proc. Natl. Acad. Sci. USA* **69**:2701.

Daugharty, H., Hopper, J. E., MacDonald, A. B., and Nisonoff, A., 1969, Quantitative investigations of idiotypic antibodies: Analysis of precipitating antibody populations, *J. Exp. Med.* **130**:1047.

Diamanstein, H., and Naher, H., 1978, Specific immune response enhancing factor in serum of immunized mice, *Nature* **271**:275.

Dorsch, S., and Ross, B., 1977, Recirculating suppressor T cells in transplantation tolerance, *J. Exp. Med.* **145**:1144.

DuClos, T. W., and Kim, B. S., 1977, Suppressor T cells: Presence in mice rendered tolerant by neonatal treatment with anti-receptor antibody or antigen, *J. Immunol.* **119**:1769.

Eardley, D. D., Hugenberger, J., McVay-Boudreau, L., Shen, F. W., Gershon, R. K., and Cantor, H., 1978, Immunoregulatory circuits among T cell sets. I. T-helper cells induce other T-cell sets to exert feedback inhibition, *J. Exp. Med.* **147**:1106.

Eichmann, K., 1975, Idiotype suppression. II. Amplification of a suppressor T cell with anit-idiotypic activity, *Eur. J. Immunol.* **5**:511.

Eichmann, K., 1978, Expression and function of idiotypes of lymphocytes, *Adv. Immunol.* **26**:195.

Eichmann, K., and Rajewsky, K., 1975, Induction of T and B cell immunity by anti-idiotypic antibody, *Eur. J. Immunol.* **5**:661.

Eig, B. M., Ju, S.-T., and Nisonoff, A., 1977, Complete inhibition of the expression of an idiotype by a mechanism of B-cell dominance, *J. Exp. Med.* **146**:1574.

Erb, P., Gasser, M., Strasser, S., Kontiainen, S., and Feldmann, M., 1978, Cellular basis of the humoral immune response in mouse and hamster, *Fed. Proc. Fed. Am. Soc. Exp. Biol.* **37**: 2032.

Evans, R. L., Breard, J. M., Lazarus, H., Schlossman, S. F., and Chess, L., 1977, Detection, isolation, and functional characterization of two human T-cell subclasses bearing unique differentiation antigens, *J. Exp. Med.* **145**:221.

Feldmann, M., Beverley, P. C. L., Dunkley, M., and Kontiainen, S., 1975, Different Ly antigen phenotypes of *in vitro* induced helper and suppressor cells, *Nature* **258**:614.

Feldmann, M., Beverly, P. C. L., Woody, J., and I. F. C. McKenzie, 1977, T–T interactions in the induction of suppressor and helper T cells: Analysis of membrane phenotype of precursor and amplifier cells, *J. Exp. Med.* **145**:793.

Fitch, F. W., 1975, Selective suppression of immune responses, *Progr. Allergy* **19**:195.

Ford, W. L., 1975, Lymphocyte migration and immune responses, *Progr. Allergy* **19**:1.

Forni, L., and Pernis, B., 1975, Interactions between Fc receptors and membrane immunoglobulins on B lymphocytes, in: *Membrane Receptors of Lymphocytes* (M. Seligman, J. L. Preud'homme, and F. M. Kourilinsky, eds.), American Elsevier, New York.

Franzl, R. E., 1962, Immunogenic sub-cellular particles obtained from spleens of antigenic-injected mice, *Nature* **195**:457.

Franzl, R. E., 1972, The primary immune response in mice. III. Retention of sheep red blood cell immunogens by the spleen and liver, *Inf. Immun.* **6**:469.

Frischknecht, H., Binz, H., and Wigzell, H., 1978, Induction of specific transplantation immune reactions using anti-idiotypic antibodies, *J. Exp. Med.* **147**:500.

Gearheart, P. J., Sigal, N. H., and Klinman, N. R., 1977, The monoclonal anti-phosphorylcholine antibody response in several murine strains: genetic implications of a diverse repertoire, *J. Exp. Med.* **147**:876.

Geczy, A. F., 1977, Histocompatibility antigens and genetic control of the immune response in guinea pigs. IV. Specific inhibition of lymphocyte proliferation by auto-anti-idiotypic antibodies, *J. Exp. Med.* **145**:1093.

Gillespie, G. V., and Barth, R. F., 1974, Cyclic variations in cell-mediated immunity to skin allografts detected by the technitium-99 microtoxicity assay, *Cell. Immunol.* **13**:472.

Golub, E. S., 1977, in: *The Cellular Basis of the Immune Response*, pp. 13–247, Sinauer Associates, Sunderland, Mass.

Hart, D. A., Wang, A.-L., Pawlak, L. L., and Nisonoff, A., 1972, Suppression of idiotypic specificities in adult mice by administration of anti-idiotypic antibody, *J. Exp. Med.* **135**:1293.

Harwell, L., Marrak, P., and Kappler, J. W., 1977, Suppressor T-cell inactivation of a helper T-cell factor, *Nature* **265**:57.

Heinemann, S., Bevan, S., Kullberg, R., Lindstrom, J., and Rice, J., 1977, Modulation of acetylcholine receptor by antibody against the receptor, *Proc. Natl. Acad. Sci. USA* **74**:3090.

Hoffmann, G. W., 1975, A theory of regulation and self-nonself dissemination in an immune network, *Eur. J. Immunol.* **5**:638.

Hopkins, W. J., 1975, Anti-thymocyte serum may enhance or suppress the response to the same antigenic determinants, *Immunology* **29**:867.

Hopkins, W. J., 1978. Restoration of suppression function in athymic mice, *Immunology* **34**:309.

Howie, S., and Feldmann, M., 1978, Immune response (Ir) genes expressed at macrophage-B lymphocyte interactions, *Nature* **273**:663.

Jacobs, S., Chang, K.-J., and Cuatrecasas, P., 1978, Antibodies to purified insulin receptor have insulin-like activity, *Science* **200**:1283.

Janeway, C. A., and Paul, W. E., 1976, The specificity of cellular immune responses in guinea pigs. III. The precision of antigen recognition by T lymphocytes, *J. Exp. Med.* **144**:1641.

Janeway, C. A., Sakato, N., and Eisen, H., 1975, Recognition of immunoglobulin idiotypes by thymus-derived lymphocytes (helper T cells/myeloma proteins/lymphocyte receptors/anti-Dnp antibodies), *Proc. Natl. Acad. Sci. USA* **72**:2357.

Jerne, N. K., 1974, Towards a network theory of the immune system, *Ann. Immunol. Inst. Pasteur* **125C**:373.

Jerne, N. K., 1976, The immune system: a web of V-domains, *Harvey Lect.* **70**:93.

Ju, S.-T., Gray, A., and Nisonoff, A., 1977, Frequency of occurrence of idiotypes associated with anti-p-azophenylarsonate antibodies arising in mice immunologically suppressed with respect to a cross-reactive idiotype, *J. Exp. Med.* **145**:540.

Julius, M. H., Augustin, A. A., and Cosenza, H., 1977, Recognition of a naturally occurring idiotype by autologous T cells, *Nature* **265**:251.

Kaplan, D. R., Quintáns, J., and Köhler, H., 1978, Clonal dominance: Loss and restoration in adoptive transfer, *Proc. Natl. Acad. Sci. USA* **75**:1967.

Kaplan, R. B., and Quintáns, J., 1979, Phosphorylcholine-specific helper T cells in mice with an X-linked defect of antibody production to the same hapten, *J. Exp. Med.* **149**:267.

Kapp, J. A., Pierce, C. W., and Benacerraf, B., 1976, Suppressive activity of lymphoid cell extracts from non-responder mice injected with the terpolymer L-glutamic acid 60-L-alanine 30-L-tyrosine 10, in *The Role of Products of the Histocompatibility Gene Complex in Immune Responses* (D. H. Katz and B. Benacerraf, eds.), pp. 569–575, Academic Press, New York.

Kappler, J. W., and Marrack, P., 1978, The role of *H-2*-linked genes in helper T-cell function. I. *In vitro* expression in B cells of immune response genes controlling helper T-cell activity, *J. Exp. Med.* **146**:1748.

Katz, D. H., and Benacerraf, B., 1976, Genetic control of lymphocyte interactions and differentiation, in: *The Role of Products of the Histocompatibility Gene Complex in Immune Responses* (D. H. Katz and B. Benacerraf, eds.), pp. 335–350, Academic Press, New York.

Kelus, A. S., and Gell, P. G., 1968, Immunological analysis of rabbit anti-antibody systems, *J. Exp. Med.* **127**:215.

Kindred, B., and Corley, R. B., 1977, A T cell-replacing factor specific for histocompatibility antigens in mice, *Nature* **268**:531.

Kluskens, L., and Köhler, H., 1974, Regulation of immune response by autogenous antibody against receptor (antibodies against phosphorylcholine/specific suppression), *Proc. Natl. Acad. Sci. USA* **71**:508.

Köhler, H., 1975, The response to phosphorylcholine dissecting an immune response, *Transpl. Rev.* **27**:26.

Köhler, H., 1979, Auto-immune-like reactions during ontogeny and operation of the immune response, in: *Workshop on Genetic Control of Autoimmune Disease* (N. R. Rose and P. E. Bigazzi, eds.), pp. 343–354, Elsevier North-Holland.

Köhler, H., and Smyk, S., 1978, Immune response to phosphorylcholine. VI. Restricted heterogeneity in inhibition of plaque formation by anti-idiotypic antibody, *Cell. Immunol.* **41**:195.

Köhler, H., Kaplan, D. R., and Strayer, D. S., 1974, Clonal depletion in neonatal tolerance, *Science* **186**:643.

Köhler, H., Rowley, D. A., DuClos, T., and Richardson, B., 1977, Complementary idiotypy in the regulation of the immune response, *Fed. Proc. Fed. Am. Soc. Exp. Biol.* **36**:221.

Köhler, H., Richardson, B. C., Rowley, D. A., and Smyk, S., 1978, Immune response to phosphorylcholine. III. Requirement of the Fc portion and equal effectiveness of IgG subclasses in antireceptor antibody-induced suppression, *J. Immunol.* **119**:1979.

Kramer, P. H., and Eichmann, K., 1977, T cell receptor idiotypes are controlled by genes in the heavy chain linkage group and the major histocompatibility complex, *Nature* **270**: 733.

Kunkel, H. G., Mannik, M., and Williams, R. C., 1963, Individual antigenic specificity of isolated antibodies, *Science* **140**:1218.

Landahl, C. A., 1976, Ontogeny of adherent cells. I. Distribution and ontogeny of A cells participating in the response to sheep erythrocytes *in vitro*, *Eur. J. Immunol.* **6**:130.

Lee, K. C., Shiozara, C., Shaw, A., and Diener, E., 1976, Requirement for accessory cells in the antibody response to T cell-independent antigens *in vitro*, *Eur. J. Immunol.* **6**:63.

Leon, M. A., and Young, N. M., 1971, Specificity for phosphorylcholine of six murine myeloma proteins reactive with pneumococcus C polysaccharide and β-lipoprotein, *Biochemistry* **10**:1424.

McKearn, T. J., 1974, Antireceptor antiserum causes specific inhibition of reactivity to rat histocompatibility antigens, *Science* **183**:94.

McKearn, T. J., Hamada, Y., Stuart, F. P., and Fitch, F. W., 1974*a*, Anti-receptor antibody and resistance to graft-versus-host disease, *Nature* **251**:648.

McKearn, T. J., Stuart, F. P., and Fitch, F. W., 1974*b*, Anti-idiotypic antibody in rat transplantation immunity. I. Production of anti-idiotypic antibodies in animals repeatedly immunized with alloantigens, *J. Immunol.* **113**:1876.

McKearn, T. J., Sarmiento, M., Weiss, A., Stuart, F. P., and Fitch, F. W., 1978, Selective suppression of reactivity to rat histocompatibility antigens by hybridoma antibodies, *Curr. Top. Microbiol. Immunol.* **81**:61.

McKearn, T. J., Weiss, A., Stuart, F. P., and Fitch, F. W., 1979, Selective suppression of humoral and cell-mediated immune response to rat alloantigens by monoclonal antibodies produced by hybridoma cell lines, *Transpl. Proc.* **11**:932.

Mackey, M. C., and Glass, L., 1977, Oscillation and chaos in physiological control systems, *Science* **197**:287.

McLachlan, S. M., Rees-Smith, B., Peterson, Y. B., Davies, T. F., and Hall, R., 1977, Thyroid-stimulating autoantibody production *in vitro*, *Nature* **270**:447.

Marchalonis, J. J., Decker, J. M., DeLuka, D., Moseley, J. M., Smith, P., and Warr, G. W.,

1976, Lymphocyte surface immunoglobulins' evolutionary origins and involvement in activation, *Cold Spring Harbor Symp. Quant. Biol.* **61**:261.

Möller, G. (ed.), 1978, *The Role of Macrophages in the Immune Response*, *Immunological Reviews*, Vol. 40, Munksgaard, Copenhagen.

Moretta, L., Mingari, M. C., and Romanzi, C. A., 1978, Loss of Fc receptors for IgG from human T lymphocytes exposed to IgG immune complexes, *Nature* **272**:618.

Mosier, D. E., and Coppleson, L. W., 1968, A three-cell interaction required for the induction of the primary immune response *in vitro*, *Proc. Natl. Acad. Sci. USA* **61**:542.

Munro, A. F., and Taussig, M. J., 1975, Two genes in the major histocompatibility complex control immune response, *Nature* **256**:103.

Oudin, J., and Michel, M., 1963, A new allotype form of rabbit serum γ-globulins apparently associated with antibody function and specificity, *C.R. Acad. Sci.* **257**:805.

Oudin, J., and Michel, M., 1969, Idiotypy of rabbit antibodies. I. Comparison of idiotypy of antibodies against *Salmonella typhi* with that of antibodies against other bacteria in the same rabbits, or of antibodies against *Salmonella typhi* in various rabbits, *J. Exp. Med.* **130**:595.

Owen, F. L., Ju, S.-T., and Nisonoff, A., 1977, Presence on idiotype-specific suppressor T cells of receptors that interact with molecules bearing the idiotype, *J. Exp. Med.* **145**:1559.

Paul, W. E., and Benacerraf, B., 1977, Functional specificity of thymus-dependent lymphocytes, *Science* **195**:1293.

Phillips, J. M., and Waldman, H., 1977, Monogamous T helper cell, *Nature* **268**:641.

Pierce, C. W., and Kapp, J. A., 1978, Functions of macrophages in antibody responses *in vitro*, *Fed. Proc. Fed. Am. Soc. Exp. Biol.* **37**:86.

Pierce, S. K., and Klinman, N. R., 1977, Antibody-specific immunoregulation, *J. Exp. Med.* **146**:509.

Pike, B. L., and Nossal, J. V., 1976, Requirement for persistent extra-cellular antigen in culture of antigen-binding B lymphocytes, *J. Exp. Med.* **144**:568.

Potter, M., and Leon, M. A., 1968, Three IgA myeloma immunoglobulins from the Balb/c mouse: Precipitation with pneumococcal C poly-saccharide, *Science* **162**:369.

Potter, M., and Lieberman, R., 1970, Common individual antigenic determinants in five of eight Balb/c IgA myeloma proteins that bind phosphorylcholine, *J. Exp. Med.* **132**:737.

Richter, P. H., 1975, A network theory of the immune system, *Eur. J. Immunol.* **5**:350.

Rodkey, L. S., 1974, Studies of idiotypic antibodies. Production and characterization of auto-anti-idiotypic antisera, *J. Exp. Med.* **139**:712.

Romball, C. G., and Weigle, W. O., 1973, A cyclical appearance of antibody-producing cells after a single injection of serum protein antigen, *J. Exp. Med.* **138**:1426.

Rosenthal, A. S., Barcinski, M. A., and Blake, J. T., 1977, Determinant selection in a macrophage dependent immune response gene function, *Nature* **267**:156.

Rosenthal, A. S., Barcinski, M. A., and Rosenwasser, L. J., 1978, Function of macrophages in genetic control of immune responsiveness, *Fed. Proc. Fed. Am. Soc. Exp. Biol.* **37**:79.

Rowley, D. A., Gowans, J. L., Atkins, R. C., Ford, W. L., and Smith, M. E., 1972, The specific selection of recirculating lymphocytes by antigen in normal and preimmunized rats, *J. Exp. Med.* **136**:499.

Rowley, D. A., Fitch, F. W., Stuart, F. P., Köhler, H., and Cosenza, H., 1973, Specific suppression of immune responses, *Science* **181**:1133.

Rowley, D. A., Cosenza, H., Leserman, L. D., and Fitch, F. W., 1975, The third cell type in the macrophage population required for the antibody response, in: *Mononuclear Phagocytes in Immunology, Infection and Pathology* (R. VanFurth, ed.), pp. 755–763, Blackwell, Oxford.

Rowley, D. A., Köhler, H., Schreiber, H., Kaye, S. T., and Lorbach, I., 1976, Suppression by autogenous complementary idiotypes: the priority of the first response, *J. Exp. Med.* **144**:946.

Rowley, D. A., Miller, G. W., and Lorbach, I., 1978, Simultaneous complementary idiotypic responses: Absence of reciprocal regulation, *J. Exp. Med.* **148**:148.

Rudikoff, S., and Claflin, J. L., 1976, Expression of equivalent clonotypes in Balb/c and A/J mice after immunization with phosphorylcholine, *J. Exp. Med.* **144**:1294.

Sakato, N., Hall, S. H., and Eisen, H. L., 1977, Restricted heterogeneity of antibodies to idiotypes of isologous immunoglobulins, *Immunochemistry* **14**:621.

Schreiber, H., DuClos, T. W., Leibson, P. J., and Rowley, D. A., 1977, Inhibition of myeloma cell growth by idiotypic-specific suppressor T-lymphocytes and anti-idiotype antibodies, *Proc. Am. Assoc. Cancer Res.* **18**:235.

Schuler, W. E., Weiler, E., and Kolb, H., 1977, Characterization of syngeneic anti-idiotypic antibody against the idiotype of Balb/c myeloma protein J558, *Eur. J. Immunol.* **7**: 649.

Sege, K., and Peterson, P. A., 1978*a*, Use of anti-idiotypic antibodies as cell-surface receptor probes, *Proc. Natl. Acad. Sci. USA* **75**:2443.

Sege, K., and Peterson, P. A., 1978*b*, Anti-idiotypic antibodies against anti-vitamin A transporting protein react with prealbumin, *Nature* **271**:167.

Shreffler, D. C., Meo, T., and David, C. S., 1976, Genetic resolution of the products and functions of I and S region genes of the mouse *H-2* complex, in *The Role of Products of the Histocompatibility Gene Complex in Immune Responses* (D. H. Katz and B. Benacerraf, eds.), pp. 3–29, Academic Press, New York.

Sidman, C. L., and Unanue, E. R., 1976, Control of B-lymphocyte function. I. Inactivation of mitogenesis by interactions with surface immunoglobulin and Fc-receptor molecules, *J. Exp. Med.* **144**:882.

Sigal, N. H., and Klinman, N. R., 1978, The B cell clonotype repertoire, *Adv. Immunol.* **26**:255.

Singer, A., Cowing, C., Hathcock, K. S., Dickler, H. B., and Hodes, R. J., 1978, Cellular and genetic control of antibody response *in vitro*. III. Immune response gene regulation of accessory cell function, *J. Exp. Med.* **147**:1611.

Sprent, J., Miller, J. F. A. P., and Mitchell, G. F., 1971, Antigen-induced selective recruitment of circulating lymphocytes, *Cell. Immunol.* **2**:171.

Stanley, E. F., and Drachman, D. B., 1978, Effect of myasthenic immunoglobulin on acetylcholine receptors of intact mammalian neuromuscular junctions, *Science* **200**:1285.

Strayer, D. S., and Köhler, H., 1976, Immune response to phosphorylcholine. II. Natural "auto"-anti-receptor antibody in neonatal Balb/c mice, *Cell. Immunol.* **25**:294.

Strayer, D. S., Cosenza, H., Lee, W., Rowley, D. A., and Köhler, H., 1974, Neonatal tolerance induced by antibody against antigen-specific receptor, *Science* **186**:640.

Strayer, D. S., Lee, W., Rowley, D. A., and Köhler, H., 1975, Anti-receptor antibody. III. Induction of long-term unresponsiveness in neonatal mice, *J. Immunol.* **114**:728.

Stuart, F. P., McKearn, T. J., and Fitch, F. W., 1974, Immunological enhancement of renal allografts, *Transpl. Proc.* **6**(4):53.

Stuart, F. P., Scollard, D. M., McKearn, T. J., and Fitch, F. W., 1976, Cellular and humoral immunity after allogeneic renal transplantation in the rat. V. Appearance of anti-idiotypic antibody and its relationship to cellular immunity after treatment with donor spleen cells and alloantibody, *Transplantation* **22**:455.

Swerkosz, J. B., Rock, K., Marrack, P., and Kappler, J. W., 1978, The role of *H-2*-linked genes in helper T-cell function. II. Isolation on antigen-pulsed macrophages of two separate populations of $F_1$ helper T cells each specific for antigen and one set of parental H-2 products, *J. Exp. Med.* **147**:554.

Szenberg, A., Marchalonis, J. J., and Warner, N. L., 1977, Direct demonstration of murine thymus-dependent cell surface endogenous immunoglobulin, *Proc. Natl. Acad. Sci. USA* **74**:2113.

Tada, T., Takemori, T., Okumura, K., Nonaka, M., and Tokuhisa, T., 1978, Two distinct types of helper T cells involved in the secondary antibody response: Independent and synergistic effects of $Ia^-$ and $Ia^+$ helper cells, *J. Exp. Med.* **147**:446.

Talal, N. (ed.), 1977, *Autoimmunity*, Academic Press, New York.

Taniguchi, M., Tada, T., and Tokuhisa, T., 1976, Properties of the antigen-specific suppressive T-cell factor in the regulation of antibody response of the mouse. III. Dual gene control of the T-cell-mediated suppression of the antibody response, *J. Exp. Med.* **144**:20.

Trenkner, E., and Riblet, R., 1975, Induction of antiphosphorylcholine antibody formation by anti-idiotypic antibodies, *J. Exp. Med.* **142**:1121.

Unanue, E. R., and Askonsas, B. A., 1968, Persistence of immunogenicity of antigen after uptake by macrophages, *J. Exp. Med.* **127**:915.

Urbain, J., Wikler, M., Franssen, J. D., and Collingnon, C., 1977, Idiotypic regulation of the immune system by the induction of antibodies against anti-idiotypic antibodies, *Proc. Natl. Acad. Sci. USA* **74**:5126.

Waddington, C. H., 1977, *Tools for Thought*, pp. 87–92, Basic Books, New York.

Ward, K., Cantor, H., and Nisonoff, A., 1978, Analysis of the cellular basis of idiotype-specific suppression, *J. Immunol.* **120**:2016.

Warren, R. W., and Davie, J. M., 1977*a*, Antigen mediation of a late-acting suppressor T-cell activity, *J. Exp. Med.* **146**:1627.

Warren, R. W., and Davie, J. M., 1977*b*, Late-acting T cell depression by high avidity IgG antibody secretions in the secondary response, *J. Immunol.* **119**:1806.

Weiss, A., and Fitch, F. W., 1978, Suppression of the plaque-forming cell response by macrophages present in the normal rat spleen, *J. Immunol.* **120**:357.

Woodland, R. T., and Wilson, D. B., 1977, The induction of specific resistance in $F_1$ hybrid rats to local graft-vs.-host reactions: Nature of the eliciting cell, *Eur. J. Immunol.* **7**:136.

Yakulis, V., Bhoopalam, N., and Heller, P., 1972, The production of anti-idiotypic antibodies to Balb/c plasmacytoma globulins in Balb/c mice, *J. Immunol.* **108**:1119.

Chapter 9

# The Biological Function of the Major Histocompatibility Complex: Hypotheses

**Daniel Meruelo**

*Irvington House Institute*
*Department of Pathology*
*New York University Medical Center*
*New York, New York 10016*

**and**

**Michael Edidin**

*Department of Biology*
*The Johns Hopkins University*
*Baltimore, Maryland 21218*

## I. INTRODUCTION

The strongest transplantation barrier and the most polymorphic gene complex in mammals, the major histocompatibility complex (MHC), has attracted enormous scientific interest during the past thirty to forty years. The MHC, which is known under a variety of names, depending on the species (Table I), has been shown to play a key role in a variety of immunological and physiological phenomena (Table II). It has become increasingly apparent that understanding the mechanisms of MHC-associated controls and responses and the sources of MHC polymorphism is of fundamental importance for a number of areas of mammalian biology.

The following review approaches such an understanding by attempting to classify and then unify all of the processes and interactions that appear to be regulated or modified by the MHC. Such classification may allow one to discern the elements common to each of the reported MHC effects. The MHC is involved

**Table I. Nomenclature and Number of Loci Associated with Selected Functions of the Major Histocompatibility Complex of Various Animals**

| | | Presence of loci controlling: | | |
|---|---|---|---|---|
| Animal | MHC designation | Major transplantation antigens | Immune responses | Elements of complement system |
| Chicken | *B* | Yes | Yes | ND[a] |
| Chimpanzee | *ChL-A* | Yes | ND | ND |
| Dog | *DL-A* | Yes | ND | ND |
| Guinea pig | *GPL-A* | Yes | Yes | Yes |
| Human | *HLA* | Yes | Yes | Yes |
| Mouse | *H-2* | Yes | Yes | Yes |
| Pig | *SL-A* | Yes | ND | ND |
| Rabbit | *RL-A* | Yes | ND | ND |
| Rat | *AgB (HI)* | Yes | Yes | ND |
| Rhesus monkey | *RhL-A* | Yes | Yes | Yes |

[a]ND, Not determined.

in six types of biological phenomena: allograft reaction *in vivo*, allograft reaction *in vitro*, genetic control of immune responses, genetic control of complement activity, genetic association with susceptibility and/or resistance to a large array of diseases, and genetic control of traits not currently classified as immunological.

These phenomena have a common thread, which can be discerned to be that products of the MHC, especially serologically detectable molecules, function at the cell surface to modify or moderate the interaction of specific cell receptors with ligands or other cells, thus enhancing or diminishing the degree of ligand-receptor interaction. In this context, the demonstrated extreme polymorphism of MHC (Snell, 1968) may have arisen because no one set of MHC products can be an optimum set of modifiers for all antigens, hormones, and other cell-surface receptors.

Whenever one deals with the enormous polymorphism of MHC, one is tempted to seek an answer for its mode of generation. This review suggests that polymorphism of MHC is generated (at least partly) when viruses, notably oncogenic viruses, integrate into the genome at or near the genes coding for MHC. For example, transcription of portions of viral genome, integrated within the MHC, together with portions of the normal genome coding for MHC antigens, may lead to synthesis and display of altered "mutant" forms of MHC antigens, which in turn would have new modifying effects on cell surfaces. In addition, transcription of integrated genomes in or near the MHC could affect the level of transcription of already existing MHC loci, thus raising the level of their products at the cell surface. If MHC products modify interactions of more specific receptors, such as antigen or hormone receptors, then changes in their

**Table II. Traits Affected by MHC Genotype**

| Trait | Reference |
|---|---|
| 1. Allograft reaction, *in vivo* and *in vitro* | Klein, 1975 |
| 2. Immune responses | Benacerraf and McDevitt, 1972; Shreffler and David, 1975 |
| 3. Levels of complement components | Allen, 1974; Alper, 1976; Zigler *et al.*, 1975; Meo *et al.*, 1975 |
| 4. Susceptibility and/or resistance to numerous diseases | Sasazuki *et al.*, 1977; Meruelo and McDevitt, 1978 |
| 5. Levels of plasma testosterone | Iványi *et al.*, 1972*b* |
| 6. Weights of steroid-sensitive organs | Iványi *et al.*, 1972*a* |
| 7. Mating behavior | Yamazaki *et al.*, 1978; Andrews and Boyse, 1978 |
| 8. Developmental effects | Erickson *et al.*, 1980; Goldman *et al.*, 1977; Boubelik *et al.*, 1975 |
| 9. Binding of viruses and bacteria to MHC antigens | Doherty *et al.*, 1976; Helenius *et al.*, 1978; Klareskog *et al.*, 1978 |
| 10. Levels of cAMP | Meruelo and Edidin, 1975*a*; Lafuse and Edidin, 1978 |
| 11. Binding of hormones to cell membranes | Meruelo and Edidin, 1975*b*; Lafuse and Edidin, 1978 |
| 12. Cell-to-cell adhesion | Lengerová *et al.*, 1977; Bartlett and Edidin, 1978 |

surface concentration, as well as in their primary structure, could lead to new effects of MHC on other cell-surface traits.

## II. ALLOGRAFT REACTION

The MHC is defined because its antigens provoke strong allograft reactions. Allografts (with the exception of the mammalian fetus) do not occur naturally. The transplantation of hearts, kidneys, and skin carried out by surgeons and experimenters is without precedent in nature. What then is the true function of histocompatibility antigens? For many years it appeared that this function would be totally unrelated to the allograft reaction. However, the discovery of the MHC-restriction phenomenon by Zinkernagel and Doherty (1974) and Shearer (1975) has cast some doubts on this argument. The new findings suggest that the individual's own MHC molecules may become alloantigens when associated with certain foreign molecules, especially viral antigens, and as such trigger a response that is indistinguishable from the classic allograft reaction. In this context, the reaction to an allogeneic-tissue transplant may be considered only a special case of the reaction to altered self.

The principal characteristic of the reaction to "altered self," first recognized in the studies of Zinkernagel and Doherty (1974), is that cytotoxic T cells generated when mice are infected with any one of many different viruses *in vivo*, have specificity not only for targets bearing the viral antigens, but also for the *H-2* (Fig. 1) type of the virus-infected cells. Effector cells are unable to lyse target cells bearing H-2 antigens unrelated to the *H-2* type of the cells that were infected by the virus [this observation has been extended to a variety of antigens other than virus (Doherty *et al.*, 1976)]. Similar observations have been made for the human MHC HLA antigens (McMichael *et al.*, 1977).

Two theories have been postulated (Doherty *et al.*, 1976) to explain the above observation: "altered self" and "dual recognition." The altered-self theory postulates that H-2 molecules associate with foreign molecules, such as virus, becoming thereby alloantigens, and as such trigger a response that is indistinguishable from the classic allograft reaction. Although there are some data in support of this concept (Freedman *et al.*, 1978), a physical bond between H-2 and virus molecules has not yet been shown by any biochemical study. Therefore, any postulated associations can, at the moment, only be taken to arise through noncovalent bonds.

"Dual recognition" mechanisms all posit a function for H-2D and H-2K molecules in bringing responding cells and targets into proximity. In its simplest form this indicates that H-2 antigens function as adhesive sites in cell interactions. A modified form of the mechanism would have H-2 antigens in proximity to and affecting the strength of adhesion at specific cellular sites. Both mechanisms have H-2 molecules serving as modifiers or modulators of cell–cell interactions, rather than serving as specific receptors in these interactions.

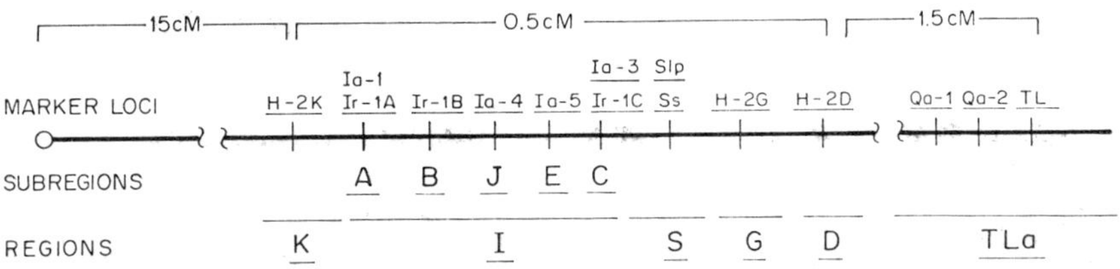


Figure 1. Partial genetic fine structure of mouse chromosome 17 (linkage group IX) showing *H-2-TLa* gene complex. This complex is divided into 6 main regions: *K*, *I*, *S*, *G*, *D*, and *TLa*. These regions are denoted by marker loci *H-2K*, *Ir-1*, *Ss*(*Slp*), *H-2G*, *H-2D*, and *TL*. The boundaries of each region are defined by intra *H-2* recombinations. The *I* region has been subdivided into five subregions by recombination: *A*, *B*, *J*, *E*, and *C*, defined by marker loci *Ir-1A*, *Ia-1*, *Ir-1B*, *Ia-4*, *Ia-5*, and *Ir-1C Ia-3* respectively. According to definitions proposed by Klein *et al.* (1974), the *K* end of the complex is the segment to the left of *Ss*. The *D* end is the segment to the right of *Ss*. Alleles are alternate genes at defined loci and "haplotype" designates the specific combination of all alleles at all loci within the complex characterizing a given mouse strain. Allele and haplotype designations are noted in lowercase letters, whereas regions, subregions, and marker loci are written with capital letters. The *TLa* region is subdivided by marker loci *Qa-1* (Stanton and Boyse, 1975), *Qa-2* (Flaherty, 1976), and *TL* (Boyse *et al.*, 1964).

## III. GENETIC CONTROL OF IMMUNE RESPONSES

MHC products are clearly stimulators of the immune system. After all, it is because of their antigenecity that they are the strongest barrier to tissue transplantation (Shreffler and David, 1975). Work on the genetic control of the immune response and on the cellular interactions involved in immunological responses strongly argues that MHC products are also involved in the generation of immunological specificity. Thus it is postulated that MHC genes and their products are part of or are associated with molecules that specifically recognize antigens and/or serve as their receptors (Benacerraf and McDevitt, 1972).

The evidence that the *H-2* complex may code for a class of molecules with a recognitive function is indirect and circumstantial. It is based mainly on two observations. First, a set of loci controlling the immune response to synthetic polypeptides, proteins, and alloantigens (the *Ir* loci) is located within the *H-2* complex (Benacerraf and McDevitt, 1972). The type of control exerted by these loci appears to be characterized by a high degree of antigen specificity. This specificity has been explained by postulating that *Ir*-gene products function as antigen receptors (Benacerraf and McDevitt, 1972). Second, the cooperation between the two classes of immunocytes (whether they be T lymphocytes, B lymphocytes, or macrophages) in generating an immune response is often found to be restricted by MHC products (Benacerraf and Katz, 1975). The specificity of this interaction can thus also be attributed, as in the case of *Ir* loci, to a recognitive capability of H-2 products, though here the products would function to recognize a second cell type rather than the antigen presented to the cell population.

*Ir*-locus control of responses to synthetic polypeptides presents two features that bear on the hypotheses to be developed in this paper. First, control of the secondary responses to most antigens rarely results in all-or-nothing responses. Instead, animals make high or low responses to the secondary antigenic challenge (Benacerraf and McDevitt, 1972). Second, a poor or low responder for one synthetic polypeptide antigen may be a good or high responder for a second antigen, while the good responder for the first antigen responds poorly to the second (Benacerraf and McDevitt, 1972). Thus, *Ir* control of immune responses appears to be exerted in modulating responses rather than in repression or induction of genes at the DNA level.

The studies indicating that a set of loci controlling the immune response to synthetic polypeptides, proteins, and alloantigens (*Ir* loci) is located within the *H-2* complex (McDevitt *et al.*, 1972) led to the postulate that the main function of these genes was to code for a receptor on the surface of T cells (Benacerraf and McDevitt, 1972). Since the original exposition of this hypothesis, much effort has been invested in the identification and isolation of the *H-2*-controlled T-cell receptor. At the biochemical level the T-cell receptor has remained very elusive. However, functional analysis of T lymphocytes has undoubtedly established the restricted range of specificity of these cells, particularly when compared with B cells. In several of these studies, Zinkernagel and Doherty (1974) have provided clear evidence of the involvement of MHC gene products in determining the specificity of T lymphocytes.

Additional studies have shown that the functional T-cell receptor may be a rather complicated structure composed of Ig idiotypes related to the variable Ig heavy chains (V/H) (Binz *et al.*, 1974*a,b*; Binz and Wigzell, 1975*a,b*; Eichmann and Rajewsky, 1975), MHC products (Doherty *et al.*, 1976), and, perhaps, interaction molecules (Benacerraf and Katz, 1975). Furthermore, it appears that the antigenic site is made up of several subsites of low affinity each (Janeway, 1976). Thus, the antigen determinant must be bound to the receptor site at several contiguous points for the cell to be activated (Janeway, 1976).

Because of the importance of MHC antigens in T-cell recognition, it would not be unreasonable to propose a model for T-cell specificity that assumes that T-cell activation is restricted by MHC products not because the latter code for T-cell receptors of different specificity or avidity, but because the latter simply modify receptor–ligand interaction at the cell surface. A simple version of this model would propose that differences in T-dependent immune responses, such as immune responses to synthetic polypeptides, do not occur because a particular *H-2* haplotype codes for a given receptor structure while another *H-2* haplotype does not. Rather, the MHC products of some haplotypes, but not others, may interact sterically or by charge–charge forces with one or more subsites of the antigen receptor (which would be coded for by genes outside the MHC), affecting the receptor's ability to bind, accept, or present antigen.

Cellular cooperation requiring I-region identity (Benacerraf and Katz, 1975) also seems to indicate a modifying function for H-2 products, or at least a function ancillary to antigen recognition. MHC restriction of cell cooperation in the immune response could be explained by mechanisms similar to those posited to act in the "dual recognition" hypothesis of MHC restriction of killer-cell–target-cell interactions, though the MHC products involved need not be the same in both instances. Such a mechanism would link interactions of immunocytes with more general cell physiology, since it appears that MHC products affect the homing *in vivo* and the adhesion *in vitro* of other cell types, including bone-marrow cells and fibroblasts (see Section VI).

## IV. GENETIC CONTROL OF COMPLEMENT LEVELS

It has been known for some time (Shreffler and David, 1972) that a locus controlling levels of a serum protein (Ss) and its allovariant Slp (Passmore and Shreffler, 1970) maps within the mouse MHC, the *H-2* complex. This fact has generally been considered an evolutionary accident, unrelated to the function of the MHC. However, it has been shown recently that the *S* region is involved in the regulation of complement activity and that Ss may be a polypeptide chain of C4 (Meo *et al.*, 1975). In addition, recent studies in man (Allen, 1974; Alper, 1976) and rhesus monkey (Zigler *et al.*, 1975) suggest that genes regulating complement activity are also associated with MHCs of these species. This may be because, as has been suggested (Klein, 1977), there has evolved a superimmunological defense system of which the MHC is only a part. Klein (1977) postulates that this supersystem evolved in mouse from an archetypal MHC gene that gave rise to the *H-2*, *T/t* and *Tla* complex, *Mls*, *Ig-L-*, and *Ig-H* chain gene complexes. If Klein is correct, the MHC–complement association found in the three species may further increase the defensive value of the MHC and immunoglobulin systems.

On the other hand, some evidence indicates that *S*-region products may be displayed as surface-membrane molecules of fibroblasts (Saunders and Edidin, 1974), and recent work (D. McClellan and M. Edidin, unpublished) indicates that cells of Ss-low and Slp animals contain appreciable levels of these proteins in their cytoplasm. Thus, the *S*-region control of complement levels is linked in two ways to the cell surface. It may be, then, that the *S* region (and its two homologues in other species) regulates the transfer of newly synthesized complement components across the plasma membrane for export. The "low" forms of genes in this region could either specify complement components of altered structure, which are not readily secreted, or specify altered accessory and perhaps MHC antigens required for proper membrane passage of the complement components. A precedent for the latter mechanism—though for stable membrane insertion rather than membrane passage of molecules—is found in the requirement for $\beta_2$ microglobulin in the display of MHC antigens (Poulik *et al.*, 1974). For example, human cells lacking a functional $\beta_2$ gene are phenotypically HLA-negative. The HLA phenotype can be rescued when such cells are fused with HLA-negative $\beta_2$-positive cells (Goodfellow *et al.*, 1975). MHC-linked regulation of complement levels could similarly be due to association of MHC products with other molecules in the cell-surface membrane.

## V. MHC ASSOCIATIONS WITH SUSCEPTIBILITY AND RESISTANCE TO DISEASE

Association between malignant disease and the *H-2* complex was first noted by Gorer (1956) and Gross (1970), who observed that all the strains showing a high incidence of spontaneous or induced leukemia had the same *H-2* haplotype ($H\text{-}2^k$). The involvement of the *H-2* complex in the Gross-virus-induced leukemogenesis was demonstrated experimentally by Lilly and his co-workers (1964). Since then *H-2* association with susceptibility or resistance to virally induced leukemias has been extensively demonstrated (Meruelo and McDevitt, 1978).

In humans, association between *HLA* and disease was first reported by Amiel

(1967). This association involved Hodgkin's disease and an *HLA-B*-locus antigen then designated 4C. Over the next ten years, a progressively larger number of diseases have been associated with HLA-A,-B,-C, or-D antigens. The most striking of these is an association between antigen B27 and ankylosing spondylitis, an association so strong that it has been utilized as an aid to clinical diagnosis (Sasazuki *et al.*, 1977). Other strong associations are also found with arthritic, perhaps autoimmune disease.

The mechanisms of action of MHC-linked loci in disease associations are not clear. Some investigators have suggested that *H-2*-linked resistance to virus-induced leukemogenesis may result from genetically controlled variation in immune responses to virus-induced antigens. This hypothesis is based on several observations. The first of these is that *Rgv-1*, a gene conferring resistance to Gross-virus-induced tumorigenesis, maps near or within the *I*-region of the *H-2* complex to which most immune-response genes have been mapped (Lilly, 1970). Furthermore, the *H-2* gene(s) have been found to influence a late event in the Friend-virus-induced disease (Lilly, 1968). No effect of *H-2*-linked genes has been detected on the initial infection by Friend virus (FV), while recovery from the virus-induced splenomegaly is significantly affected by MHC genotype. These findings have suggested that MHC control occurred at a point after malignancy had ensued, and a likely candidate for a defense mechanism operating at such an advance stage of the disease is an immunological one (McDevitt and Bodmer, 1972; Lilly and Pincus, 1973).

Support for this hypothesis was provided by studies of Aoki *et al.* (1966) demonstrating that serum levels of anti-Gross-virus antibodies were higher in mice homozygous or heterozygous for the resistant *H-2* haplotype that in animals homozygous for the susceptible *H-2* type. Similar findings were provided by Sato *et al.* (1973) in studies of resistance to certain leukemias derived from BALB/c mice. Furthermore, Blank *et al.* (1976) have found that animals of the *H-2*-resistant haplotype can generate a cell-mediated cytotoxic (CMC) response to FV-induced tissue-culture-adapted tumor cells, whereas mice of the susceptible *H-2* type cannot. More recently, direct evidence has been obtained for the involvement of *Ir*-type mechanisms in control of the spontaneous AKR leukemia (Meruelo *et al.*, 1980*b*).

Difficulties with the hypothesis that *Ir*-type mechanisms alone are involved in resistance to all virus-induced neoplasias arise from mapping studies. Genes conferring resistance to FV radiation-induced leukemia virus (RadLV) and mammary-tumor virus map in the *H-2D* region of the complex (Meruelo and McDevitt, 1978). However, almost all *Ir* genes mapped to date are found to the left of *H-2D*, in the *I* region of the complex. The situation is, in fact, analogous to *HLA*-disease associations in which some diseases are associated with *HLA-D* ("*I* region") and others with *HLA-A* ("*D* region") and *HLA-B* ("*K* region") (Sasazuki *et al.*, 1977).

It has, therefore, become important to determine the mechanism(s) by which *H-2D*-linked genes confer resistance to MuLV-induced neoplasias. Some data are currently available to approach such an understanding. In mice infected with RadLV, as was previously observed for Friend virus (Lilly, 1968), *H-2D*-linked genetic control apparently does not influence initial virus replication, but instead alters virus proliferation and spread (Meruelo *et al.*, 1978). It has been observed that immediately after RadLV inoculation dramatic changes in the quantitative expression of H-2 antigens can be detected on the cell surface of the great majority of thymocytes (Meruelo *et al.*, 1978). Increases in expression of H-2D antigens occur in resistant but not susceptible mice, suggesting that the elevated antigen levels might be involved in resistance to the disease. This suggestion finds added support in the discovery that elevated H-2-antigen expression in resistant virus-infected mice is necessary to trigger a strong CML response capable of eliminating virus-infected cells (Meruelo, 1979).

*In vitro* experiments with human peripheral T cells immunized to influenza virus (McMichael *et al.*, 1978) indicate that even when target lymphocytes share HLA antigens with sensitizing cells and with their attacker cells—that is, in conditions where good lysis is expected (McMichael and Askonas, 1978)—lysis cannot always be achieved. One specificity in particular, HLA-A2, is always associated with poor or no lysis of targets matched with their attackers for this antigen (McMichael, 1978).

The results on H-2 antigens and resistance to RadLV tumorigenesis indicate that H-2 antigens may be quantitatively important in enhancing the attack of T cells on virus-infected targets. The results with human lymphocytes reinforce this suggestion, though here the T-cell killing is affected by the particular specificity displayed on killer and target cells rather than by the quantity of HLA. If such mechanisms are at work, they point again to a function for products of MHC in modifying reactions at the cell surface. Such a modifying function for MHC determinants could also be invoked to explain the association of particular antigens with human diseases, at least those of immune origin and perhaps others caused by infectious agents.

## VI. GENETIC CONTROL OF TRAITS NOT CURRENTLY CLASSIFIED AS IMMUNOLOGICAL

MHC haplotypes have been associated with a number of traits, in whole animals and in single cells, that appear not to be immunological in nature. These traits may be divided into six groups: plasma testosterone and weights of steroid-sensitive organs (seminal vesicle, testes, thymus, and lymph nodes); mating behavior; developmental effects; binding of viruses and bacteria to MHC antigens;

cell levels of cyclic AMP (cAMP) and binding of hormones to cell membranes; and cell-to-cell adhesions. In all but two of these it appears that MHC affects interactions at the cell surface.

Androgen-dependent organs of the mouse vary in weight with the *H-2* haplotype of the strains examined (Iványi *et al.*, 1972; Gregorova *et al.*, 1973, 1975, 1977). Higher levels of plasma testosterone and testosterone-binding globulin are associated with the haplotype that determines the weights of lower organs (Iványi *et al.*, 1972*a*,*b*). When castrated males of high- and low-weight strains were compared they were also found to differ in their vesicular-gland responses to limited doses of testosterone (Micková and Iványi, 1975). An attempt was made to analyze the trait in fully segregating backcrosses, but it appears that loci outside the MHC also affect the quantitative traits examined. The MHC effect could be on the stimulation of Leydig cells, the producers of testosterone, by polypeptide hormones whose receptors lie at the cell surface, but the data on castrates and on the reciprocal relation between plasma-testosterone levels and organ weights indicate that the target cells and organs are also affected. Since the manner in which steroids permeate the cell surface is not clear, we cannot readily construct a mechanism for MHC effects on this permeation. If the MHC effects are exerted directly on cytosol receptors for steroids, then a rethinking of the functional unity of MHC products will be required. On the other hand, there is a suggestion that steroid action on the plasma membrane may be required in some instances (Godeau *et al.*, 1978).

Our remarks on mechanisms must also apply to the complicated patterns of mating preference shown by inbred MHC-congenic mice when offered matings with mice of various MHC haplotypes (Yamazaki *et al.*, 1978; Andrews and Boyse, 1978). One might trace the MHC effect to cell-surface olfactory receptors, but the phenomenon is too complex to allow, at present, mechanistic analysis at the molecular level.

Two developmental effects have been mapped to the mouse MHC. The induction of cleft palate in progeny of pregnant females given cortisone is a function of *H-2* type of the fetuses. Like the other MHC effects described, the effect is not absolute; animals of all haplotypes are susceptible and other loci affect the frequency of cleft palate as well (Biddle and Fraser, 1977). The MHC effect here may be indirect, via an influence of *H-2* on levels of cAMP in the palate. Erickson and co-workers (1980) feel that the *H-2*, rather than directly affecting the glucorticoid receptors, as had been suggested (Goldman *et al.*, 1977) affects the cAMP levels, which in turn, in some way affect the palate's response to glucorticoids.

The second developmentally associated MHC effect is that of *H-2* (together with two other loci) on expression of H-2 antigens in erythrocytes of neonatal mice (Boubelik *et al.*, 1975). Animals of some *H-2* haplotypes produce erythrocytes that at birth are agglutinable by anti-H-2 antibodies, whereas animals of other *H-2* haplotypes produce erythrocytes that are not agglutinable until three days after birth. The molecular basis for this MHC-linked trait has been barely explored (Boubelik and Lengerová, 1977), but it does appear that the majority of the erythrocytes in newborn mice of both haplotypes are fully differentiated; there are low and constant proportions of reticulocytes in animals of both haplotypes (T. Spack and M. Edidin, unpublished), and the change in agglutinability does not appear to be due to new synthesis of H-2, or to major replacement of one cell population by another. The *H-2* effect here could be similar to the effect postulated for complement components, an effect on correct insertion of molecules in a membrane. Late-maturing cells would then carry forms of H-2 that require long times to orient correctly in the erythrocyte surface. Alternatively, hormonal or other stimulation of newborn erythrocytes might have differential effects on cells bearing different sets of H-2 antigens. Cell agglutinability would then be a function not of the amount of antigen displayed but of the efficacy of hormones in causing alterations in cell shape or rigidity allowing agglutination.

Recently it has been reported that Semliki Forest virus spike proteins interact specifically with mouse and human MHC antigens (Helenius *et al.*, 1978). The virus seems to utilize the antigens as receptors. Perhaps this utilization represents evolutionary adaptation by the virus, not to an arbitrary surface glycoprotein but rather to molecules that already function as surface receptors. A similar interpretation might be put on the finding that some, but not all, bacteria examined bind HLA-containing liposomes (Klareskog, 1978), though they do not bind pure phospholipid liposomes.

Liver cyclic-AMP levels clearly are a function of *H-2* haplotype in mouse (Meruelo and Edidin, 1975*a*). The greatest differences are only about two-fold, but these differences segregate in crosses between cAMP high and low strains, both when congenic strains are crossed and when fully segregating crosses are made (W. Lafuse, D. Meruelo, and M. Edidin, in preparation). Preliminary work on this indicates that the differences in cAMP are a function of stimulation of adenylate cyclase by peptide hormones, and that fluoride stimulation and basal levels of enzyme activity did not vary with *H-2* haplotype. Cyclic nucleotide phosphodiesterase also did not differ in extracts made from cAMP-high and -low livers (Meruelo, 1974; Meruelo and Edidin, 1975*b*). These findings have been borne out by a direct demonstration that the binding of both glucagon and insulin to liver membranes varies with the *H-2* haplotype of the membrane donors. Animals whose livers have higher levels of cAMP have higher-affinity binding sites for both hormones than those with lower cAMP content in liver (Lafuse, 1978; Lafuse and Edidin, 1978). Binding of both hormones is inhibited by anti-*H-2* antisera. It appears then that there is a direct effect of *H-2* on binding of glucagon, a major determinant of liver cyclic AMP levels, and also an effect, of similar magnitude, on binding of insulin, a hormone whose effects are not apparently mediated by cAMP. These data again suggest that either MHC loci code for hormone receptors, or that MHC products, initially recognized as antigens, interact with specific hormone receptors to modify their interaction with hormones. cAMP levels of spleen and kidney have also been examined and in these tissues too there is a hierarchy of cAMP levels associated with *H-2* haplotypes, though this hierarchy is not the same as in liver (Lafuse, 1978). This is consistent with differences between the tissues in the hormones whose action given rise to steady-state levels of cAMP. Erickson and his colleagues have also examined cAMP levels in mouse sperm and in the tongues and palates of 15-day-old mouse embryos. While no differences associated with *H-2* could be found for sperm (Erickson *et al.*, 1979), there were *H-2*-associated differences found between palatal shelves and tongues (Erickson *et al.*, 1980). The data overall are consistent with a mechanism of MHC-product action similar to that found in liver—an influence on the binding of specific hormones to the cell surface. This influence might even take the form of a competitive binding of hormone, if MHC antigens structurally mimic hormone receptors, as suggested by Svejgard and Ryder (1976).

The earliest indication that MHC products might function in cell-to-cell adhesion came from the studies cited in Section III, on the requirements for *H-2* matching in cell-to-cell cooperation in the immune response. In this case, interacting cells could not be isolated and the association of these cells was inferred from measurements of the ensuing immune responses. More direct measurements of *H-2* effects on cell association, measured either as cell homing *in vivo* or cell adhesion *in vitro*, generally support a function for *H-2* in mediating or modifying cell-to-cell adhesion. Lengerová and colleagues (1977) showed that *H-2*-matched erythropoietic cells function better in irradiated hosts than do cells mismatched at *H-2*. They also found in an *in vitro* adhesion assay (the assay measured the collection of single cells on a monolayer of peritoneal or bone-marrow-derived cells) that *H-2* matching of cells enhanced adhesion (Zelený *et al.*, 1978). McClay and Gooding (1978), on the other hand, could not find an *H-2* effect on adhesion of single fetal-brain or liver cells to aggregates matched for cell type but of different *H-2* types, though H-2 antigens were expressed on these cells. Their failure to find an *H-2* effect may be due to differences in the assay used, or to the fact that they did not compare *H-2* effects in congenic strains, but instead examined cells of strain C3H and C57BL/10, which differ at many other loci. There is some evidence that loci outside the MHC may abrogate the effects of *H-2* both on cAMP levels and on cell adhesion (see below). This experiment would be worth repeating with fetal cells from congenic animals.

Bartlett and Edidin (1978) have shown that there are *H-2*-associated differences in the rate of collection of labeled single cells by fibroblast monolayers from *H-2*-congenic strains. An *H-2* effect could also be shown in fully segregating backcross fetuses between "high-" and "low-"collection-rate strains, and anti-*H-2* antisera—but not other antisera binding to the cells—interfered with single-cell collection. The *H-2* hierarchy established for fetal-derived fibroblasts was not the same as that derived for adult-derived fibroblasts. Also, non-MHC loci in one group of congenic strains, on the C57BL/10 background, abolished the *H-2* effect unless cells were first treated with neuraminidase or were suspended in serum containing medium during the assay. In these experiments, as in the experiments on hormone binding, there are clear effects of MHC apparently by modifying the degree or strength of cell-to-cell contacts during adhesion. Also, in parallel with the work on cAMP, *H-2* effects are a function of the tissues or cells examined and the conditions under which the assay is performed. Overall, the results are congruent with those for cell-to-cell cooperation in immune responses and with some aspects of MHC restriction of killer-cell–target-cell interactions. Snell (1980) has recently discussed aspects of MHC products' function in cell-to-cell association in immune responses and immunocyte interactions.

## VII. FURTHER ANALYSES OF THE IMPORTANCE OF MHC ANTIGENS AND GENES

From what has been said thus far, it is possible to begin to see an approach to unifying the function of MHC gene products and to understanding the great polymorphism of the complex in terms of its adaptive value. However, there is a second key question: How is MHC polymorphism generated? In answer to this question several findings will first be described and then integrated into a model for generation of polymorphism.

### A. Frequency of *H* Mutations

The first relevant observation concerns the extraordinary mutation rate associated with genes of the mouse MHC. The most unstable *H-2* allele is *H-2K*$^b$, with a mutation rate of $5.5 \times 10^{-4}$ generation (Melvold and Kohn, 1974). This rate exceeds that reported for any other mammalian locus (Klein, 1975).

This extraordinary mutation rate could be accounted for by several simple explanations. A trivial explanation would be that the *H-2K*$^b$ is not a single locus but a cluster of many loci with similar functions. However, the eight known mutants of this allele fail to complement each other (Melvold and Kohn, 1974), suggesting that the mutations have all occurred at the same locus. Another explanation for the high rate is that the mutations are regulatory rather than structural. The problem with this interpretation is that all eight mutations are of the loss-and-gain type, and it is difficult to understand how a regulatory mutation can effect this type of antigenic change.

Of all *H* mutations thus far detected, 98% are of the gain (or loss-and-gain) type and 2% are of the loss type (Klein, 1975). Bailey (1966) has suggested that the preponderance of the gain (or loss-and-gain) type mutations either is an artifact of the method used for detection of *H* mutations or, alternatively, *H* mutations might actually result from the incorporation of viral genomes into germinal cells. According to Bailey, such incorporation would be often accompanied by the appearance of new transplantation antigens in the cell membrane of the somatic cells descending from the "infected" germinal cells. In support of this hypothesis, Bailey (1966) cites his observation, confirmed by others (Kohn and Melvold, 1974), that the spontaneous mutation rate is significantly influenced by environmental conditions; for example, maintenance of mice in "less isolated" environments (i.e., mice exposed to viral infections). This observation is important only because the variation in spontaneous mutation rate as a result of environmental conditions is a peculiarity of the *H* system; the mutation rates at non-*H* (e.g., coat-color) loci are relatively stable under different environmental conditions (Searle, 1972, 1974).

Three additional pieces of circumstantial data suggest that the notion of virus integration in chromosome 17 may have validity. Ever since thymus-leukemia antigens (TLa) were first described, suggestions have been made about their possible origin in a viral genome integrated in chromosome 17. This was generally supported by the fact that $TL^-$ to $TL^+$ phenotypic conversion was always diagnostic of malignancy (Stockert *et al.*, 1971). Recently this notion has come into question (Stockert and Old, 1977), principally because the molecular weight of the antigens on SDS gels in 45,000 rather than the molecular weight expected for any known viral glycoprotein. However, very recently Elder *et al.* (1978) have shown that the *env* product of MuLV, although 70,000 in molecular weight, is derived by glycosylation from a 45,000-molecular-weight protein. Further support for TLa as virally-specified antigen has been provided by Gazdar *et al.* (1977) and Ruddle *et al.* (1978) through work on somatic-cell hybrids. Their studies indicate that all hybrid clones capable of replicating ecotropic MuLV virus retain chromosomes 5, 15, and 17, suggesting that these chromosomes may contain genes important in virus replication, or may possibly contain sites necessary for integration. Chromosome 17 is the site of the mouse MHC including TLa.

Heron *et al.* (1978) have suggested that increased H-2D-antigen expression after RadLV may result from the production and effect of interferon. However, this possibility has been previously tested and ruled out (Meruelo and McDevitt, 1978; Meruelo *et al.*, 1980*a*). In view of these findings, the above-discussed suggestion on virus–genome integration in chromosome 17 will be explored further.

The integration hypothesis would explain the observation that RadLV causes dramatic and very prolonged (lasting at least nine weeks after virus infection) increases in H-2D synthesis immediately after virus injection (Meruelo *et al.*, 1978). According to this hypothesis, viruses can integrate near *H-2D* or *H-2K*, and

RadLV preferentially integrates near *H-2D*, increased *H-2* expression then would result because the cellular transcription apparatus, under virus control, would preferentially transcribe virus-genome sequences and adjacent *H-2D* sequences. A hypothesis postulating linked transcription of virus and *H-2D* sequences is in accord with other published data. Thus Freedman *et al.* (1978) have recently shown an association of *H-2D* with long-term production and release *in vitro* of both infectious virus and viral proteins.

Additional evidence consistent with this integration hypothesis comes from the following observations. First, ultraviolet inactivation (5020 $ergs/mm^2$) of virus—which lowers infectivity to less than 0.01% without affecting core or envelope viral proteins (Declève *et al.*, 1977)—is sufficient to prevent RadLV-induced increased synthesis and expression of H-2 antigens (D. Meruelo and J. Kramer, unpublished). Ultraviolet-damaged RNA may not be transcribed into DNA and may be unable to integrate.

Second, most radiation-induced C57BL/Ka thymic lymphomas do not express viral antigens detectable by immunofluorescence or radioimmune-competition assay (Ihle *et al.*, 1976*a*,*b*), despite the fact that RadLV, a virus with thymotropic-leukemogenic properties (Kaplan, 1967), can usually be recovered from such tumors by passage of cell-free extracts *in vivo* (Lieberman and Kaplan, 1959). Declève *et al.* (1977) have suggested that this paradox can be resolved by the hypothesis that RadLV is initially activated by X irradiation in a replication-defective form (RadLV-O), in which only the oncogenic segment (*lmf*) of the RadLV genome is expressed (and this would go undetected by immunofluorescence of radioimmune-competition assay, which use antibodies directed at non-*lmf*-derived antigens) and that RadLV acquires infectivity *in vivo* secondarily, possibly by a recombination mechanism (Elder *et al.*, 1978). Studies by Chazan and Haran-Ghera (1976) have shown that X irradiation treatment sufficient to induce thymic lymphomas increases the number of high *H-2*-bearing cells in the thymus. This set of observations may be taken to indicate that the activation of the *lmf* is sufficient to observe increased *H-2* expression in the thymus.

This postulate requires that the oncogenic segment of RadLV interact with *H-2D* gene(s) to increase transcription and translation. The question is then: By what mechanism? If the *lmf* for RadLV bears some close nucleotide resemblance to the gene(s) coding for H-2.4 (the private specificity of $H\text{-}2D^d$), this close structural resemblance over a long stretch of nucleotides would facilitate integration of the virus *lmf* in chromosome 17. Once integrated, the *lmf* can be transcribed either with *H-2D* genes or with other viral genes (*env*, *pro*, and *gag*). If *lmf* is transcribed simultaneously with *H-2D* genes, increased H-2D-antigen expression will be observed (because of the preferential transcription and translation of virus-associated genes, the rate of synthesis of the associated *H-2D* genes should be faster). On the other hand, if the viral genes are transcribed simultaneously with *lmf*, *H-2D* transcription or synthesis may be shut off to permit production of fully infectious virus particles. In this connection, it has been shown that H-2-antigen synthesis is shut off when high quantities of complete infectious virus are being produced (Meruelo, 1979).

One important assumption of this hypothesis is that the *lmf* gene for RadLV bears resemblance to the private specificities of *H-2D*$^d$ and not *H-2D*$^s$ or *H-2D*$^q$. The reason for this is that RadLV infection leads to increased *H-2D*$^d$ expression but not to increased expression of *H-2D*$^s$ and *H-2D*$^q$. Furthermore, preliminary observations suggest that the private, not public, specificities determine *H-2D*-increased expression (D. Meruelo, unpublished). The private specificities of *H-2D* can be coded for only by a small hypervariable segment of the molecule, since too much homology exists between products of distinct *H-2D* alleles (Nathenson and Cullen, 1974; Silver and Hood, 1976). Therefore, another logical corollary of this hypothesis is that the *lmf* is represented by a short nucleotide sequence. This concept is not farfetched in view of the fact that it has been suggested that *lmf* may be associated with a small protein of the *env* gene (Chien *et al.*, 1978). Even a small region of genetic material can play a key role in determining genetic rearrangements. For example, it has recently been shown (Brack *et al.*, 1978) that a DNA segment known as the J region, coding for only 13 or so amino acids, may play a determining role in the generation of antibody diversity.

If integration of viruses can occur within a sequence coding for H-2D or H-2K antigens, then such antigens would appear as mutant forms. Such integration might also account for killer-cell MHC restriction, at least when the killers are directed against virus-infected cells. H-2 molecules with portions coded for by viral genomes would be altered structurally and antigenically. Of course, this cannot be the only way in which viral and other antigens associate with *H-2*, since attacks on hapten–cell conjugates are *H-2*-restricted (Shearer, 1975), and the binding to bacteria is restricted by MHC antigens even when these are inserted into artificial membranes not by synthesis but by fusion (Klareskog *et al.*, 1978). Some of the MHC-restriction experiments have also been carried out with viruses that do not integrate (Doherty *et al.*, 1976).

On the other hand, the hypothesis of integration of viral genomes' causing antigenic changes in H-2 molecules would explain some reports of inappropriate H-2 and Ia-like antigenic specificities of foreign haplotypes on tumor cells (Garrido *et al.*, 1976*a,b*), since inappropriate public and private specificities may appear because of altered transcription following virus integration. The evolutionary implications of such a mechanism in terms of its generation of diversity is discussed below.

### B. Adaptive Value of *H-2* Polymorphism

Until now we have simply stated that MHC genes are characterized by a high degree of polymorphism. This statement has been made without taking time to set forth current genetic concepts of polymorphism.

Genetic polymorphism is defined as the occurrence together, in the same habitat, of two or more discontinuous forms or phases of an allele in such proportions that the rarest one cannot be maintained merely by recurrent mutations (Snell, 1968). It was originally thought that the proportion of polymorphic genes in a population was extremely low, and that all polymorphisms resulted from a selective advantage (Snell, 1968). It was considered unthinkable until a relatively short time ago that different allelic forms of a gene could be maintained in the absence of any effect on survival of the individual. Recently, however, the use of electrophoretic and immunological methods has uncovered the existence of a large number of polymorphic loci. Polymorphism in at least 26 loci is average for a mouse population; the average individual is heterozygous in at least 8.5% of its loci (Selander, 1970). In other species estimates of polymorphic loci are even higher. The unexpectedly high frequency of polymorphisms in natural populations has raised the issue of whether a selectionist interpretation is suited to explain all genetic polymorphism. There is now a school of thought that postulates that most polymorphisms arise and can be maintained by numerous mutations, because many of these are neutral (Klein, 1975). Polymorphisms probably, however, result from a mixture of selectively advantageous and neutral mutations.

Even when viewed in the context of widespread genetic polymorphisms, MHC polymorphism remains exceptional. Among the 500 or so known loci in the mouse, none has been found to be even remotely close to *H-2* in its polymorphism. This unusual polymorphism is no experimental artifact, nor does it appear unusual simply because techniques for detection of other complex loci are not as sensitive (Klein, 1975).

MHC products, at least MHC antigens, are well exposed on the cell surface and appear in large numbers relative to those other receptors that have been measured. For example, MHC antigens elicit very strong immune reactions, and they are cleaved off the membrane easily by enzymes. They are then ideally suited to modify interactions between ligands arriving on the membrane and their surface receptors. They may then, to borrow a term from Jerne (1971), serve as generators of diversity of all responses to all ligands at the cell surface, and not merely in immunological interaction.

But how can H-2 molecules act? We have previously postulated that *H-2*, and its homologue in other species, plays significant roles in generating biochemical individuality by modifying cell-surface interactions and reactions (Meruelo and Edidin, 1975*a*,*b*). Though the many processes involving interactions at the cell surface that have been found to be affected by *H-2* genotype may be due to the role of still more genes within the *H-2* region affecting membrane phenotype, it seems more plausible that a relatively small number of loci exert a wide range of effects on membrane function, especially in view of the expected percentage of active DNA present in this segment of chromosome (Shreffler and David, 1975).

A model of *H-2* modifying the interaction of a variety of molecules and ligands with their specific receptors on the cell surface would be consistent with the quantitative nature of all *H-2*-associated responses noted so far, instead of the all-or-none effects expected of more direct genetic control. This model implies that there need not be always high or always low responses associated with a particular *H-2* genotype. The modification of binding by H-2 antigens would be expected to vary with the chemistry of the substances bound, and the expected interaction could not be predicted until the detailed chemistry of H-2 antigens *in situ* is completely understood.

## VIII. CONCLUSION

The present chapter is an attempt to give an alternate interpretation of the available data regarding MHC genes. It has attempted to bring together into a cohesive theory much of what is known today. The state of the field is such that most of the pieces of the puzzle are missing, and consequently a great deal of speculation has been inserted in order to complete the picture. For every interpretation given, there are probably a dozen others that are equal or better. The choice between alternatives was subjective, and therefore probably biased. In addition, a number of distinct hypotheses have been linked together in this writing as a matter of predilection, while the validity of each of these is clearly independent of the others.

Had these concepts been postulated privately, they might have been useful as guides to future experiments; however, published as they are, they will probably serve only to embarrass their authors by their errors. There is, nevertheless, an outside chance that they can help or stimulate others, even if it is to disprove these concepts.

## ACKNOWLEDGMENTS

We wish to thank Dr. Allen Mayer for his comments and suggestions and Mses. Marlene Chavis and Beverly Coopersmith for their patience and their excellent secretarial assistance. The research reported herein was supported by National Institutes of Health Grants CA 22247 (D. M.) and AI-14584 (M. E.), American Cancer Society Grant IM-163 (D. M.), a grant from the Irma T. Hirsch Foundation (D. M.), and a Training Grant from the Department of Biology and the Johns Hopkins University. This is contribution 1031 from the Department of Biology, the Johns Hopkins University.

## IX. REFERENCES

Allen, F. H., 1974, Linkage of HL-A and GBG, *Vox Sang* **27**:382.

Alper, C. A., 1976, Inherited structural polymorphism in human C2: evidence for genetic linkage between C2 and BF, *J. Exp. Med.* **114**:1111.

Amiel, J. L., 1967, Study of leucocyte phenotypes in Hodgkin's disease, in: *Histocompatibility Testing* (E. S. Curtoni, P. L. Matius, and R. M. Tosi, eds.), pp. 79–81, Munksgaard, Copenhagen.

Andrews, P. W., and Boyse, E. A., 1978, Mapping of an *H-2* linked gene that influences mating preference in mice, *Immunogenetics* **6**:265.

Aoki, T., Boyse, E. A., and Old, L. J., 1966, Occurrence of natural antibody to the G (Gross) leukemia antigen in mice, *Cancer Res.* **26**:1415.

Bailey, D. W., 1966, Heritable histocompatibility changes: Lysogeny in mice? *Transplantation* **4**:482.

Bartlett, P. F., and Edidin, M., 1978, Effect of *H-2* gene complex in rates of fibroblast intercellular adhesion, *J. Cell. Biol.* **77**:377.

Benacerraf, B., and Katz, D. H., 1975, The histocompatibility-linked immune response genes, *Adv. Cancer Res.* **21**:121.

Benacerraf, B., and McDevitt, H. O., 1972, Histocompatibility-linked immune response genes, *Science* **175**:273.

Biddle, F. G., and Fraser, F. C., 1977, Genetics of cortisone-induced cleft-palate in mouse-embryonic and maternal effects, *Genetics* **85**:289.

Binz, H., and Wigzell, H., 1975*a*, Shared idiotypic determinants in B and T lymphocytes reactive against the same antigenic determinants. I. Demonstration of similar or identical idiotypes on IgG molecules and T cell receptors with specificity for the same alloantigens, *J. Exp. Med.* **142**:197.

Binz, H., and Wigzell, H., 1975*b*, Shared idiotypic determinants on B and T lymphocytes reactive against the same antigenic determinants. IV. Isolation of two groups of naturally-occurring idiotypic molecules with specific antigen-binding activity in the serum and urine of normal rats, *Scand. J. Immunol.* **4**:591.

Binz, H., Lindenman, J., and Wigzell, H., 1974*a*, Cell bound receptors for alloantigens on normal lymphocytes. I. Characterization of receptors carrying cells by the use of antibodies to alloantigens, *J. Exp. Med.* **139**:877.

Binz, H., Lindenman, J., and Wigzell, H., 1974*b*, Cell bound receptors for alloantigens on normal lymphocytes. II. Antialloantibody serum contains specific factors reacting with relevant immunocompetent T lymphocytes, *J. Exp. Med.* **140**:731.

Blank, K. K., Freedman, H. A., and Lilly, F., 1976, T lymphocyte response to Friend virus induced tumor cell lines in mice of strains congenic at *H-2*, *Nature* **260**:250.

Boubelik, M., and Lengerová, A., 1977, Analysis of genetic differences in early versus late agglutinability with H-2 antibodies of neonatal mouse erythrocytes, *J. Immunogenet.* **4**:341.

Boubelik, M., Lengerová, A., Bailey, D. W., and Matousek, V., 1975, A model for genetic analysis of programmed gene expression as reflected in the development of membrane antigens, *Dev. Biol.* **47**:206.

Boyse, E. A., Old, L. J., Luell, S., 1964, Genetic determination of the TL (thymus–leukemia) antigen in the mouse, *Nature* **201**:779.

Brack, C., Hinama, M., Lenhard-Schuller, R., and Tonegawa, S., 1978, Complete immunoglobulin gene is created by somatic recombination, *Cell* **15**:1.

Chazan, R., and Haran-Ghera, N., 1976, The role of thymus subpopulations in "T" leukemia development, *Cell. Immunol.* **23**:356.

Chien, Y.-H., Verma, I. M., Shih, T. Y., Scolnik, E. M., and Davidson, N., 1978, Heteroduplex analysis of the sequence relation between the RNA's of mink cell focus–inducing and murine leukemia viruses, *J. Virol.* **28**:352.

Declève, A., Lieberman, M., Ihle, J. N., Kaplan, H. S., 1977, Biological and serological characteristics of C-type RNA viruses isolated from C57BL/Ka strain of mice. 3. Characterization of isolates and their interactions in vitro and in vivo, in: *Radiation-induced Leukemogenesis and Related Viruses* (J. F. Duplan, ed.), pp. 247–264, North-Holland, Amsterdam.

Doherty, P. C., Blanden, R. V., and Zinkernagel, R. M., 1976, Specificity of virus-immune effector T cells for H-2K or H-2D compatible interactions: implications for H-antigen diversity, *Transpl. Rev.* **29**:89.

Eichmann, K., and Rajewsky, K., 1975, Induction of T and B cell immunity by anti-idiotypic antibody, *Eur. J. Immunol.* **5**:661.

Elder, J. H., Gautsch, J. W., Jensen, F. C., and Lerner, R. A., 1978, Multigene family of endogenous retroviruses: recombinant origin of diversity, *J. Natl. Cancer Inst.* **61**:625.

Erickson, R. P., Butley, M. S., Martin, S. R., and Betlack, C. J., 1979, Variation among inbred strains of mice in adenosine 3′:5′ cyclic monophosphate levels of spermatozoa, *Genet. Res.* **33**:129.

Erickson, R. P., Butley, M. S., and Sing, C. F., 1980, A role for adenosine 3′:5′ cyclic monophosphate in the *H-2* determined component of genetic susceptibility to steroid-induced cleft palate, *J. Immunogenet.* (in press).

Flaherty, L., 1976, The TLa region of the mouse: identification of a new serologically defined locus, Qa-2, *Immunogenetics* **3**:533.

Freedman, H. A., Lilly, F., Strand, M., and August, J. T., 1978, Variations in viral gene expression in Friend virus-transformed cell lines congenic with respect to the *H-2* locus, *Cell* **13**:33.

Garrido, F., Schirrmacher, V., and Festenstein, H., 1976*a*, *H-2* like specificities of foreign haplotypes appearing on a mouse sarcoma after vacania virus infection, *Nature* **259**:228.

Garrido, F., Festenstein, H., and Schirrmacher, V., 1976*b*, Further evidence for depression of *H-2* and *IA* like specificities of foreign haplotypes in mouse tumor cell lines, *Nature* **261**:705.

Gazdar, A. F., Oie, H., Lalley, P., Moss, W., Minna, J. D., and Francke, U., 1977, Identification of mouse chromosomes required for murine leukemia virus replication, *Cell* **11**:949.

Godeau, J. F., Schorderet-Slatkine, S., Hubert, P., and Baulier, E. E., 1978, Induction of maturation in *Xenopus laevis* oocytes by a steroid linked to a polymer, *Proc. Natl. Acad. Sci. USA* **75**:235.

Goldman, A. S., Katsumata, M., Yuffe, S. J., and Gasser, D. L., 1977, Palatal cytosol corticol-binding protein associated with cleft palate susceptibility and *H-2* genotype, *Nature* **265**:643.

Goodfellow, P., Jones, E., van Heyningen, V., Solomon, E., Bobrow, M., Migiano, V., and Bodmer, W. F., 1975, The β-2 microglobulin gene is on chromosome #15 and not in the *HL-A* region, *Nature* **254**:267.

Gorer, P. A., 1956, Some recent work on tumor immunity, *Adv. Cancer Res.* **4**:149.

Gregorová, S., and Iványi, P., 1973, *H-2* associated genetic differences in androgen dependent traits: The effect of castration and testosterone injections, *Folia Biol.* **19**:337.

Gregorová, S., Iványi, P., and Gutman, E., 1975, Genetic differences in Levatorani muscle weight between inbred and congenic mouse strains, *Physiol. Bohemosl.* **24**:321.

Gregorová, S., Iványi, P., Simonova, D., and Micková, M., 1977, *H-2* associated differences in androgen-influenced organ weights of A strains and C57BL/10 mouse strains and their crosses, *Immunogenetics* **4**:301.

Gross, L., 1970, *Oncogenic Viruses* (2nd ed.), Pergamon Press, Oxford.

Helenius, A., Morin, B., Fries, E., Simons, E., Robinson, P., Schirrmacher, V., Terhorst, C., and Strominger, J. L., 1978, Human (HLA-A and HLA-B) and murine (H-2K and H-2D) histocompatibility antigens are cell surface receptors for Semliki Forest virus, *Proc. Natl. Acad. Sci. USA* **75**:3846.

Heron, I., Hekland, M., and Berg, K., 1978, Enhanced expression of β2-microglobulin and HLA antigens on human lymphoid cells by interferon, *Proc. Natl. Acad. Sci. USA* **75**: 6215.

Ihle, J. N., McEwan, R., and Bengali, K., 1976*a*, Radiation leukemia in C57BL/6 mice. I. Lack of serological evidence for the role of endogenores ecotropic viruses in pathogenesis, *J. Exp. Med.* **144**:1391.

Ihle, J. N., Joseph, D. R., Pazmino, N. H., 1976*b*, Radiation leukemia in C57BL/6 mice. II. Lack of ecotropic virus expression in the majority of lymphomas, *J. Exp. Med.* **144**: 1406.

Iványi, P., Gregorová, S., Micková, M., 1972*a*, Genetic difference in thymus, lymph node, testes and vesicular gland weights among inbred mouse strains, association with the major histocompatibility (H-2) system, *Folia Biol.* **18**:81.

Iványi, P., Hampl, R., Starka, L., Micková, M., 1972*b*, Genetic association between *H-2* gene and testosterone metabolism in mice, *Nature New Biol.* **283**:280.

Janeway, C., 1976, The specificity of T lymphocyte responses to chemically defined antigens, *Transplant. Rev.* **29**:165.

Jerne, N. K., 1971, The somatic generation of immune recognition, *Eur. J. Immunol.* **1**:1.

Kaplan, H. S., 1967, On the natural history of the murine leukemias: Presidential address, *Cancer Res.* **37**:1321.

Klareskog, L., Banck, G., Forsgren, A., and Peterson, P. A., 1978, Binding of HLA antigen-containing liposomes to bacteria, *Proc. Natl. Acad. Sci. USA* **75**:6197.

Klein, J., 1975, *Biology of the Mouse Histocompatibility Complex*, Springer-Verlag, New York.

Klein, J., 1977, Evolution and function of major histocompatibility system—Facts and speculations, in: *Major Histocompatibility Systems in Man and Animals* (D. Götze, ed.), pp. 339–378, Springer-Verlag, Berlin.

Klein, J., Festenstein, F., McDevitt, H. O., Shreffler, D. C., Snell, G. D., and Stempfling, J. H., 1974, Genetic nomenclature for the *H-2* complex of the mouse, *Immunogenetics* **1**:184.

Kohn, H. I., and Melvold, R. W., 1974, Spontaneous histocompatibility mutations detected by dermal grafts: Significant changes in rate over a 10 year period in the mouse H-system, *Mutat. Res.* **24**:163.

Lafuse, W., 1978, The Role of the *Histocompatibility-2* Locus in Modifying Cyclic-AMP Levels, Ph.D. thesis, the Johns Hopkins University, Baltimore.

Lafuse, W., and Edidin, M., 1978, H-2 haplotype affects binding of glucagon to mouse liver plasma membranes, *Fed. Proc. Fed. Am. Soc. Exp. Biol.* **37**:1600.

Lengerová, A., Zelevý, V., Haskorec, M., and Hilgert, I., 1977, Search for the physiological function of *H-2* gene products, *Eur. J. Immunol.* **7**:62.

Lieberman, M., Kaplan, H. S., 1959, Leukemogeneic activity of filtrates from radiation-induced lymphoid tumors of mice, *Science* **130**:387.

Lilly, F., 1968, The effect of histocompatibility-2 type in response to the Friend leukemic virus in mice, *J. Exp. Med.* **127**:465.

Lilly, F., 1970, The role of genetics in Gross virus leukemogenesis, *Bibl. Haematol.* **36**:213.

Lilly, F., and Pincus, T., 1973, Genetic control of murine viral leukomogenesis, *Adv. Cancer Res.* **17**:1231.

Lilly, F., Boyse, E. A., and Old, L. J., 1964, Genetic basis of susceptibility to viral leukemogenesis, *Lancet* **2**:1207.

McClay, D. R., and Gooding, L. R., 1978, Involvement of histocompatibility antigens in embryonic cell recognition events, *Nature* **274**:367.

McDevitt, H. O., and Bodmer, W. F., 1972, Histocompatibility antigens, immune responsiveness and susceptibility to disease, *Am. J. Med.* **52**:1.

McDevitt, H. O., Deak, B. D., Shreffler, D. C., Klein, J., Stimpfling, J. H., and Snell, G. D., 1972, Genetic control of the immune response: mapping of the Ir-1 locus, *J. Exp. Med.* **135**:1259.

McMichael, A. J., 1978, HLA restriction of human cytotoxic T lymphocytes specific for influenza virus: poor recognition of virus associated with HLA A2, *J. Exp. Med.* **148**: 1458.

McMichael, A. J., and Askonas, B. A., 1978, Influenza specific cytotoxic T cells in man: induction and properties of the cytotoxic cell, *Eur. J. Immunol.* (in press).

McMichael, A. J., Ting, A., Zweerink, H. J., and Askonas, B. A., 1977, HLA restriction of cell mediated lysis of influenza virus-infected human cells, *Nature* **270**:524.

Melvold, R. W., and Kohn, H. I., 1975, Histocompatibility gene mutation rates: H-2 and *non*-H-2, *Mutat. Res.* **27**:415.

Meo, T., Krasteff, T., and Shreffler, D. C., 1975, Immunochemical characterization of murine H-2 controlled Ss (serum substance) protein through identification of its human homologue is the fourth component of complement, *Proc. Natl. Acad. Sci. USA* **72**: 4536.

Meruelo, D., 1974, Modulation of Cyclic AMP Levels by the *Histocompatibility-2* Locus, Ph.D. thesis, The Johns Hopkins University, Baltimore, MD.

Meruelo, D., 1979, A role for elevated H-2 antigen expression in resistance to neoplasia caused by radiation-induced leukemic virus: enhancement of effective tumor surveillance by killer lymphocytes, *J. Exp. Med.* **149**:898.

Meruelo, D., and Edidin, M., 1975*a*, Association of mouse liver adenosine 3′:5′-cyclic monophosphate (cyclic AMP) level with *histocompatibility-2* genotype, *Proc. Natl. Acad. Sci. USA* **72**:2644.

Meruelo, D., and Edidin, M., 1975*b*, Modulation of hormonal effects on adenyl cyclose by the *Histocompatibility-2* (H-2) locus, *Fed. Proc. Fed. Am. Soc. Exp. Biol.* **34**:979.

Meruelo, D., and McDevitt, H. O., 1978, Recent studies on the role of the immune response in resistance to virus-induced leukemias and lymphomas, *Sem. Hemat.* **15**:399.

Meruelo, D., Nimelstein, S., Jones, P., Lieberman, M., and McDevitt, H. O., 1978, Increased synthesis and expression of H-2 antigens as a result of radiation leukemia virus infection: a possible mechanism for *H-2* linked control of virus-induced neoplasia, *J. Exp. Med.* **147**:470.

Meruelo, D., Sonnenfeld, G., McDevitt, H. O., and Merigan, T., 1980*a*, Effect of Type I and Type II interferons on murine lymphocyte surface antigen expression. Induction or selection? (submitted for publication).

Meruelo, D., Flieger, N., Smith, D., and McDevitt, H. O., 1980*b*, *In vivo* or *in vitro* treatments with anti I-J abolish immunity to AKR leukemia (manuscript in preparation).

Micková, M., and Iványi, P., 1975, Influence of *H-2* system on sensitivity of vesicular glands to testosterone hormone, *Folia Biol.* **21**:435.

Nathenson, S. G., and Cullen, S. E., 1974, Biochemical properties and immunochemical genetic relations of mouse H-2 alloantigens, *Biochem. Biophys. Acta* **344**:1.

Passmore, H. C., and Shreffler, D. C., 1970, A sex linked serum protein variant in the mouse: inheritance and association with the *H-2* region, *Biochem. Genet.* **4**:351.

Poulik, M. D., Ferrone, S., Pellegrino, M. A., Sevier, D. E., Oh, S. K., and Reisfeld, R. A., 1974, Association of HL-A antigens and $\beta$2-microglobulin: Concepts and questions, *Transpl. Rev.* **21**:106.

Ruddle, N. H., Conta, B. S., Leinwand, L., Kozak, C., Ruddle, F., Besmer, P., and Baltimore, D., 1978, Assignment of the receptor for ecotropic murine leukemia virus to mouse chromosome 5, *J. Exp. Med.* **148**:451.

Sasazuki, T., McDevitt, H. O., and Grumet, F. C., 1977, The association between genes in the major histocompatibility complex and disease susceptibility, *Ann. Rev. Med.* **28**: 425.

Sato, H., Boyse, E. A., Aoki, T., Iritani, C., and Old, L. J., 1973, Leukemia-associated transplantation antigens related to murine leukemia virus. the X. 1 system: Immune response controlled by a locus linked to *H-2*, *J. Exp. Med.* **138**:593.

Saunders, D. A., and Edidin, M., 1974, Sites of localization and synthesis of Ss protein in mice, *J. Immunol.* **112**:2210.

Searle, A. G., 1972, Spontaneous frequencies of point mutations in mice, *Humangenetik* **16**:33

Searle, A. G., 1974, Mutation induction in mice, *Adv. Rad. Biol.* **4**:131.

Selander, R. K., 1970, Biochemical polymorphism in populations of the house mouse and old-field mouse, in: *Variation in Mammalian Populations*, Symposia of the Zoological Society of London No. 26 (R. J. Berry and H. N. Southern, eds.), pp. 73–91, Academic Press, New York.

Shearer, G. M., 1975, Cell-mediated cytotoxicity to trinetrophenyl-modified syngeneic lymphocytes, *Eur. J. Immunol.* **4**:527.

Shreffler, D. C., and David, C. S., 1972, Studies on recombination within mouse H-2 complex. I. Three recombinants which position Ss locus within complex, *Tissue Antigens* **2**:232.

Shreffler, D. C., and David, C. S., 1975, The H-2 major histocompatibility complex and the I immune response region: genetic variation, function and organization, *Adv. Immunol.* **20**:125.

Silver, J., and Hood, L., 1976, Preliminary amino acid sequences of transplantation antigens: Genetic and evolutionary implications, in: *Contemporary Topics in Molecular Immunology*, Vol. 5 (H. N. Eisen and R. A. Reisfeld, eds.), pp. 35–68, Plenum Press, New York.

Snell, G. D., 1968, The *H-2* locus of the mouse: Observations and speculations concerning its comparative genetics and its polymorphisms, *Folia Biol.* **14**:335.

Snell, G., 1980, The major histocompatibility complex: Its evolution and involvement in cellular immunity, *Harvey Lect.* (in press).

Stanton, T. H., and Boyse, E. A., 1976, A new serologically defined locus, Qa-1, in the TLa region of the mouse, *Immunogenetics* **3**:525.

Stockert, E., and Old, L J., 1977, Preleukemic expression of TL antigens in x-irradiated C57BL/6 mice, *J. Exp. Med.* **146**:271.

Stockert, E. L., Old, L. J., and Boyse, E. A., 1971, the $G_{IX}$ system: A cell surface alloantigen associated with murine leukemia virus: Implications regarding chromosomal integration of the viral genome, *J. Exp. Med.* **133**:1334.

Svejgard, A., and Ryder, L. P., 1976, Interaction of HLA molecules with non-immunological ligands as an explanation of HLA and disease associations, *Lancet* **2**:547.

Yamazaki, K., Yamaguchi, M., Andrews, P. W., Peake, B., and Boyse, E. A., 1978, Mating preferences of F2 segregates of crosses between MHC-congenic mouse strains, *Immunogenetics* **6**:253.

Zelený, V., Matousek, V., and Lengerová, A., 1978, Intercellular adhesiveness of *H-2* identical and *H-2* disparate cells, *J. Immunogenet.* **5**:41.

Zigler, J. B., Alper, C. B., Balmer, H., 1975, Properidin factor B and histocompatibility loci linked in rhesus monkey, *Nature* **254**:609.

Zinkernagel, R. M., and Doherty, P. C., 1974, Restriction of in vitro T cell-mediated cytotoxicity in lymphocytic choriomeningitis within a syngeneic or semi-allogeneic system, *Nature* **248**:701.

*Chapter 10*

# *Molecular Interactions and Recognition Specificity of Surface Receptors*

**John J. Marchalonis**

*Cancer Biology Program*
*NCI Frederick Cancer Research Center*
*Frederick, Maryland 21701*

## I. INTRODUCTION

Virtually all cells express some capacity to recognize and respond to external molecular stimuli. One system that has been subjected to extensive study is the recognition of an antigen by immunologically competent lymphocytes. This is a phenomenon in which cell-surface receptor molecules bind "non-self" ligands in a specific manner. This binding initiates a chain of molecular events that underlie lymphocyte activation and interaction among immunocytes, with the eventual results being the production of specific effector thymus-derived (T) or bone-marrow-derived (B) cells. The capacity to discriminate between "self" and "non-self" is not restricted to vertebrate species, although the receptors and mechanisms evolved by plants (Clarke and Knox, 1978) and invertebrate species (Jenkin, 1976) apparently differ from those of the vertebrate immune system (Marchalonis, 1977*a*). Available data suggest that surface glycoproteins are involved in such recognition events, and the possible similarities and differences governing cell-surface recognition in these three systems and in embryonic development are problems of great current interest.

In this chapter I will raise critical issues regarding (1) definition of surface recognition, (2) structural and thermodynamic properties of molecules implicated in primary binding and cell activation, and (3) events correlated with primary binding of ligands to cell-surface receptors. I will develop the hypothesis that specific primary binding of ligand to cell-associated receptors occurs by processes that are identical to those exhibited by the same molecules in free solution. In order to accomplish this goal, it is necessary to consider molecules possibly involved in recognition, structural relationships among surface receptors, binding parameters of receptors and molecules in solution, and molecular properties of the combining sites of probable receptor molecules. The manner by which the receptors are attached to the membrane must also be considered, because, although the combining site for ligand is apparently accessible to the solution, the receptor molecule must be tightly associated with the hydrophobic environment of the plasma membrane, either through association with an adapter or because of the presence of a hydrophobic anchoring sequence. I will restrict discussion to studies with lectins and antibodies, because these are molecules that show remarkable binding specificity for defined ligands, they can be associated with plasma membranes, and detailed information on their structures and combining properties is available. Although receptors for polypeptide hormones can also be specific cell-surface-associated molecules (Cuatrecasas and Hollenberg, 1976; Flier *et al.*, 1977), a complete discussion of their properties is beyond the scope of this chapter.

## II. GROUND RULES

Three general points, which bear upon all of the recognition/activation/differentiation systems to be considered below, are as follows:

1. Cells do not recognize cells.
2. Rather, molecules on the surface of cells recognize molecules on other cells or in solution.
3. Molecule–molecule binding is specific, but it does not guarantee cell activation and differentiation.

Evidence that binding of ligand to cells in a specific manner does not necessarily result in activation comes from studies involving binding of antiimmunoglobulin (Ig) antibodies to murine B cells (Greaves *et al.*, 1974), binding of concanavalin A to B cells (Greaves *et al.*, 1974), and binding of antilymphocyte globulin to B cells (Decker *et al.*, 1977). In all of these cases, the B cells are rich in surface receptors for the particular ligands, but direct combination does not result in cell stimulation. "Recognition" must be considered in terms of two sequential phenomena: (1) primary binding of ligand and (2) the events of cell activation and differentiation. In the case of lymphocytes, some workers define primary binding as being equivalent to specific recognition (Marchalonis, 1977*a*; Marchalonis and Warr, 1979), whereas others include specific immune differentiation (Paul and Benacerraf, 1977) in their definition of recognition. As illus-

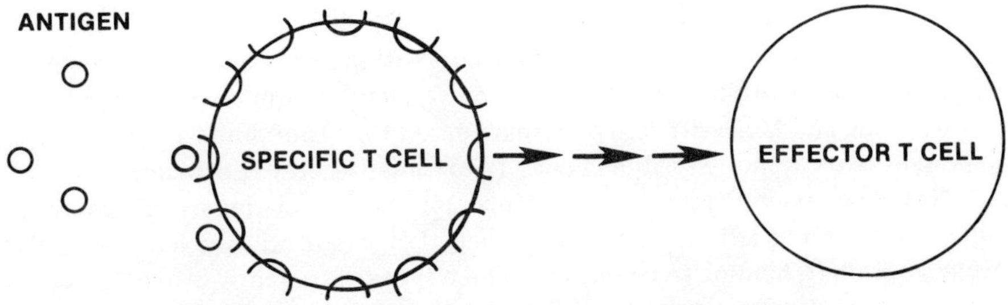


| PRIMARY BINDING | "SPECIFIC IMMUNE DIFFERENTIATION" |
|---|---|
| DIFFUSION-CONTROLLED REACTION | REQUIRES METABOLIC ENERGY |
| DEPENDENT UPON AFFINITY OF RECEPTOR | SHOWS "H-LINKED" RESTRICTION |
| DOES NOT SHOW "H-LINKED" RESTRICTION | PARTIAL LIST OF EVENTS INVOLVED: RECEPTOR REDISTRIBUTION; ACTIVATION; T/T COOPERATION; T/M$\phi$ COOPERATION; T/B COOPERATION; Ia-ASSOCIATED FACTORS; $Ca^{++}$ INFLUX; OTHERS |
| RAPID (Occurs within seconds) | INTERMEDIATE TO SLOW (Few minutes to many hours) |

Figure 1. Scheme listing the events involved in primary binding of antigen by an antigen-specific T cell and those involved in activation and differentiation into an effector T cell.

trated in Fig. 1, primary binding is a diffusion-controlled process, which is governed by the laws of thermodynamics, whereas differentiation requires an unknown series of cellular and biochemical events. The model depicted here represents events involved in the elaboration of antigen-specific effector T cells. Even with effector cells such as cytotoxic T cells, the processes of binding to target and lysis are distinct (Fishelson and Berke, 1978). It is suggested that major-histocompatibility-complex- (MHC-) associated surface structures might exert their effects following primary binding of ligand, because anti-*H-2* sera block specific T-cell differentiation when given 8 hr following interaction with antigen (Bluestein, 1974). Moreover, MHC-associated effects have been shown to operate at the levels of T-B (Katz and Benacerraf, 1975) and T–macrophage (Benacerraf,

1978; Erb and Feldmann, 1975) interactions. By contrast, ligand binding is a rapid diffusion-controlled reaction that occurs within a few minutes (Yahara and Edelman, 1972; Curtain *et al.*, 1978). Moreover, neither primary antigen binding (Hämmerling and McDevitt, 1974; Bernard *et al.*, 1977) nor primary delayed-type hypersensitivity responses (Miller *et al.*, 1976) are markedly *H*-dependent.

This diagram emphasizes problems inherent in extrapolating from the end result of cell differentiation, e.g., the existence of cytotoxic killer cells to the initial event of primary binding (recognition). Three types of currently available experimental approaches bear directly upon primary receptors, namely, (1) experiments testing codistribution of antigens and putative receptors (Roelants *et al.*, 1973, 1974; DeLuca *et al.*, 1978, 1979), (2) isolation of specific-binding proteins from the membrane (Marchalonis, 1976*a*,*b*), and (3) inhibition of primary binding (Warner, 1974).

## III. CELL-SURFACE MOLECULES IMPLICATED AS RECEPTORS

In principle, recognition molecules associated with the cell surface can be produced endogenously by the cell in question or can be passively absorbed from the serum. In the latter case, specific surface molecules such as the Fc receptors of lymphocytes (Warner, 1974; Dickler, 1976), macrophages (Berken and Benacerraf, 1966; Warner, 1974), and mast cells (Metzger, 1977; Conrad *et al.*, 1975) are frequently involved as adaptors that bind the exogenously produced molecule and display it in proper orientation on the cell surface. Although the bulk of currently available data derives from studies with Igs—notably, IgG subclasses for monocytes and lymphocytes and IgE for mast cells of mammals—non-Ig recognition molecules might also be present on the surface of mammalian cells. Two examples of this situation are C-reactive protein, which can serve as an opsonin for mammalian phagocytes (Kindmark, 1971), and circulating invertebrate agglutinins, which can impart a recognition specificity to invertebrate amoebocytes (Jenkin, 1976).

Table I gives a partial listing of endogenously synthesized surface molecules that have been implicated in specific-recognition events at the cell surface. It is now well established that B cells of mammals express two types of Igs on their surface: 7 S IgM (mIgM for membrane-associated IgM) in mammals (Marchalonis and Cone, 1973; Vitetta and Uhr, 1973; Warr and Marchalonis, 1977) and nonmammalian species studied (Warr, Chapter 6, this volume), and IgD or a similar molecule in man and rodents (Vitetta and Uhr, 1975; Warr and Marchalonis, 1977). It is noteworthy that Igs bearing the isotypic determinants of the murine IgD-like protein have not been found in serum (J. W. Goding, G. W. Warr, and J. J. Marchalonis, unpublished observations). This Ig might, thus, be restricted to

**Table I. Recognition Molecules**

| Receptor | Cell | Specificity | Molecular arrangement | Comments |
|---|---|---|---|---|
| 7 S IgM[a] | B cell | Antigen | $(L\mu)_2$ | s-s-Bonded tetramer |
| IgD[b] | B cell | Antigen | $(L\delta)_2$ | s-s-Bonded tetramer |
| IgM (t)[c] | T cell | Antigen | $L(\tau)_2L$ | s-s-Bonded heavy-chain dimer |
| IgT | | | | |
| H antigens[d] | All cells | ?–Cell interaction | $(H)\ (\beta_2M)$ | Noncovalent dimer |
| $\beta_2$ microglobulin[e] | All cells | ?–Cell interaction | | |
| Ia antigen[d] | Lymphocytes, macrophages, skin, sperm | ?–Cell interaction | $\alpha\beta$ | Some s-s-bonded dimers |
| Discoiden I[f] | Slime-mold aggregate | *N*-Acetyl-galactosamine–cell interaction | $(Sub)_4$ | Noncovalent tetramer of identical subunits of mass 26,000 |
| Limulus hemagglutinin[g] | Amoebocytes? | *N*-Acetyl-neuraminic acid–*N*-acetylgalatosamine | $(Sub)_{18}$ | Noncovalent multimer of subunits of mass 22,000 |
| Concanavalin A[h] | Jack bean seed | α-D-Mannose–α-D-glucose | $(Sub)_4$ | Tetramer of four identical subunits of mass 26,000 |

[a] Marchalonis and Cone, 1973; Vitetta and Uhr, 1973.
[b] Vitetta and Uhr, 1975; Warr and Marchalonis, 1977.
[c] Moseley *et al.*, 1977; Marchalonis and Warr, 1979; Cone and Janeway, 1977.
[d] Vitetta and Capra, 1978.
[e] Poulik, 1976.
[f] Frazier *et al.*, 1975.
[g] Marchalonis and Edelman, 1968*a*.
[h] Lis and Sharon, 1973.

the lymphocyte surface where it binds antigen (Marchalonis, 1976*b*; Goding and Layton, 1976), but serves an unknown function in activation. Murine IgD has been suggested as a triggering receptor (Vitetta and Uhr, 1975), and this and other hypotheses are currently under investigation (Cooper and Dayton, 1977).

Although the 7 S IgM of human and murine B cells is strongly associated with the plasma membrane, it is apparently not an integral membrane protein (Melcher and Uhr, 1977). Its solubility properties are not markedly different from those of the hydrophilic circulating Igs (Cone and Marchalonis, 1974; Melcher and Uhr, 1977); labeling of membrane vesicles indicates that it does not span the plasma membrane (Walsh and Crumpton, 1977); and its heavy chain, like that of serum $\mu$, possesses a C-terminal tyrosine residue (McIlhinney *et al.*, 1978). According to these observations, it is necessary to invoke an "adapter" (Marchalonis, 1976*a*) or Fc-receptor-like component to account for the strong association of endogenously synthesized IgM with the B-cell plasma membrane. The requirement for such a component is reinforced by reports that the distribution of surface Ig on B cells is nonrandom (Loor, 1977; Perelson, 1978) and correlates with the arrangement of submembrane contractile proteins (Schreiner and Unanue, 1976). The concept of an adaptor for B-cell surface Ig has been discussed previously and an "activation complex" consisting of a sensor element (mIgM), a transducer (the adaptor), and an effector element (unknown enzyme or contractile element on the inner face of the membrane) has been proposed (Marchalonis, 1976*a*). Support for involvement of contractile elements derives from the recent finding of Flanagan and Koch (1978) that cross-linked surface Ig attaches to actin. This hypothesis will be presented in a more general form below.

The existence of an Ig-like molecule on T cells has been disputed for the past decade. It is now clear, however, that T cells can express and synthesize a molecule that shares variable-region (Binz and Wigzell, 1977; Rajewsky and Eichmann, 1977; Warr *et al.*, 1979) and Fab-region (Szenberg *et al.*, 1977; Marchalonis *et al.*, 1978; Hämmerling *et al.*, 1976; Jones *et al.*, 1976; Warr *et al.*, 1978) determinants with serum Igs, but most probably represents an isotype not found in serum or on the B-cell surface (Marchalonis, 1975; Moseley *et al.*, 1977; Cone and Janeway, 1977; Cone, 1978). Figure 2 illustrates the Ig-like surface components of murine T and B cells as visualized by transmission immunoelectron-microscopy with purified chicken antibodies to the $(Fab')_2$ fragment of mouse IgG. Table II gives a list of evidence supporting the conclusions that chicken antibodies specific for the Fab fragment of murine IgG react only with Ig-polypeptide determinants and that the Ig-like surface molecule recognized by these antibodies is most probably involved in primary recognition of antigen.

B-cell surface molecules are of the form L-s-s-$\mu$-s-s-$\mu$-s-s-L and L-L-s-s-$\delta$-s-s-$\delta$-s-s-L, where s-s represents disulfide bonds. The Ig-like T-cell molecule can be represented as (L) $\tau$-s-s-$\tau$ (L), indicating that the covalent unit is a disulfide-bonded dimer of heavy chains ($\tau$), while the light chains are not covalently associated

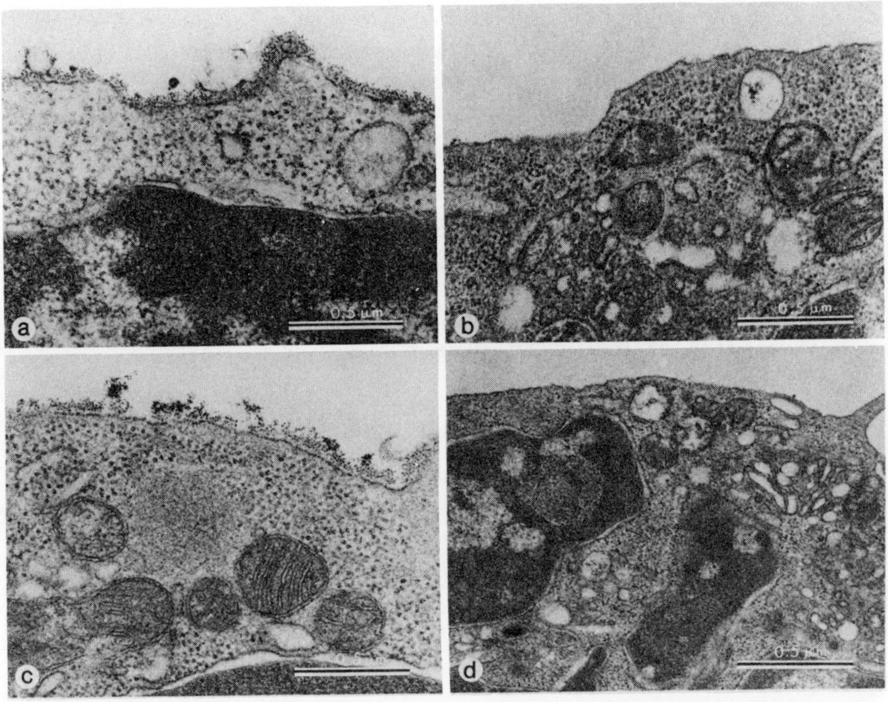

Figure 2. Visualization by transmission immunoelectronmicroscopy of surface Igs on murine thymus lymphocytes and "nude" spleen lymphocytes by chicken antibodies to mouse Fab. (a) C57BL thymus lymphocyte reacted with chicken anti-Fab, followed by ferritin-labeled rabbit antibody to chicken IgY. (b) C57BL thymus lymphocyte reacted with normal-chicken IgY, followed by ferritin-labeled rabbit antichicken IgY. (c) B cell of *nu/nu* spleen reacted with rabbit antimouse Fab, followed by ferritin-labeled rabbit antichicken IgY. (d) B cell reacted with normal-chicken IgY, followed by ferritin-labeled rabbit antichicken IgY. Notice the layer of ferritin immediately external to the plasma membrane in a and c. Binding of chicken anti-Fab was abolished by absorption with insolubilized κ chains or IgG. I am grateful to Drs. C. Bucanna and L. Hoyer for providing the photographs. The specific antibody was prepared as described by Szenberg *et al.* (1977) and absorbed according to Marchalonis *et al.* (1978). Conditions for immunoelectronmicroscopy are given in Marchalonis *et al.* (1978).

(Moseley *et al.*, 1977). Studies in progress on the covalent structure of the Ig-like T-cell molecule indicate that CNBr -cleavage or tryptic digestion of $^{125}$I-labeled light chain produces peptides resembling those of κ chains, as resolved by ion-exchange chromatography (Moseley *et al.*, 1979*b*). Figure 3 gives a comparison by polyacrylamide-gel electrophoresis in SDS-containing buffer of isolated heavy chains of normal mouse IgG, the IgM myeloma MOPC 104E, the IgA myeloma MOPC 315, the T lymphoma WEHI 22, and the T lymphoma WEHI 7. The T-cell

**Table II. Evidence That Chicken Antibodies to $(Fab')_2$ Fragments of Murine IgG Recognize Only Immunoglobulin Polypeptide Determinants and That the Surface Molecules Recognized Are Involved in Primary Recognition of Antigen**

| Observation | References |
|---|---|
| 1. Immunizing antigens lack carbohydrate | *a–c* |
| 2. Inhibiting antigens lack carbohydrate | *a–c* |
| 3. Antibodies react only with lymphocytes | *a, b, d* |
| 4. Absorption with nonlymphoid alloantigen-bearing cells does not remove reactivity to lymphocytes | *b, d* |
| 5. Antibody to Fab blocks binding of antigen by specific B and T cells | *e* |
| 6. Antibody to Fab codistributes with antigen on antigen-binding T and B cells | *e* |
| 7. Antibody to Fab does not codistribute with anit-Thy 1 or anti-*H*-2 | *e* |
| 8. Antibody to Fab blocks binding of arsonate hapten by idiotype-bearing IgG antibody to this hapten | *f* |
| 9. Components resembling immunoglobulin polypeptide chains are isolated from T and B cells | *b, c* |
| 10. Components resembling $B_2M$ and histocompatibility antigens are not isolated | *b, c* |

[a] Szenberg *et al.*, 1977.
[b] Marchalonis *et al.*, 1978.
[c] Warr *et al.*, 1978.
[d] Marchalonis *et al.*, 1979*a*.
[e] DeLuca *et al.*, 1978*b*.
[f] Warr *et al.*, 1979.

Ig heavy chains migrate in the region between $\mu$ and $\gamma$. Comparisons of radioiodinated tryptic peptides of the $\mu$, $\gamma$, $\alpha$, and T-lymphoma heavy chains were performed by simultaneous resolution of double-labeled peptides by ion-exchange chromatography on Dowex 50W X2. As shown in Fig. 4, WEHI 22 heavy chain is markedly distinct from gamma chain in its peptide profile, but shows 40–50 % of tyrosine-containing peptides with $\mu$ and $\alpha$ chains (Moseley *et al.*, 1979*a*). Two-dimensional "mapping" techniques show that the T-cell polypeptide chains are distinct from $\beta_2$ microglobulin and viral glycoproteins.

Studies based upon the use of antiidiotype antibodies to isolate heavy-chain dimers (140,000 MW; monomer approx. 70,000) but not light chains (Binz and Wigzell, 1978), might be explained by the above structure of the T-cell Ig because the antiidiotypic reagents used recognize $V_H$-specific determinants. Investigators using antisera reactive with light chain (Cone, 1976; Cone and Brown, 1976) and Fab-region (Szenberg *et al.*, 1977; Moseley *et al.*, 1977) determinants have isolated a heavy chain of similar mass and variable amounts of light chain. T-cell Ig differs markedly from B cells in its solubility properties (Cone and Marchalonis, 1974; Cone, 1976; Haustein and Goding, 1975; Smith *et al.*, 1975), and this observation has been an important factor in claims by some workers that they are unable to isolate the molecule (Vitetta *et al.*, 1972) under conditions of

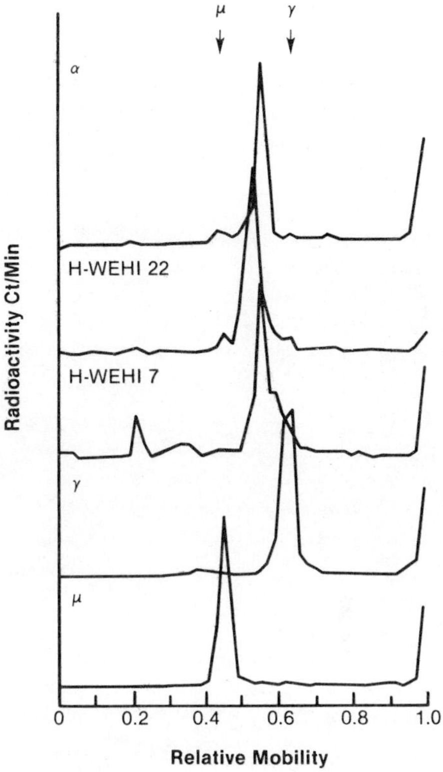


Figure 3. Comparison by SDS-PAGE of reduced BALB/c IgA (α), T-lymphoma WEHI-22, T-lymphoma WEHI-7, MγG (γ), and MOPC 104E MγM (μ), on 8% gels. Peak counts for the heavy chains were respectively $12 \times 10^4$ ct/min; $18 \times 10^3$ ct/min; $14 \times 10^3$ ct/min; $16 \times 10^4$ ct/min; and $14 \times 10^4$ ct/min. These gels give maximal resolution in the heavy-chain region. The light chains run off the gels under these circumstances. Notice that the T-lymphoma heavy chains migrate somewhat faster than μ and resemble α chains in their mobility in this system. T-lymphoma Ig was isolated from $^{125}$I-labeled culture fluid with the use of specific immunoadsorbents prepared from rabbit antibodies to normal-mouse serum IgM. T-cell Ig was isolated via an Fd-region cross-reaction (Moseley *et al.*, 1977).

high detergent concentrations. It is worthwhile pointing out that no one has ever isolated T-cell Ig using the high detergent concentrations of Vitetta *et al.* (1972), but numerous laboratories have isolated Ig-like molecules from T cells using solvents and conditions devised for T cells (see Cone, 1978, and Marchalonis and Warr, 1979, for reviews). Cone *et al.* (1977) have shown that T-cell Ig differs from IgM and IgD in its capacity to bind nonionic detergent. The T-cell molecule acts like an integral membrane protein when analyzed by gradient ultracentrifugation in detergent, whereas mIgM and mIgD act like serum molecules and sediment as 7 S units (Cone *et al.*, 1977). T-cell Ig may, therefore, be more deeply integrated into the plasma membrane than the B-cell molecules. Either it would require an adaptor distinct from those on B cells or else it might even lack the requirement for an adaptor.

Evidence of the involvement of molecules encoded by the MHC in specific T-cell recognition derives from (1) demonstration of MHC-associated restriction in the generation of cytotoxicity to virally infected cells (Zinkernagel and Doherty, 1977), (2) restriction of responses to hapten-modified cells (Shearer *et al.*, 1977),

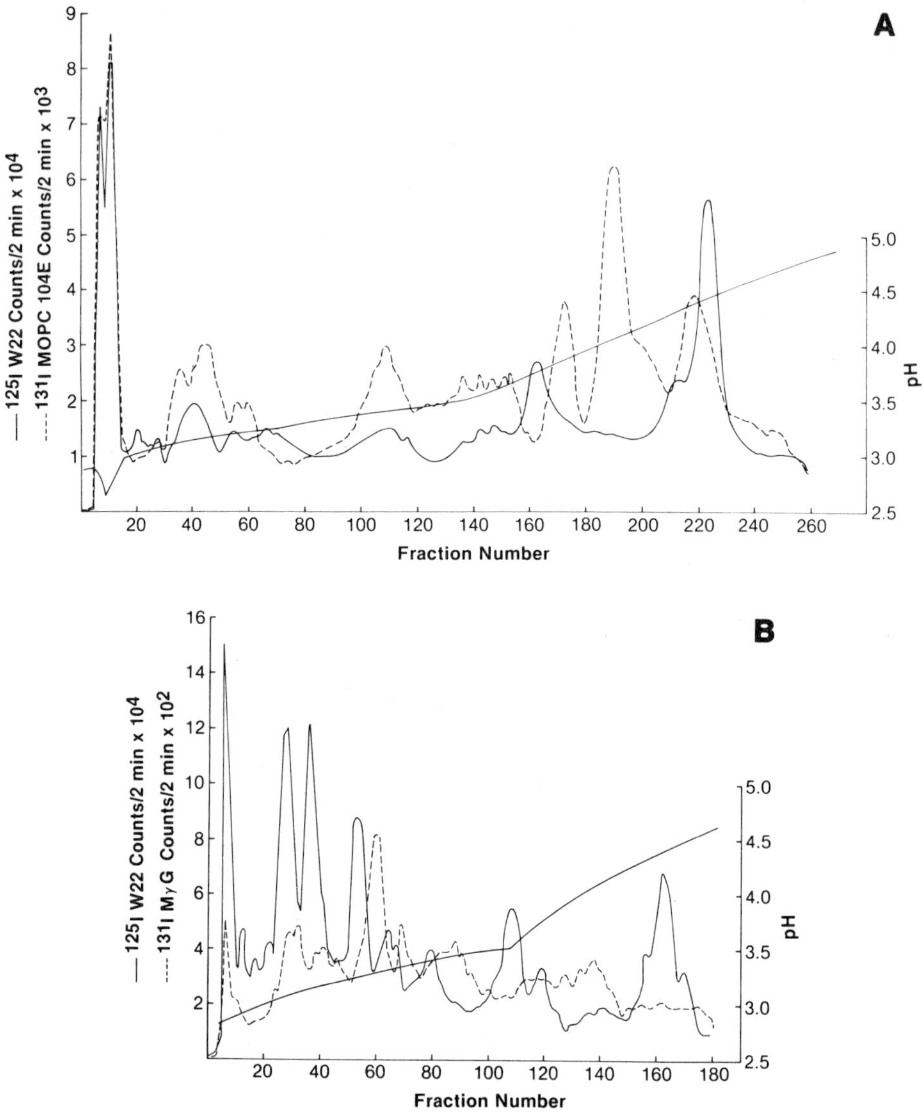


Figure 4. Simultaneous comparisons of the $^{125}$I-labeled tyrosine-containing tryptic peptides of heavy chain of the T-lymphoma WEHI-22 and heavy chains of serum immunoglobulins. Comparison of the tryptic peptides of [$^{125}$I]-WEHI 22 heavy chain (———) with: [$^{131}$I]-MOPC 104E $\mu$ (----) (A); [$^{131}$I]-M$\gamma$G – $\gamma$ (----) (B); and [$^{131}$I]-MOPC 315 – $\alpha$ (----) (C). Peptides were eluted from Dowex 50W × 2 cation-exchange resin at 40°C with a pyridine acetate gradient from 0.02 M pyridine pH 3.0 to 0.2 M pyridine pH 5.0 (Moseley *et al.*, 1979*a*).

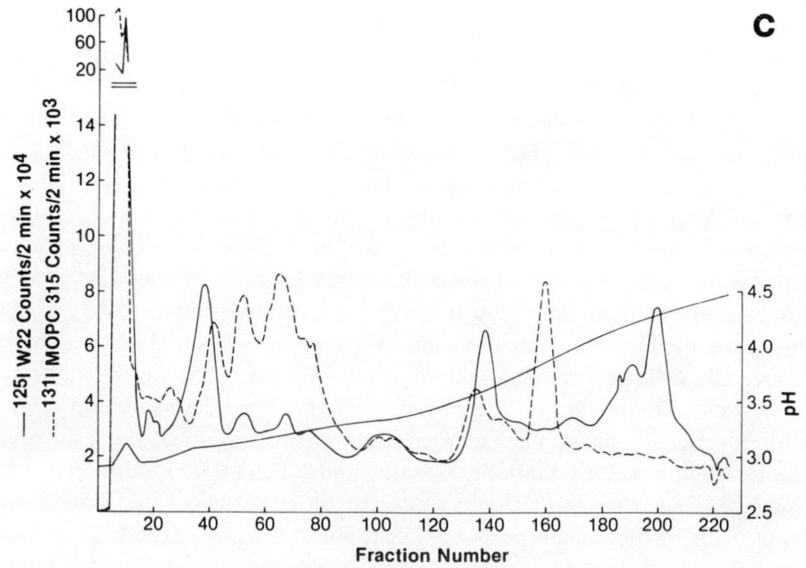


Figure 4. (*Continued*)

and (3) the reported existence of T-cell-generated antigen-specific soluble non-Ig factors bearing I-region determinants that amplify (Munro and Taussig, 1975) or suppress (Tada *et al.*, 1977) B-cell responses. Considerable evidence exists to suggest that MHC-associated markers, notably histocompatibility antigens (H antigens) and immune-response gene products (Ia antigens), are not primary receptors for antigen (Marchalonis *et al.*, 1974; Klein, 1976), but probably function during the activation and differentiation phases of the specific T-cell response (Katz and Benacerraf, 1975; Marchalonis *et al.*, 1974; Schwartz, 1978; Benacerraf, 1978). HL-A antigens have a mass of approximately 44,000 daltons and are integral membrane proteins (Walsh and Crumpton, 1977). Treatment of cells with papain cleaves the molecules into an N-terminal, carbohydrate-bearing fragment of about 36,000 daltons and a membrane-spanning C-terminal fragment of 8000 daltons (Terhorst *et al.*, 1977). The first 5000 daltons of the low-molecular-weight fragment are enriched with hydrophobic amino acids, whereas the C-terminal 3,000-dalton piece is hydrophilic in amino-acid content. H antigens generally occur in noncovalent association with $\beta_2$ microglobulin ($\beta_2$M), a polypeptide of 100 residues (approx. mass 12,000 daltons) that exhibits weak homology with the C$\gamma$3 domain of IgG (Vitetta and Capra, 1978). The $\beta_2$M/HL-A complex usually consists of one molecule of each, but artifactual dimers of the form $\beta_2$M/H-s-s-H/$\beta_2$M have been observed. Possible homologies among membrane molecules will be discussed below.

Ia antigens, like H antigens, are integral-membrane glycoproteins containing fragments that span the plasma membrane (Snary *et al.*, 1977). Two types of polypeptide have been found. One has an apparent mass of 33,000 daltons ($\alpha$ chain), while the second chain ($\beta$) has a mass of 28,000 daltons. Neither of these chains shows homology to H-2, $\beta_2$M, or Ig, although human and mouse Ia antigens are clearly homologous (Vitetta and Capra, 1978; Silver *et al.*, 1977).

The molecules listed above are definitely membrane-associated and some structural data are available for each of them. It is of interest that $\mu$ and $\delta$ chains (Hunt and Marchalonis, 1974), H antigens (Snary *et al.*, 1977), and Ia antigens (Cullen *et al.*, 1974) are glycoproteins that bind lectins such as concanavalin A or lentil lectin. $\beta_2$M and light chains lack appreciable carbohydrate. Lectins themselves comprise a broad category of receptor molecules found to be associated with plasma membranes of mammalian liver (Stockert *et al.*, 1974), embryonic chicken cells (Mir-Lechaire and Barondes, 1978), and cells of the slime mold *Dictyostelium discoideum* (Frazier *et al.*, 1975). These lectins exhibit clear specificity for certain sugars (Table I), and moreover, certain of them apparently promote specific cell interactions. Balsamo and Lilien (1975) found that soluble factors prepared from neural retina or cerebral-lobe tissue cultures bound specifically to cells of the same type and brought about cell aggregation. These factors showed specificity for *N*-acetylgalactosamine. Two distinct developmentally regulated lectins were found in the slime mold (Frazier *et al.*, 1975). Neither is present when the cells are in the vegetative (feeding) stage. Both lectins increase in the cohesive differentiating aggregate, but the ratio of discoiden II to discoiden I is greater at early than at late differentiation stages. Two distinct developmentally related lectins have recently been found in chick embryonic muscle cells (Mir-Lechaire and Barondes, 1978). The possibility, thus, must be entertained that surface molecules showing binding specificities for various sugar moieties arise at different stages of development and may be instrumental in initiating specific cellular recognition. Since it has been suggested that products of the MHC might play a role in cell–cell interactions in development (Miller and Vadas, 1977) and in immune collaboration (Katz and Benacerraf, 1975), the types of specificity involved might parallel those of the lectins described here. Moreover, many of the antigens to which non-Ig Ia-antigen-bearing suppressor factors bind are rich in carbohydrate (e.g., keyhole limpet hemocyanin) and will bind standard lectins such as Con A (Smith and Revel, 1971). Recent work from this laboratory (J. M. Decker and J. J. Marchalonis, unpublished) shows that both T and B lymphocytes of mice possess surface molecules that exhibit lectinlike properties, e.g., they bind to heavily glycosylated proteins such as fetuin and mucine and not to nonglycosylated proteins.

## IV. STRUCTURAL RELATIONSHIPS AMONG SURFACE RECEPTORS

The possibility exists that all surface glycoproteins of mammalian cells share a common evolutionary ancestry, and more specific questions regarding homolo-

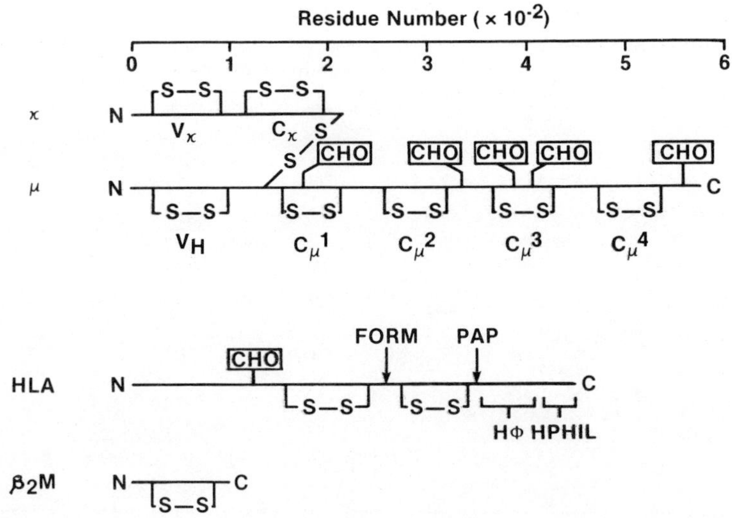


Figure 5. Schematic representations of $\kappa$ chain, $\mu$ chain, HLA, and $\beta_2$M sequences, indicating approximate positions of disulfide bonds (s-s) and carbohydrate moieties (CHO). FORM and PAP indicate respectively the positions at which formic acid and papain cleave HL-A (Terhorst *et al.*, 1977). H$\Phi$, hydrophobic stretch of sequence. HPHIL, hydrophilic stretch of sequence.

gies among Igs, H antigens, and $\beta_2$M have been pursued. Figure 5 presents a comparison among $\kappa$ chain, $\mu$ chain, HL-A, and $\beta_2$M. $\beta_2$M is approximately the size of an Ig domain and possesses an internal disulfide bond. It shows weak homology with the C$\gamma$3 domain of human $\gamma$ chain (Cunningham *et al.*, 1972). HL-A has two internal disulfide-bonded loops separated by approximately the same number of amino acid residues as occur within Ig domains. It possesses a portion that penetrates the plasma membrane and consists of a hydrophilic tail and a hydrophobic stretch (8000 daltons).

Tables III, IV, and V illustrate comparisons among the N-terminal amino acid sequences of Ig polypeptide chains, HL-A, and two agglutinins that were chosen to represent well-characterized lectins of an invertebrate (Finstad *et al.*, 1974) and a plant (Reeke *et al.*, 1974). It is clear that Ig chains show considerable homology among vertebrate species, e.g., $V_H$ of shark shows 6 identities in the first 10 residues with the heavy chain of mouse antibody to the arsonate hapten. By contrast, no homology is shown with the N-terminal sequences of HL-A, *Limulus* HA, and Con A, although on occasion one residue of identity owing to statistical fluctuation is noted. The dangers of drawing conclusions regarding specificity from limited sequence data by alignment or deletions "to maximize homology" are illustrated in Table VI. Both chicken $V_\lambda$ and Con A have N-terminal alanyl residues. When these are aligned, 30% identity is seen.

Although the N-termini of Igs and H antigens do not show significant homol-

**Table III. $V_{\kappa}$ versus HL-A and Agglutinin Sequence**

| | Residue number | | | | | | | | | |
|---|---|---|---|---|---|---|---|---|---|---|
| | 1 | 2 | 3 | 4 | 5 | 6 | 7 | 8 | 9 | 10 |
| Shark[a] | ASP | | THR | MET | THR | GLU | SER | PRO | PRO | VAL |
| Mouse (MOPC 41)[b] | ASP | ILE | GLN | MET | THR | GLN | SER | PRO | SER | SER |
| Human[c] (AG) | ASP | ILE | GLN | MET | THR | GLN | SER | PRO | SER | SER |
| HL-A-A2[d] | GLY | SER | HIS | SER | MET | ARG | TYR | PHE | PHE | THR |
| *Limulus*[e] HA | LEU | PRO | SER | GLY | | ILE | PRO | SER | | VAL |
| Con A[f] | ALA | ASP | THR | ILE | VAL | ALA | VAL | GLU | LEU | ASP |

[a] Sledge *et al.*, 1974.
[b] Gray *et al.*, 1967.
[c] Titani *et al.*, 1969.
[d] Vitetta and Capra, 1978.
[e] Finstad *et al.*, 1974.
[f] Reeke *et al.*, 1974.

**Table IV. $V_{\lambda}$ versus HL-A and HA Sequence**

| | Residue number | | | | | | | | | |
|---|---|---|---|---|---|---|---|---|---|---|
| | 1 | 2 | 3 | 4 | 5 | 6 | 7 | 8 | 9 | 10 |
| Chicken[a] | – | – | ALA | LEU | THR | GLN | PRO | ALA | SER | – |
| Mouse (RPC 20)[b] | PCA | ALA | VAL | VAL | THR | GLN | GLN | SER | ALA | – |
| Human (HS 92)[c] | PCA | SER | VAL | LEU | THR | GLN | PRO | PRO | SER | – |
| HL-A-A2[d] | GLY | SER | HIS | SER | MET | ARG | TYR | PHE | PHE | THR |
| *Limulus*[e] HA | LEU | PRO | SER | GLY | | ILE | PRO | SER | | VAL |
| Con A[f] | ALA | ASP | THR | ILE | VAL | ALA | VAL | GLU | LEU | ASP |

[a] Kubo *et al.*, 1971. Aligned to maximize homology to λ chains.
[b] Cesari and Weigert, 1973.
[c] Hood and Ein, 1968.
[d] Vitetta and Capra, 1978.
[e] Finstad *et al.*, 1974.
[f] Reeke *et al.*, 1974.

**Table V. $V_H$ versus HL-A and Agglutinin Sequence**

| | Residue number | | | | | | | | | |
|---|---|---|---|---|---|---|---|---|---|---|
| | 1 | 2 | 3 | 4 | 5 | 6 | 7 | 8 | 9 | 10 |
| Shark[a] | GLU | ILE/VAL | VAL | LEU | THR | GLN | PRO | GLX | ALA | GLX |
| Mouse (Anti-ARS)[b] | GLU | VAL | GLN | LEU | GLN | GLN | SER | GLY | ALA | GLU |
| Human ($V_H$III)[c] | GLU | VAL | GLN | LEU | VAL | GLU | SER | GLY | GLY | GLY |
| H-LA-A2[d] | GLY | SER | HIS | SER | MET | ARG | TYR | PHE | PHE | THR |
| *Limulus*[e] HA | LEU | PRO | SER | GLY | | ILE | PRO | SER | | VAL |
| Con A[f] | ALA | ASP | THR | ILE | VAL | ALA | VAL | GLU | LEU | ASP |

[a]Sledge *et al.*, 1974.
[b]Marchalonis *et al.*, 1979*b*.
[c]Kabat *et al.*, 1976.
[d]Vitetta and Capra, 1978.
[e]Finstad *et al.*, 1974.
[f]Reeke *et al.*, 1974.

ogy, the N-terminal residue of the acid-cleaved fragment of HL-A (see Fig. 2) shows striking homology with Ig-variable-region sequences in the region of the second half-cysteine involved in forming the internal disulfide-bonded loop (Terhorst *et al.*, 1977; Ploegh *et al.*, 1978). Segrest and Feldmann (1974) performed a computer search of various protein sequences for hydrophobic stretches comparable to the membrane-spanning region of glycophorin, the major transmembrane glycoprotein of human erythrocytes. Such stretches did not occur in Ig-constant regions, but strongly hydrophobic sequences were found in the V regions of human $\mu$ (Ou) and murine $\lambda$ (MOPC 104E) chains. These hydrophobic sequences were closely C-terminal to the half-cysteine residues 92 and 88, re-

**Table VI. Chicken $V_\lambda$ versus Concanavalin A ("Shifted")**

| | Residue number | | | | | | | | | |
|---|---|---|---|---|---|---|---|---|---|---|
| | 1 | 2 | 3 | 4 | 5 | 6 | 7 | 8 | 9 | 10 |
| Chicken[a] | ALA | LEU | THR | GLN | PRO | ALA | SER | – | VAL | SER |
| Con A[b] | ALA | ASP | THR | ILE | VAL | ALA | VAL | GLU | LEU | ASP |

[a]Kubo *et al.*, 1971. Aligned in residue order as sequenced.
[b]Reeke *et al.*, 1974.

**Table VII. Amino Acid Sequence Comparison of HLA-B7 13,000 $M_r$ Acid Cleavage Fragment with Immunoglobulin Chains, Papain Human Growth Hormone, and Bovine Ribonuclease**

| HLA-B7[a] | μ(ou)[b] | MOPC 104E λ[c] | Papain[d] | Growth hormone[e] | RNA′ se[f] |
|---|---|---|---|---|---|
| Asp | | Lys | | Ser | Gln |
| Pro | Leu | Ala | | His | His |
| Lys | Ile | Ala | | Asn | Met |
| Arg | Met | Leu | | Asp | Asp |
| Thr | Ile | Thr | | Asp | Ser |
| Val | Asn | Gly | | Ala | Ser |
| Thr | Val | Ala | | Leu | Thr |
| Arg | Asn | Gln | | Leu | Ser |
| Pro | Pro | Thr | | Lys | Ala |
| Ile/Leu | Val | Glu | | Asn | Ala |
| Asp | Asp | Asp | Asp | Tyr | Ser |
| Glu | Thr | Glu | Arg | Gly | Ser |
| Ala | Ala | Ala | Arg | Leu | Ser |
| Ile/Leu | Thr | Ile | Ser | Leu | Asn |
| | Tyr | | | | |
| Tyr | Tyr | Tyr | Try | Tyr | Tyr |
| ( )[g] | Tyr | Phe | Gly | ( ) | ( ) |
| Cys | 92 Cys | 88 Cys | 63 Cys | 164 Cys | Cys |
| Ala | Ala | Ala | Asn | Phe | Asn |
| Ile/Leu | ↓ HØ Region | Leu ↓ HØ Region | | | |

[a] Data of Terhorst *et al.*, 1977.
[b] Data of Putnam *et al.*, 1973. Aligned to give maximum identity. Tyr 89 is considered an extra residue and moved out of sequence.
[c] Data of Appella, 1971.
[d] Data of Mitchell *et al.*, 1970.
[e] Data of Li *et al.*, 1969. A gap has been inserted between Tyr and Cys 164.
[f] Data of Smyth *et al.*, 1963. A gap has been inserted between Tyr and Cys.
[g] ( ) indicates introduction of a gap in sequence to maximize homology.

spectively, which closed the intradomain disulfide-bonded loops. As shown in Table VII, impressive sequence identity occurs in the region of the half-cysteine immediately preceding the hydrophobic region. This situation parallels that found in HL-A, where the acid cleavage fragment closely precedes the hydrophobic stretch that penetrates the membrane. Similar sequences are also found in completely non-Ig-type molecules such as papain, growth hormone, and ribonuclease, and might reflect a particular folding pattern of these molecules about certain cysteine residues. If this conjecture proves true, HL-A and Igs are not homologous in an evolutionary sense, but rather show some convergence in certain regions of the molecule. Further sequence and molecular-conformation data are required to test this possibility.

Although no evidence of direct homology between *Limulus* HA, Con A, and Igs has been found, it is interesting that the lectin subunits are approximately the same size as light chains. The three lectins considered here form noncovalently associated multimers. Agglutinins of other invertebrate species, e.g., the oyster (Acton *et al.*, 1969), are constructed in a manner similar to that of the horseshoe crab.

## V. BINDING PARAMETERS OF RECEPTORS

The primary binding phase of recognition is a diffusion-controlled process that occurs rapidly and in strict accordance with the laws of thermodynamics. Although the receptors considered above, namely, lectins and Igs, are not homologous molecules, a comparison of the energetics of their binding reactions should provide useful information on the forces involved in primary binding of specific ligands by proteins. As a model for the combination of a protein with a known ligand, and as an illustration of the binding of a protein to cell-membrane structures, I will present some data on the binding of Con A to murine (CBA) thymus lymphocytes. As illustrated in Fig. 6, thymus cells bind about $4 \times 10^6$ molecules of lectin (MW 100,000), with an affinity ($K$) of approximately $5 \times 10^6$ liters/mole at 4°C. Under comparable conditions, B cells bound about $2 \times 10^6$ molecules/cell, with an affinity of $6 \times 10^6$ liters/mole. The binding could be completely inhibited by the sugar α-methyl-mannopyranoside. Consistent with a diffusion-controlled process, binding was rapid and temperature-dependent. Eighty percent of the saturation value was achieved in less than 10 minutes at 37°C, while 50% of saturation was achieved in the same time interval at 4°C (J. J. Marchalonis and J. Pye, unpublished observations). Similar binding data have been obtained by other workers (Yahara and Edelman, 1972).

In order for the binding to occur, the change in free energy of the reaction must be $<0$. The expression for Gibbs free energy is as follows:

$$\Delta F = \Delta H - T\Delta S$$

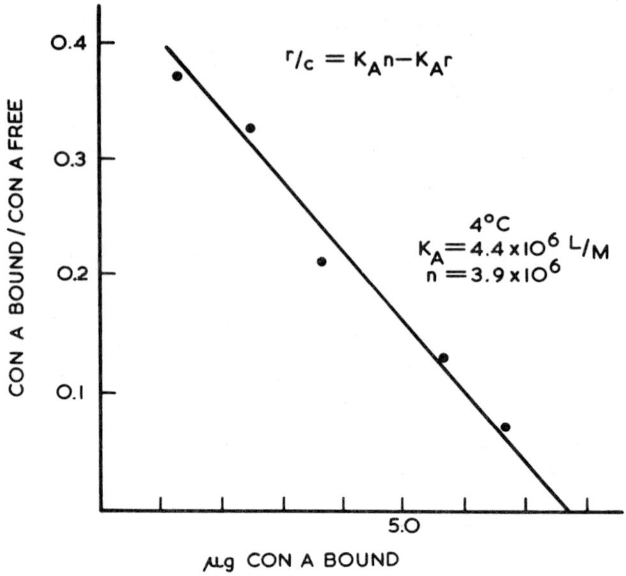


Figure 6. Scatchard plot illustrating binding of concanavalin A (Con A) to murine (CBA) thymus lymphocytes. Binding was quantified with $^{125}$I-labeled Con A. Unpublished data of J. J. Marchalonis and J. Pye.

where $\Delta F$ is the change in free energy, $\Delta H$ is the change in enthalpy or heat of the reaction, $T$ is absolute temperature, and $\Delta S$ is the entropy change. In a reaction such as that considered above, $\Delta F$ can be calculated directly from the binding constant, $\Delta H$ from the slope of plots of ln $K$ versus $1/T$ and, then, $\Delta S$ from the equation given here. Table VIII illustrates these parameters for the binding of Con A to mannosyl moieties on thymus cells. This binding is characterized by a large negative $\Delta F$, a small heat term, and a large positive entropy. The driving

**Table VIII. Thermodynamic Parameters of Binding of Con A to T Cells[a]**

| Temperature (°C) | $K$ (liters/mole) | $\Delta F$ (kcal/mole) | $\Delta H$ (kcal/mole) | $\Delta S$ (cal/deg · mole) |
|---|---|---|---|---|
| 4° (277°K) | $4.77 \times 10^6$ | −8.43[b] | 0.47[c] | 32.1[d] |
| 20° (293°K) | $2.97 \times 10^6$ | −8.65 | | 31.1 |
| 37° (310°K) | $2.70 \times 10^6$ | −9.09 | | 30.8 |

[a]Unpublished data of Marchalonis and Pye.
[b]$\Delta F = -RT \ln K$.
[c]From slope of plot of ln $K$ versus $1/T$.
[d]From $\Delta F = \Delta H - T\Delta S$.

force in this reaction, thus, is the entropy change, and the binding can be characterized as a hydrophobic interaction (Kauzmann, 1959). The large positive entropy change results from the loss of bound water, which then increases its translational degrees of freedom. It is noteworthy that the binding constant for combination of Con A with cell-surface receptors is two orders of magnitude greater than that for binding of the free sugar (Yariv *et al.*, 1968). This result illustrates the profound effect of multivalency on apparent affinity of binding.

Although antibodies and Con A are not structurally related molecules, we might ask whether the binding of antigen and antibody resembles the above example in its energetic properties. Precise studies have been carried out on the binding of purified antibodies to haptens (Eisen and Karush, 1949; Karush, 1962) and to small proteins such as insulin (Berson and Yalow, 1959). At this time, T and B cells have been shown to share antigenic determinants found on the idiotypic V-region portions of serum antibodies (Binz and Wigzell, 1977; Rajewsky and Eichmann, 1977), but binding-affinity studies have not been performed on isolated surface receptors of either cell type. In one case, however, a small subpopulation of isolated B-cell surface Ig was found to bind specifically to the dinitrophenyl hapten (Marchalonis, 1976*b*). As shown in Table IX, antibody populations of different specificity can differ markedly in their enthalpy and entropy changes, even though $\Delta F$ is large and negative. The binding to *m*-azophenylarsonate and insulin is a clear example of entropy-driven hydrophobic reactions. The combination with *p*-azophenyl-β-lactoside, by contrast, shows a small negative entropy change and is driven by the change in the heat term. This effect probably results from the formation of hydrogen bonds between the hapten and combining-site residues (Karush, 1962).

The large entropy change in the binding of insulin to its antibody is noteworthy because this represents an interaction between two proteins, and the energetics of the process are very similar to those encountered in other specific protein–protein interactions. Chothia and Janin (1975) have studied the formation of insulin dimers, the binding of trypsin inhibitor to trypsin, and the forma-

**Table IX. Thermodynamic Parameters of Antigen–Antibody Binding**

| Antibody to | $K$ (liters/mole) | $\Delta F$ (kcal/mole) | $\Delta H$ (kcal/mole) | $\Delta S$ (e.u./mole) | $T$ (°C) |
|---|---|---|---|---|---|
| *m*-Azophenylarsonate[a] | $3 \times 10^5$ | −9.8 | −0.8 | 20.0 | 23 |
| *p*-Azophenyl-β-lactoside[b] | $1.6 \times 10^5$ | −9.5 | −9.7 | −0.8 | 25 |
| Insulin[c] | $1 \times 10^9$ | −15.4 | −3.6 | 38.0 | 37 |

[a] Data of Eisen and Karush, 1949.
[b] Data of Karush, 1957.
[c] Data of Berson and Yalow, 1959.

tion of dimers between hemoglobin $\alpha$ and $\beta$ chains. Their data indicate that hydrophobicity is the major factor that stabilizes protein–protein interactions, and they estimate that each subunit must bury about 600 $Å^2$ of surface area, a contribution that can be derived from only a small number of amino-acid residues (about 10). Although comparable data on the formation of Igs from light and heavy chains and on the combination of $\beta_2$M and HL-A are unavailable, the formation of these specific protein pairs most probably is a hydrophobic interaction of similar nature. Chothia and Janin (1975) point out that the hydrophobic contribution to protein–protein interaction is nonspecific and that proper formation of hydrogen bonds and Van der Waals contacts requires complementarity of the protein surfaces involved. The surfaces must be able to pack closely together, with the polar atoms properly positioned to make hydrogen bonds. The Van der Waals and polar interactions contribute little stability to the formed complex, but these interactions provide the specificity needed in determining which proteins may recognize one another.

## VI. COMBINING SITES OF LECTINS AND ANTIBODIES

Although plant lectins and vertebrate antibodies are not evolutionary homologues, both types of molecules exhibit marked specificity for sugars, and in the case of antibodies, for other low-molecular-weight compounds. Furthermore, the binding reactions in both cases are those between a protein and a small ligand that occur in accordance with the thermodynamics of diffusion-controlled reactions. At present, detailed knowledge exists of the combining site for sugars on Con A (Reeke *et al.*, 1974) and of the antigen combining site on antibodies (Saul *et al.*, 1978), so it is possible to make a comparison of these binding sites.

Con A consists of four identical subunits of mass 26,000 daltons, each of which contains one binding site for D-glucopyranoside (Edelman, 1972; Becker *et al.*, 1971). In the intact tetramer, 4 sugar molecules occupy symmetrically equivalent positions. The iodine atom of *o*-iodophenyl $\beta$-D-glucopyrasanoside was shown by X-ray crystallographic studies to be located within a relatively narrow, but deep, pocket, of approximate dimensions $6 \times 7.5 \times 18$ Å, and to be surrounded by hydrophobic amino acids (Edelman, 1972; Becker *et al.*, 1971). Although the combining sites of other lectins have not been investigated in such detail, it appears that multimeric lectins contain one binding site per monomeric unit (Lis and Sharon, 1973). Binding of sugars can induce conformational changes that result in cooperative interactions among subunits. The sugar-combining sites of Con A are identical and have an affinity of approx. $3 \times 10^4$ liters/mole for $\alpha$-D-mannopyranoside (Yariv *et al.*, 1968; So and Goldstein, 1968).

The combining site for antigen is also a pocket of essentially hydrophobic character, in which hydrophobic and charged amino acid residues contribute the fine specificity. Antibodies can vary greatly in affinity with antigen, from approx. $10^4$ liters/mole to $>10^{10}$ liters/mole, depending upon the particular antibody population. The size of the combining site as judged by X-ray crystallographic analysis is about 15 × 6 Å, with a depth of approx. 6 Å (Poljak *et al.*, 1977). The combining site of antibodies differs from that of lectins in mode of formation because interaction between the variable regions of the heavy and light chains is required to form the pocket. In particular, the contact residues that impart the particular specificity for antigen are contributed by the hypervariable regions of the particular $V_H$ and $V_L$ combination (Padlan *et al.*, 1977).

The requirement for both $V_H$ and $V_L$ determinants can be illustrated with the use of murine IgG antibody of restricted heterogeneity raised against the arsonate (ARS) hapten. Such antibodies bear a cross-reactive idiotypic determinant (Tung and Nisonoff, 1975). In our hands, immunization of A/J mice with ARS-derivatized *Limulus* hemocyanin under conditions devised by Tung and Nisonoff (1975) resulted in production of IgG2 antibody of restricted heterogeneity, as assessed by zone electrophoresis, isoelectric focusing, and N-terminal amino acid sequence analysis. Of the first 30 residues of the $\kappa$ chain (of $V_\kappa$I subgroup), only 1 position showed more than 1 amino acid. The first 12 residues of the heavy chain gave a single sequence (Marchalonis *et al.*, 1979*b*). These sequences were identical to the dominant sequences obtained by Capra *et al.* (1975, 1977) for the cross-reactive anti-ARS idiotype-bearing IgGl molecule. A rabbit antiserum specific for the idiotypic determinant of the anti-ARS molecule was raised. This antiidiotype blocked the capacity of the antibody to combine with the arsonate hapten, and was probably directed against combining-site determinants. The requirement for specific light- and heavy-chain contributions to the idiotype is shown in Table X, which presents data obtained with the use of anti-ARS antibody and normal IgG and their polypeptide-chain combinations, to inhibit specific precipitation of the idiotype-bearing molecule. Normal IgG and its constituent chains do not inhibit the precipitation. The anti-ARS $\gamma$ chain gives appreciable inhibition alone and in combination with normal light chain, but recombination with specific anti-ARS light chain is required to give inhibition comparable to that of the original intact anti-ARS antibody. These data exactly parallel classic studies (Fougereau *et al.*, 1964) showing that light and heavy chains of the proper specificity are required to form the combining site of antibodies. As observed here, heavy-chain preparations alone or in combination with pooled light chains show some antibody activity, but admixture of antibody light and heavy chains brings about optimal recovery of antibody activity. The present antiidiotype results are of some interest because the cross-reactive anti-ARS idiotype has been reported on T cells specific for the arsonate hapten (Goodman *et al.*, 1978). If the existence of this idiotype on T cells proves to be definite, it suggests that the combining sites of T-cell receptors, B-cell receptors, and serum

**Table X. Inhibition of Precipitation of Anti-ARS Antibody by Antiidiotypic Reagents[a]**

| Preparation | Relative amount of immunoglobulin giving 50% inhibition of precipitation (pmole) |
|---|---|
| Normal MIgG | NSI[b] |
| Normal MigG $\gamma$ chains | NSI |
| Normal MIgG L chains | NSI |
| Idiotype-bearing anti-ARS antibody | 1.0 |
| Idiotype-anti-ARS anti-$\gamma$ chain | 6.4 |
| Idiotype-anti-ARS anti-L chain | 53.6 |
| Normal $\gamma$/normal L recombinant | NSI |
| Normal $\gamma$/anti-ARS L recombinant | 17.8 |
| Anti-ARS $\gamma$/normal L recombinant | 2.5 |
| Anti-ARS $\gamma$/anti-ARS L recombinant | 0.7 |

[a]Data of Marchalonis *et al.* (1979*b*).
[b]NSI, no significant inhibition at any concentration of inhibitor.

Igs are formed in the same manner from $V_H$ and $V_L$ determinants. Much evidence has been advanced supporting the presence of Ig idiotypes on antigen-specific T cells, but antigenic (Rajewsky and Eichmann, 1977), biochemical (Binz and Wigzell, 1977), and genetic (Binz *et al.*, 1976) data indicate that the idiotype-bearing T-cell receptor consists predominantly or solely of heavy chains. The presence of light chains on T cells has, however, been supported by studies involving: inhibition of antigen binding (Warner, 1974); direct visualization and isolation (Szenberg *et al.*, 1977; for reviews see Marchalonis, 1975, Cone and Janeway, 1977, and Cone, 1978); and demonstration of mRNA-specifying $\kappa$ chain in the vast majority of thymus cells (Storb, 1978). I would suggest that more detailed analyses of idiotype-bearing T-cell receptors will disclose the presence of $V_L$ determinants. See Warr (this volume) for further discussion of the Ig T-cell receptor.

Studies of the size of the combining site (Roubal *et al.*, 1974), the energetics of binding of antigen (Clem and Small, 1967; Ambrosius and Fiebig, 1972), and limited N-terminal sequence data (Sledge *et al.*, 1974) suggest that this structure is conserved in vertebrate evolution (Marchalonis, 1977*a*). This conclusion is not surprising, because Igs of all vertebrate species—including the primitive cyclostomes (Marchalonis and Edelman, 1968*b*) and elasmobranchs (Marchalonis and Edelman, 1965; Clem and Small, 1967)—contain light and heavy chains comparable to those of mammalian antibodies, and the basic unit of Ig structure is the light-chain–heavy-chain pair (Marchalonis, 1977*a*). It should be noted that certain Igs in lower species (Marchalonis and Edelman, 1968*b*; Steiner *et al.*, 1975) and mammals (Grey *et al.*, 1968; Warner and Marchalonis, 1972) consist of light and heavy chains without disulfide linkages between these chains.

## VII. PRIMARY BINDING AND SUBSEQUENT EARLY MEMBRANE EVENTS

Primary binding of lectins to lymphocytes and the subsequent early membrane events provide useful models for study of initial events of recognition. As described above, murine T and B cells bind approx. $5 \times 10^6$ molecules of Con A per cell, with affinity constants of about $4 \times 10^6$ liters/mole, a value that is 2 orders of magnitude greater than that of Con A for free monosaccharide, even though rigorous specificity is maintained for the sugar. Binding of Con A or antibodies (Yahara and Edelman, 1972; Curtain *et al.*, 1978) to lymphocytes occurs extremely rapidly, in a manner consistent with a diffusion-controlled process.

Studies with spin-labeled probes indicated that this binding results in the aggregation of membrane glycosphingolipids in the vicinity of ligand receptor clusters (Curtain *et al.*, 1978; Curtain, 1979), accompanied by a decrease in the ordering of the phospholipids in the bulk of the membrane. These changes occur so rapidly that they are essentially completed by the time the first measurement can be made (Fig. 7). The membrane-lipid parameters revert to control values approximately 1 h after ligand binding, correlating with receptor redistribution and loss. Production of cAMP occurs with a substantial lag following the membrane-lipid changes, although increased levels of cAMP are readily observed within 15 min after ligand addition.

Figure 7 shows that a strong correlation exists between membrane-lipid changes and the mitogenic response to Con A by human peripheral-blood lymphocytes. The aggregation of glycosphingolipids and the decrease in phospholipid ordering are not, however, strict correlates of mitogenesis, because nonmitogenic ligands that bind to lymphocytes also produce changes comparable in magnitude to those depicted here. For example, antilymphocyte globulin (a T-cell mitogen) and Con A (a T-cell mitogen) both bind to B cells to a degree similar to that observed for T cells and cause membrane-lipid changes similar to those shown here (Curtain *et al.*, 1978). They do not, however, stimulate DNA synthesis. The results illustrated here for quantitative studies involving spin-labeled probes parallel those obtained in previous studies using fluorescein-labeled mitogens and antibodies to investigate redistribution of mitogenic and nonmitogenic lectins. It was found that capping occurs with mitogenic and nonmitogenic lectins and there was no correlation between degree of capping and mitogenesis (Ahmann and Sage, 1974; Greaves *et al.*, 1972; Taylor *et al.*, 1971; Schreiner and Unanue, 1976; Nicolson *et al.*, 1977).

Use of ALG and Con A to stimulate T cells and to isolate membrane receptors suggests that the triggering component for Con A is most likely a glycoprotein of approximate mass 180,000 daltons (Decker *et al.*, 1977). This molecule is illustrated in Fig. 8. Con-A-binding surface proteins comprise a variety of glycoproteins, including this component, H antigens (Snary *et al.*, 1977), Ia anti-

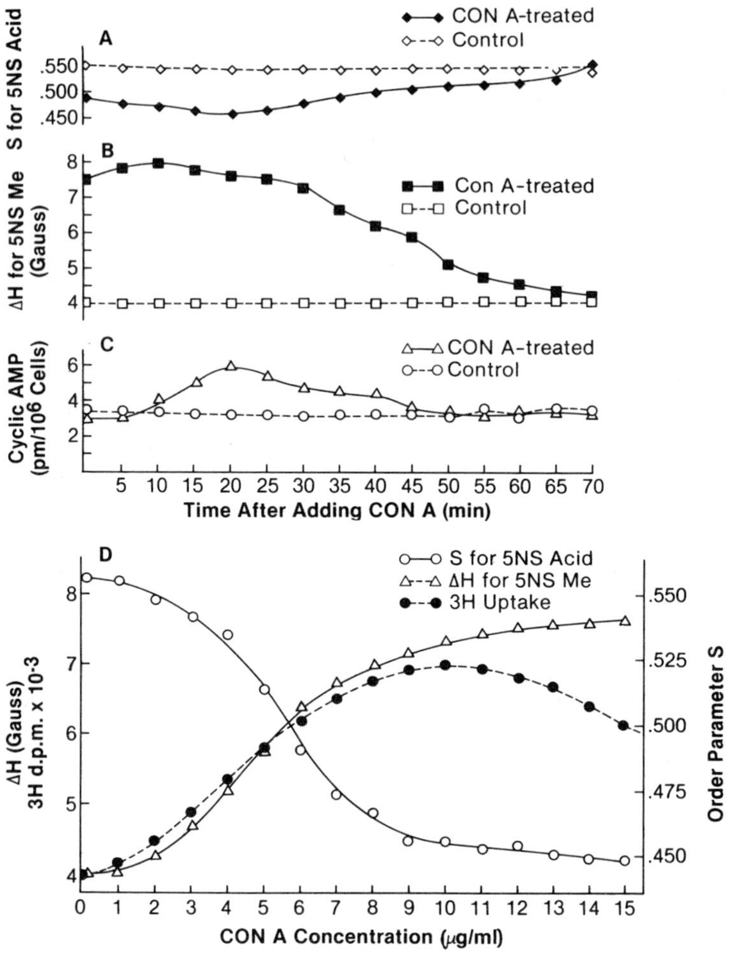


Figure 7. Molecular parameters of the binding of concanavalin A (Con A) to murine thymus lymphocytes. (A) The order parameter S as a function of time following binding of Con A measured for thymus lymphocytes containing spin-labeled stearic acid with the nitroxide group in the 5 position. A decrease in this parameter reflects an increase in ordering (or viscosity). (B) The probe–probe interaction parameter $\Delta H$ (in gauss) as a function of time following binding of Con A for thymus lymphocytes containing the spin-labeled methyl ester of stearic acid with the nitroxide group in the 5 position. This parameter increases as restriction increases. Both spin-labeled probes insert into the plasma membrane with the hydrophilic group, carboxyl- or methyl-ester, exposed to the solvent. (C) Kinetics of appearance of cAMP following binding of Con A. (D) Comparison of dosage of Con A required for mitogenesis ($[^3H]$thymidine uptake) with changes in the probe–probe interaction parameter ($\Delta H$) and the order parameter $S$. Data of Curtain *et al.* (1978).

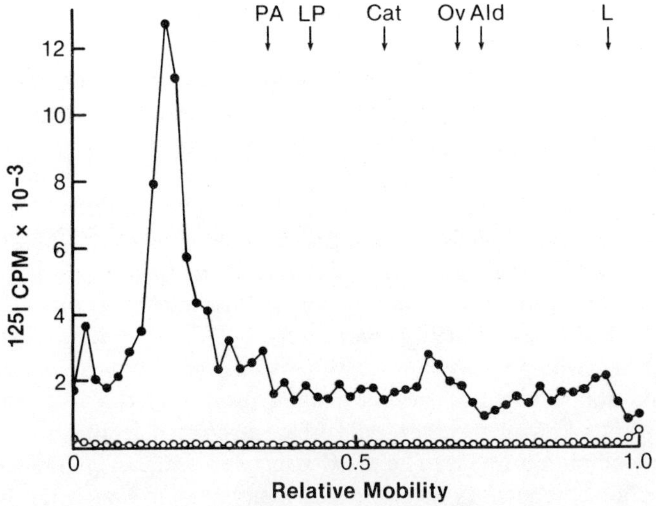


Figure 8. Radioiodinated surface glycoprotein recognized by horse antiserum to mouse thymus cells resolved by polyacrylamide-gel electrophoresis in SDS. •——•, specifically precipitated component; ○——○, control precipitate (normal-horse IgG plus rabbit antiserum to horse IgG); 10% acrylamide, reduced sample. L, light chain (MW 23,000); ALD, aldolase (MW 40,000); Ov, ovalbumin (MW 43,000); Cat, catalase (MW 60,000); LP, lactoperoxidase (MW 77,500); PA, phosphorylase A (MW 94,000). Data of Decker *et al.* (1977).

gens (Cullen *et al.*, 1974), Thy 1 (Letarte-Muirhead *et al.*, 1975), and Igs (Hunt and Marchalonis, 1974). The component that is precipitable with ALG also binds to Con A. Furthermore, treatment of T cells with nonstimulatory doses of ALG blocks stimulation with optimal doses of Con A, and nonstimulatory (superoptimal) doses of Con A block stimulation by ALG.

These data indicate that primary binding of a specific ligand to cell-surface acceptors and that certain subsequent membrane-modulation events are not sufficient to guarantee cell division and differentiation. The biochemistry of early membrane events following ligand binding is discussed in detail elsewhere (Decker and Marchalonis, 1978).

## VIII. CONCLUSIONS: PRIMARY BINDING AND ACTIVATION

I have given illustrations to develop the concept that primary binding of ligand by cell-associated receptors is in principle identical to the process that occurs for the same molecules in solution. In support of this hypothesis, it is possible to isolate hapten-binding cell-surface Igs (Marchalonis, 1976*b*), as well as serum Igs (Marchalonis and Warr, 1978) strictly on the basis of binding affinity with the specific hapten. The membrane-associated receptor differs from the molecule in solution, however, because either it is adapted to bind tightly to the lipid matrix of the plasma membrane or it is strongly bound to an "adapter" molecule, which is itself an integral membrane protein. Comparisons of endogenously produced B-cell membrane Igs with the passively adsorbed Igs of macrophages, mast cells, and B cells indicate that a specific "adapter" (here, $F_c$ receptor) is most probably required to allow binding of the Ig molecule to the plasma membrane in the proper orientation for specific combination with antigen (Marchalonis, 1976*a*; Loor, 1977; Ramasamy, 1976). It is likely that amoebocytes interacting with hemolymph agglutinins possess receptors for a portion of the molecule not involved in specific combination with the sugar moiety. At present it is not known whether cell-surface-associated lectins are integral or peripheral membrane proteins. The MHC-associated antigens particularly HL-A, have hydrophobic sequences that span the membrane, although the N-terminal glycosylated portion, like that of glycophorin (Furthmayr, 1978), is exposed to the aqueous external environment. The lectins and antibodylike molecules exhibit exquisite binding specificity for defined ligands, whereas the MHC-associated molecules *per se* have not been shown to bind ligands in a similar fashion. They possibly function in cell–cell interactions (Katz and Benacerraf, 1975; Benacerraf, 1978) and in molecular interactions and regulatory events required for cell activation and differentiation to occur (Marchalonis *et al.*, 1974). In particular, they may be involved in the regulation of self-tolerance (Marchalonis *et al.*, 1974; Schwartz, 1978), or in the amplification of the response following primary recognition (Marchalonis *et al.*, 1974).

The initial binding of ligand to cells is extremely rapid, occurring within a few minutes. In fact, changes in lipid viscosity that immediately follow binding of Con A to surface accepters occur so rapidly that the effect is maximal within the 2 min required to make the first measurement (see Fig. 4). Subsequent events of activation and differentiation include production of cyclic AMP (Fig. 4 and Parker, 1974), synthesis of nonhistone chromatin proteins (Decker and Marchalonis, 1978; Decker *et al.*, 1977), MHC-mediated effects (Bluestein, 1974), and cell–cell interactions (Feldmann, 1977), all of which show a lag ranging from minutes (cAMP) to many hours (MHC effects; DNA synthesis). Since primary binding of ligand is not always sufficient for activation and differentiation to occur, and the degree of differentiation achieved by an activated cell is conditioned by interaction with other cells and cell-free factors, it has been proposed that cell-surface receptors are part of a recognition–activation complex (Marchalonis, 1976*a*). In the case of antigen recognition, the variable regions of surface Ig would constitute the specific sensor element on B and T cells, and an adaptor or $F_c$-receptor-type molecule associated with the heavy-chain C regions could serve as a transducer molecule. This transducer might span the membrane and interact with an effector element that then would transmit a signal to the nucleus. This type of model might explain signal transmission by the endogenously synthesized Igs of B cells and by passively bound Igs of monocytes and mast cells. It is possible that MHC-associated markers might make up part of the recognition–activation complex. The mast cell–IgE system might well serve as an excellent model for the study of early events of antigen-mediated cell differentiation using the events of degranulation (Raff and Lawson, 1977). Other surface receptors might themselves be integral-membrane proteins and an adapter might not be required. Binding of ligand to such receptors might induce a conformational change, allowing them to interact with effector units that are mobile in the plane of the membrane (Cuatrecasas and Hollenberg, 1976). Although our knowledge of the structural properties of lymphocyte primary receptors for antigen is increasing, the biochemical mechanisms by which ligand binding initiates differentiation in this system remain largely obscure, and details of the molecular events of cell–cell interactions are eagerly awaited.

## ACKNOWLEDGMENTS

I thank Drs. J. D. Capra, H. L. Ploegh, and J. L. Strominger for preprints of unpublished work.

This research was sponsored by the National Cancer Institute under contract number N01-CO-75380 with Litton Bionetics, Inc.

## IX. REFERENCES

Acton, R. T., Bennett, J. C., Evans, E. E., and Schrohenloher, R. E., 1969, Physical and chemical characterization of oyster hemagglutinin, *J. Biol. Chem.* **244**:4128.

Ahmann, G. B., and Sage, H. J., 1974, Binding of purified lectins to guinea pig lymphocytes, *Cell. Immunol.* **13**:407.

Ambrosius, H., and Fiebig, H., 1972, Evolution of antibody affinity, in: *L'Étude Phylogénique et Ontogénique de la Résponse Immunitaire et son Apport à la Théorie Immunologique* (P. Liacopoulos and J. Panijel, eds.), pp. 135–146, Inserm, Boulogne.

Appella, E., 1971, Amino acid sequence of two mouse immunoglobulin lambda chains, *Proc. Natl. Acad. Sci. USA* **68**:590.

Balsamo, J., and Lilien, J., 1975, The binding of tissue specific adhesive molecules to the cell surface. A molecular basis for specificity, *Biochemistry* **14**:167.

Becker, J. W., Reeke, G. N., Jr., and Edelman, G. M., 1971, Location of the saccharide binding site of concanavalin A, *J. Biol. Chem.* **246**:6123.

Benacerraf, B., 1978, A hypothesis to relate the specificity of T lymphocytes and the activity of I region-specific Ir genes in macrophages and B lymphocytes, *J. Immunol.* **120:** 1809.

Berken, A., and Benacerraf, B., 1966, Properties of antibodies cytophilic for macrophages, *J. Exp. Med.* **123:**119.

Bernard, C. C. A., Roberts, I. M., and Mackay, I. R., 1977, Experimental autoimmune encephalomyelitis in mice antigen binding lymphocyte to basic protein of myelin insusceptible and resistance strains, *J. Immunogenetics* **4:**277.

Berson, S. A., and Yalow, R. S., 1959, Quantitative aspects of the reaction between insulin and insulin binding antibody, *J. Clin. Invest.* **38:**1996.

Binz, H., and Wigzell, H., 1978, Antigen binding, idiotypic T-lymphocyte receptors, in: *Contemporary Topics in Immunobiology*, Vol. 7: *T Cells* (O. Stutman, ed.), pp. 113–177, Plenum Press, New York.

Binz, H., Wigzell, H., and Bazin, H., 1976, T-cell idiotypes are linked to immunoglobulin heavy chain genes, *Nature* **264:**639.

Bluestein, H., 1974, Alloantiserum-mediated suppression of histocompatibility linked Ir-gene controlled immunoresponses, *J. Exp. Med.* **140:**481.

Capra, J. D., Tung, A. S., and Nisonoff, A., 1975, Structural studies on induced antibodies with defined idiotypic specificities. I. The heavy chains of anti-*p*-azophenylarsonate antibodies from A/J mice bearing a cross reactive idiotype, *J. Immunol.* **114:**1548.

Capra, J. D., Klapper, D. G., Tung, A. S., and Nisonoff, A., 1977, Identical hyperavailable regions in light chains of differing $V_{\kappa}$ subgroups, *Cold Spring Harbor Symp. Quant. Biol.* **41:**847.

Cesari, I. M., and Weigert, M., 1973, Mouse lambda-chain sequences, *Proc. Natl. Acad. Sci. USA* **70:**2112.

Chothia, C., and Janin, J., 1975, Principles of protein–protein recognition, *Nature* **256:**705.

Clarke, A., and Knox, R. B., 1978, Cell recognition in flowering plants, *Q. Rev. Biol.* **53:**3.

Clem, L. W., and Small, P. A., Jr., 1967, Phylogeny of immunoglobulin structure and function, *J. Exp. Med.* **125:**893.

Cone, R. E., 1976, Factors influencing the isolation of membrane immunoglobulins from T and B lymphocytes, *J. Immunol.* **116:**847.

Cone, R. E., 1978, The search for the T cell antigen receptor, in *Progress in Immunology III*, pp. 8–17, Australian Academy of Science, Canberra.

Cone, R. E., and Brown, W., 1976, Isolation of membrane associated immunoglobulins from T lymphocytes by non-ionic detergents, *Immunochemistry* **13:**571.

Cone, R., and Janeway, C., 1977, The T cell receptors, in: *Immune System: Genetics and Regulation* (E. E. Sercarz, L. A. Herzenberg, and C. F. Fox, eds.), pp. 175–178, Academic Press, New York.

Cone, R. E., and Marchalonis, J. J., 1974, Surface proteins of thymus-derived lymphocytes and bone-marrow-derived lymphocytes: Selective isolation of immunoglobulin and the theta antigen by non-ionic detergents, *Biochem. J.* **140:**345.

Cone, R. E., Hoessli, D., and Rosenstein, R. W., 1977, Analysis of detergent-extracted immunoglobulins of T and B lymphocytes by ultracentrifugation and column chromatography, *Immunochemistry* **14:**345.

Conrad, D. H., Bazin, H., Sehon, A. H., and Froese, A., 1975, Binding parameters of the interaction between rat IgE and rat mast cell receptors, *J. Immunol.* **114:**1688.

Cooper, M. D., and Dayton, D. H., 1977, *Development of Host Defenses*, Raven Press, New York.

Cuatrecasas, P., and Hollenberg, M. D., 1976, Membrane receptors and hormone action, *Adv. Prot. Chem.* **30:**251.

Cullen, S. E., David, C. S., Shreffler, D. C., and Nathenson, S. G., 1974, Membrane molecules determined by the H-2 associated immune response region: Isolation and some properties, *Proc. Natl. Acad. Sci. USA* **71:**648.

Cunningham, B. A., Wang, J. L., Pflumm, M. N., and Edelman, G. M., 1972, Isolation and proteolytic cleavage of the intact subunit of concanavalin A, *Biochemistry* **11**:3233.

Curtain, C. C., 1979, Lymphocyte surface modulation and glycosphingolipids, *Immunology* **36**:805.

Curtain, C. C., Looney, F. D., Marchalonis, J. J., and Raison, J. K., 1978, Changes in lipid ordering and state of aggregation in lymphocyte plasma membranes after exposure to mitogens, *J. Membr. Biol.* **44**:211.

Decker, J. M., and Marchalonis, J. J., 1978, Molecular events in lymphocyte activation: Role of nonhistone chromosomal proteins in regulating gene expression, in: *Contemporary Topics in Molecular Immunology*, Vol. 7 (R. A. Reisfeld and F. P. Inman, eds.), pp. 365–413, Plenum Press, New York.

Decker, J. M., Warr, G. W., and Marchalonis, J. J., 1977, A membrane glycoprotein which binds antilymphocyte globulin and concanavalin A is implicated in stimulation of murine T lymphocytes, *Biochem. Biophys. Res. Commun.* **74**:1536.

DeLuca, D., Warr, G. W., and Marchalonis, J. J., 1978, Phylogenetic origins of immune recognition: Lymphocyte surface immunoglobulins and antigen binding in the genus *Carassius* (Teleostii), *Eur. J. Immunol.* **8**:525.

DeLuca, D., Warr, G. W., and Marchalonis, J. J., 1979, Codistribution of antigen and Fab determinants on thymic antigen-binding cells, in: *Function and Structure of the Immune System* (W. Müller-Ruchholtz and H. K. Müller-Hermelink, eds.), pp. 165–171, Plenum Press, New York.

Dickler, H. B., 1976, Lymphocyte receptors for immunoglobulin, *Adv. Immunol.* **24**:167.

Edelman, G. M., 1972, The covalent and three dimensional structure of concanavalin A, *Proc. Natl. Acad. Sci. USA* **69**:2580.

Eisen, H. N., and Karush, F., 1949, The interaction of purified antibody with homologous hapten: antibody valence and binding constant, *J. Am. Chem. Soc.* **71**:363.

Erb., P., and Feldmann, M., 1975, The role of macrophages in the generation of helper cells. II. The genetic control of the macrophage T cell interaction for helper cell induction with soluble antigen, *J. Exp. Med.* **142**:460.

Feldmann, M., 1977, Cell interactions in the immune response *in vitro* in: *The Lymphocyte: Structure and Function* (J. J. Marchalonis, ed.), pp. 279–307, Marcel Dekker, New York.

Finstad, J., Good, R. A., and Litman, G. W., 1974, The erythrocyte agglutinin from *Limulus polyphemus* hemolymph: Molecular structure and biological function, *Ann. N.Y. Acad. Sci.* **234**:170.

Fishelson, Z., and Berke, G., 1978, T lymphocyte-mediated cytolysis: Dissociation of the binding and lytic mechanisms of the effector cell, *J. Immunol.* **120**:1121.

Flanagan, J., and Koch, G. L. E., 1978, Cross-linked surface Ig attaches to actin, *Nature* **273**:278.

Flier, J. S., Kahn, C. R., Jarrett, D. B., and Roth, J., 1977, The immunology of the insulin receptor, in: *Immunology of Receptors* (B. Cinader, ed.), pp. 477–489, Marcel Dekker, New York.

Fougereau, M., Olins, D. E., and Edelman, G. M., 1964, Reconstitution of antiphage antibodies from L and H polypeptide chains and the formation of interspecies molecular hybrids, *J. Exp. Med.* **120**:349.

Frazier, W. A., Rosen, S. D., Reitherman, R. W., and Barondes, S. A., 1975, Purification and comparison of two developmentally regulated lectins from *Dictyostylium discoideum*, *J. Biol. Chem.* **250**:7714.

Furthmayr, H., 1978, Structural comparison of glycophorins and immunochemical analysis of genetic variants, *Nature* **271**:519.

Goding, J. W., and Layton, J. E., 1976, Antigen-induced co-capping of IgM and IgD-like receptors on murine B cells, *J. Exp. Med.* **144**:852.

Goodman, J. W., Fong, S., Lewis, G. K., Kamin, R., Nitecki, D. E., and der Balean, G., 1978, Antigen structure and lymphocyte activation, *Immunol. Rev.* **39**:36.

Gray, W. R., Dreyer, W. J., and Hood, L., 1967, Mechanism of antibody synthesis size differences between mouse kappa chains, *Science* **155**:465.

Greaves, M. F., Bauminger, S., and Janossy, G., 1972, Lymphocyte activation. III. Binding sites for phytomitogens on lymphocyte subpopulations, *Clin. Exp. Immunol.* **10**:537.

Greaves, M. F., Janossy, G., Feldmann, M., and Doenhoff, M., 1974, Polyclonal mitogens and the nature of B lymphocyte activation mechanisms, in: *The Immune System: Genes, Receptors and Signals* (E. E. Sercarz, A. R. Williamson, and C. F. Fox, eds.), pp. 271–297, Academic Press, New York.

Grey, H. M., Abel, C. A., Yount, W. J., and Kunkel, H. G., 1968, A subclass of human $\gamma$A-globulins ($\gamma A_2$) which lacks the disulfide bonds linking heavy and light chains, *J. Exp. Med.* **128**:1223.

Hämmerling, G. J., and McDevitt, H. O., 1974, Antigen binding T and B lymphocytes. II. Studies on the inhibition of antigen-binding to T and B cells by anti-immunoglobulin and anti-H-2 sera, *J. Immunol.* **112**:1726.

Hämmerling, U., Mack, C., and Pickel, H. G., 1976, Immunofluorescence analysis of Ig determinants of mouse thymocytes and T cells, *Immunochemistry* **13**:525.

Haustein, D., and Goding, J. W., 1975, Surface immunoglobulin heavy chains of murine splenocytes and thymocytes are different, *Biochem. Biophys. Res. Commun.* **65**:483.

Hood, L., and Ein, D., 1968, Immunoglobulin lambda chain structure: Two genes, one polypeptide chain, *Nature* **220**:764.

Hunt, S., and Marchalonis, J. J., 1974, Radioiodinated lymphocyte surface glycoproteins: Concanavalin A binding proteins include surface immunoglobulin, *Biochem. Biophys. Res. Commun.* **61**:1227.

Jenkin, C. R., 1976, Factors involved in the recognition of foreign material by phagocytic cells from invertebrates, in: *Comparative Immunology* (J. J. Marchalonis, ed.), pp. 80–97, Blackwell, Oxford.

Jones, V. E., Graves, H. E., and Orlans, E., 1976, The detection of $(Fab')_2$-related surface antigens in the thymocytes of children, *Immunology* **30**:281.

Kabat, E. A., Wu, T. T., and Bilofsky, H., 1976, *Variable Regions of Immunoglobulin Chains*, Medical Computer Systems, Cambridge, Mass.

Karush, F., 1957, The interaction of purified anti-β-lactoside antibody with haptens, *J. Am. Chem. Soc.* **79**:3380.

Karush, F., 1962, Immunologic specificity and molecular structure, *Adv. Immunol.* **2**:1.

Katz, D. H., and Benacerraf, B., 1975, The function and interrelationships of T cell receptors, Ir genes and other histocompatibility gene products, *Transpl. Rev.* **22**:175.

Kauzmann, W., 1959, Some factors in the interpretation of protein denaturation, *Adv. Prot. Chem.* **14**:1.

Kindmark, C.-O., 1971, Stimulating effect of C-reactive protein on phagocytosis of various species of pathogenic bacteria, *Clin. Exp. Immunol.* **8**:941.

Klein, J., 1976, An attempt at an interpretation of the mouse H-2 complex, in: *Contemporary Topics in Immunobiology*, Vol. 5 (W. O. Weigle, ed.), pp. 297–336, Plenum Press, New York.

Kubo, R. T., Rosenblum, I. Y., and Benedict, A. A., 1971, Amino terminal sequences of heavy and light chains of chicken anti-dinitrophenyl antibody, *J. Immunol.* **107**:1781.

Letarte-Muirhead, M., Barclay, A. N., and Williams, A. F., 1975, Purification of the Thy-1 molecule, a major cell surface glycoprotein of rat thymocytes, *Biochem. J.* **151**:685.

Li, C. H., Dixon, J. S., and Liu, W.-K., 1969, Human pituitary growth hormone, *Arch. Biochem. Biophys.* **133**:70.

Lis, H., and Sharon, N., 1973, The biochemistry of plant lectins (phytohemagglutinins), *Ann. Rev. Biochem.* **42**:541.

Loor, F., 1977, Structure and dynamics of the lymphocyte surface, in relation to differentiation, recognition and activation, *Progr. Allergy* **23:**1.

McIlhinney, R. A. J., Richardson, N. E., and Feinstein, A., 1978, Evidence for a C-terminal tyrosine residue in human and mouse B-lymphocyte membrane $\mu$-chains, *Nature* **272:** 555.

Marchalonis, J. J., 1975, Lymphocyte surface immunoglobulin, *Science* **190:**20.

Marchalonis, J. J., 1976*a*, Surface immunoglobulin of B and T lymphocytes: Molecular properties, association with the cell membrane, in: *Contemporary Topics in Molecular Immunology*, Vol. 5 (H. N. Eisen and R. A. Reisfeld, eds.), pp. 125–160, Plenum Press, New York.

Marchalonis, J. J., 1976*b*, Isolated radioiodinated surface immunoglobulins of murine bone marrow derived lymphocytes which bind the 2,4-dinitrophenyl hapten, *Immunochemistry* **13:**667.

Marchalonis, J. J., 1977*a*, Antigen recognition by T lymphocytes: Status of the minimal hypothesis, *Ricerca* **7:**1.

Marchalonis, J. J., 1977*b*, *Immunity in Evolution*, Harvard University Press, Cambridge, Mass.

Marchalonis, J. J., and Cone, R. E., 1973, Biochemical and physiological properties of lymphocyte surface immunoglobulin, *Transpl. Rev.* **44:**3.

Marchalonis, J. J., and Edelman, G. M., 1965, Phylogenetic origins of antibody structure. I. Multichain structure of immunoglobulins in the smooth dogfish (*Mustelus canis*), *J. Exp. Med.* **122:**601.

Marchalonis, J. J., and Edelman, G. M., 1968*a*, Isolation and characterization of a natural hemagglutinin from *Limulus polyphemus*, *J. Mol. Biol.* **32:**453.

Marchalonis, J. J., and Edelman, G. M., 1968*b*, Phylogenetic origins of antibody structure. III. Antibodies in the primary immune response of the sea lamprey, *Petromyzon marinus*, *J. Exp. Med.* **127:**891.

Marchalonis, J. J., and Moseley, J. M., 1978, The immunoglobulin-like T cell receptor problem in: *Proceedings VI International Conference on Lymphatic Tissues and Germinal Centers in Immune Reactions*, in press.

Marchalonis, J. J., and Warr, G. W., 1978, Phylogenetic origins of immune recognition: Naturally occurring DNP-binding molecules in cordate sera and hemolymph, *J. Dev. Comp. Immunol.* **2:**443.

Marchalonis, J. J., and Warr, G. W., 1979, Antigen receptors on thymus-derived lymphocytes, in: *Cancer Biology Reviews*, Vol. 1 (J. J. Marchalonis, M. G. Hanna, Jr., and I. J. Fidler, eds.), pp. 1–47, Marcel Dekker, New York.

Marchalonis, J. J., Morris, P. J., and Harris, A. W., 1974, Speculations on the functions of the products of immune response genes, *J. Immunogenetics* **1:**63.

Marchalonis, J. J., Bucana, C., Hoyer, L., Warr, G. W., Hanna, M. G., Jr., and Szenberg, A., 1978, Visualization of a guinea pig T lymphocyte surface component cross-reactive with immunoglobulin, *Science* **199:**433.

Marchalonis, J. J., Warr, G. W., Bucana, C., and Hoyer, L., 1979*a*, The immunoglobulin-like T cell receptor. I. *In situ* demonstration of immunoglobulin Fab-region determinants in rodent T cells, *J. Immunogenet.*, in press.

Marchalonis, J. J., Warr, G. W., Smith, P., Begg, G. S., and Morgan, F. J., 1979*b*, Structural and antigenic studies of an idiotype-bearing murine antibody to the arsonate hapten, *Biochemistry* **18:**560.

Melcher, U., and Uhr, J. W., 1977, Density differences between membrane and secreted immunoglobulins of murine splenocytes, *Biochemistry* **16:**145.

Metzger, H., 1977, Early molecular events in immunoglobulin E mediated mast cell exocytosis, in: *Immune System: Genetics and Regulation* (E. E. Sercarz, L. A. Herzenberg, and C. F. Fox, eds.), pp. 679–690, Academic Press, New York.

Miller, J. F. A. P., and Vadas, M. A., 1977, The major histocompatibility complex influence on immune reactivity and T-lymphocyte activation, *Scand. J. Immunol.* **6**:771.

Miller, J. F. A. P., Vadas, M. A., Whitelaw, A., and Gamble, J., 1976, Role of major histocompatibility complex gene products in delayed-type hypersensitivity, *Proc. Natl. Acad. Sci. USA* **73**:2486.

Mir-Lechaire, F.-J., and Barondes, S. H., 1978, Two distinct developmentally regulated lectins in chick embryo muscle, *Nature* **272**:256.

Mitchell, R. E. J., Chaiken, I. M., and Smith, E. L., 1970, The complete amino acid sequence of papain, *J. Biol. Chem.* **245**:3485.

Moseley, J. M., Marchalonis, J. J., Harris, A. W., and Pye, J., 1977, Molecular properties of T lymphoma immunoglobulin. I. Serological and general physicochemical properties, *J. Immunogenet.* **4**:233.

Moseley, J. M., Beatty, E. A., and Marchalonis, J. J., 1979*a*, Molecular properties of T-lymphoma immunoglobulin. II. Peptide composition of the heavy chain, *J. Immunogenet.* **6**:1.

Moseley, J. M., Beatty, E. A., and Marchalonis, J. J., 1979*b*, Molecular properties of T-lymphoma immunoglobulin, III. Peptide composition of the light chain, *J. Immunogenet.* **6**:19.

Munro, A. J., and Taussig, M. J., 1975, Two genes in the major histocompatibility complex control immune responses, *Nature* **256**:103.

Nicolson, G. L., Poste, G., and Tae, H. J., 1977, The dynamics of cell membrane organization, in: *Dynamic Aspects of Cell Surface Organization* (G. Poste and G. L. Nicolson, eds.), pp. 1–73, North-Holland, Amsterdam.

Padlan, E. A., Davies, D. R., Pecht, I., Gevol, D., and Wright, D., 1977, Model-building studies of antigen binding sites: The hapten-binding site of MOPC-315, *Cold Spring Harbor Symp. Quant. Biol.* **41**:627.

Parker, C. W., 1974, in: *Cyclic AMP, Cell Growth and the Immune Response* (L. Lichtenstein and C. Parkers, eds.), p. 35, Springer-Verlag, New York.

Paul, W. E., and Benacerraf, B., 1977, Functional specificity of thymus-dependent lymphocytes, *Science* **195**:1293.

Perelson, A. S., 1978, Spatial distribution of surface immunoglobulin on B lymphocytes: Local ordering, *Exp. Cell. Res.* **112**:309.

Ploegh, H. L., Orr, H. T., Robb, R., and Strominger, J. L., 1978, Structure of HLA antigens, in: *Biological Markers of Neoplasia* (R. Ruddon, ed.), pp. 201–211, Plenum Press, New York.

Poljak, R. J., Amzel, L. M., Chen, B. L., Chiu, Y. Y., Phizackerley, C. K., Saul, F., and Yserum, X., 1977, Three dimensional structure and diversity of immunoglobulins, *Cold Spring Harbor Symp. Quant. Biol.* **41**:639.

Poulik, M. D., 1976, in: *Trace Components of Plasma: Isolation and Clinical Significance*, pp. 155–177, Alan R. Liss, Inc., New York.

Putnam, F. W., Florent, G., Paul, C., Shinoda, T., and Shimizer, A., 1973, Complete amino acid sequence of the mu heavy chain of a human IgM immunoglobulin, *Science* **182**: 287.

Raff, M. C., and Lawson, D., 1977, Membrane events in cell signalling, in: *Immune System: Genetics and Regulation* (E. E. Sercarz, L. A. Herzenberg, and C. F. Fox, eds.), pp. 669–678, Academic Press, New York.

Rajewsky, K., and Eichmann, D., 1977, Antigen receptors of T helper cells, in: *Contemporary Topics in Immunobiology*, Vol. 7: *T Cells* (O. Stutman, ed.), pp. 69–112, Plenum Press, New York.

Ramasamy, R., 1976, Attachment of the antigen receptor to the B cell membrane, *Immunochemistry* **13**:705.

Reeke, G. N., Becker, J. W., Cunningham, B. A., Gunther, G. R., Wang, J. L., and Edelman, G. M., 1974, Relationships between structure and activities of concanavalin A, *Ann. N.Y. Acad. Sci.* **234**:369.

Roelants, G. E., Forni, L., and Pernis, B., 1973, Blocking and redistribution ("capping") of antigen receptors on T and B lymphocytes by anti-immunoglobulin antibody, *J. Exp. Med.* **137**:1060.

Roelants, G. E., Ryden, A., Hagg, L.-B. and Loor, F., 1974, Active synthesis of immunoglobulin receptors for antigen by T lymphocytes, *Nature* **247**:106.

Roubal, W. T., Etlinger, H. M., and Hodgins, H. O., 1974, Spin-label studies of a hapten-combining site of rainbow trout antibody, *J. Immunol.* **113**:309.

Saul, F. A., Amzel, L. M., and Poljak, R., 1978, Preliminary refinement and structural analysis of the Fab fragment from human immunoglobulin N at 2.0 Å resolution, *J. Biol. Chem.* **253**:585.

Schreiner, G. F., and Unanue, E. R., 1976, Membrane and cytoplasmic changes in B lymphocytes induced by ligand-surface immunoglobulin interaction, *Adv. Immunol.* **24**:37.

Schwartz, R. H., 1978, Editorial: A clonal deletion model for Ir gene control of the immune response, *Scand. J. Immunol.* 7:3.

Segrest, J. P., and Feldmann, R. J., 1974, Membrane proteins: Amino acid sequence and membrane penetration, *J. Mol. Biol.* 87:853.

Shearer, G. M., Schmitt-Verhulst, A.-M. and Rehn, T. G., 1977, Significance of the major histocompatibility complex as assessed by T cell mediated lympholysis involving syngeneic stimulating cells, in: *Contemporary Topics in Immunobiology*, Vol. 7: *T Cells* (O. Stutman, ed.), pp. 221–243, Plenum Press, New York.

Silver, J., Cecka, J. M., McMillan, M., and Hood, L., 1977, Chemical characterization of products of the *H-2* complex, *Cold Spring Harbor Symp. Quant. Biol.* **41**:369.

Sledge, C., Clem, L. W., and Hood, L., 1974, Antibody structure: Amino terminal sequences of nurse shark and light and heavy chains, *J. Immunol.* **112**:941.

Smith, S., and Revel, J. P., 1971, Mapping of concanavalin A binding sites on the surface of several cell types, *Dev. Biol.* 27:434.

Smith, W. I., Ladoulis, C. T., Misra, D. N., Gell, T. J. III, and Bazin, H., 1975, Lymphocyte plasma membranes. III. Composition of lymphocyte plasma membranes of normal and immunized rats, *Biochim. Biophys. Acta* **382**:506.

Smyth, D. G., Stein, W. H., and Moore, S., 1963, The sequence of amino acid residues in bovine pancreatic ribonuclease revisions and confirmations, *J. Biol. Chem.* **238**:227.

Snary, D., Barnstable, C., Bodmer, W. F., Goodfellow, P., and Crumpton, J. J., 1977, Human Ia antigens-purification and molecular structure, *Cold Spring Harbor Symp. Quant. Biol.* **41**:379.

So, L. L., and Goldstein, I. J., 1968, Protein carbohydrate interaction, *J. Biol. Chem.* **243**: 2003.

Steiner, L. A., Mikoryak, C. A., Lopes, A. D., and Green, C., 1975, Immunoglobulins in ranid frogs and tadpoles, in: *Immunologic Phylogeny* (W. H. Hildemann and A. A. Benedict, eds.), pp. 173–183, Plenum Press, New York.

Stockert, R. J., Morell, A. G., and Scheinberg, I. H., 1974, Mammalian hepatic lectin, *Science* **186**:365.

Storb, U., 1978, Direct demonstration of immunoglobulin κ chain RNA in thymus T cells by *in situ* hybridization, *Proc. Natl. Acad. Sci. USA* 75:2905.

Szenberg, A., Marchalonis, J. J., and Warner, N. L., 1977, Direct demonstration of endogenous murine T-cell surface immunoglobulin, *Proc. Natl. Acad. Sci. USA* 74:2113.

Tada, T., Taniguchi, M., and David, C. S., 1977, Suppressive and enhancing T cell factors as I-regions gene products properties and the subregion assignment, *Cold Spring Harbor Symp. Quant. Biol.* **41**:119.

Taylor, R. B., Duffies, P. H., Raff, M. C., and de Petris, S., 1971, Redistribution and pinocytosis of lymphocyte surface immunoglobulin molecules induced by anti-immuoglobulin antibody, *Nature New Biol.* **233**:225.

Terhorst, C., Robb, R., Jones, C., and Strominger, J. L., 1977, Further structural studies of the heavy chain of HLA antigens and its similarity to immunoglobulins, *Proc. Natl. Acad. Sci. USA* **74**:4002.

Titani, K., Shinoda, T., and Putnam, F. W., 1969, The amino acid sequence of a K type Bence Jones protein, *J. Biol. Chem.* **244**:3550.

Tung, A. J., and Nisonoff, A., 1975, Isolation from individual A/J mice of anti-*p*-azophenylarsonate antibodies bearing a cross-reactive idiotype, *J. Exp. Med.* **141**:112.

Vitetta, E. S., and Capra, J. D., 1978, The protein products of the murine 17th chromosome: Genetics and structure, *Adv. Immunol.* **26**:147.

Vitetta, E. S., and Uhr, J. W., 1973, Synthesis, transport, dynamics, and fate of cell surface Ig and alloantigens in murine lymphocytes, *Transplant. Rev.* **14**:50.

Vitetta, E. S., and Uhr, J. W., 1975, Immunoglobulin receptors revisited, *Science* **189**:964.

Vitetta, E. S., Bianco, C., Nussenzweig, V., and Uhr, J. W., 1972, 1972, Cell surface immunoglobulin. IV. Distribution among thymocytes, bone marrow cells, and their derived populations, *J. Exp. Med.* **136**:81.

Walsh, F. S., and Crumpton, M. J., 1977, Orientation of cell-surface antigens in the lipid bilayer of lymphocyte plasma membrane, *Nature* **269**:307.

Warner, N. L., 1974, Membrane immunoglobulins and antigen receptors on B and T lymphocytes, *Adv. Immunol.* **19**:67.

Warner, N. L., and Marchalonis, J. J., 1972, Structural differences in mouse IgA myeloma proteins of different allotypes, *J. Immunol.* **109**:657.

Warr, G. W., and Marchalonis, J. J., 1977, Lymphocyte surface immunoglobulins: detection, characterization and occurrence in diseases of the lymphoid system, *Crit. Rev. Clin. Lab. Sciences* **7**:185.

Warr, G. W., Marton, G., Szenberg, A., and Marchalonis, J. J., 1978, Reactions of chicken antibodies with immunoglobulins of mouse serum and T cells, *Immunochemistry* **15**: 615.

Warr, G. W., DeLuca, D., and Marchalonis, J. J., 1979, The immunoglobulin-like T cell receptor. III. Binding of the arsonate hapten by idiotype-bearing T cells and antibody is blocked by avian antibody to $(Fab')_2$, *Mol. Immunol.*, in press.

Yahara, I., and Edelman, G. M., 1972, Restriction of the mobility of lymphocyte immunoglobulin receptors by concanavalin A, *Proc. Natl. Acad. Sci. USA* **69**:608.

Yariv, J., Kalb, A. J., and Levitzki, A., 1968, The interaction of concanavalin A with methyl alpha-D-glucopyranoside, *Biochim. Biophys. Acta* **165**:303.

Zinkernagel, R. M., and Doherty, P. C., 1977, Major transplantation antigens, virsues, and specificity of surveillance T cells, in: *Contemporary Topics in Immunobiology*, Vol. 7: *T Cells* (O. Stutman, ed.), pp. 179–220, Plenum Press, New York.

# *Index*

| | | | |
|---|---|---|---|
| | | | |
| | | | |
| | | | |
| | | | |
| | | | |
| | | | |
| | | | |
| | | | |
| | | | |
| | | | |
| | | | |
| | | | |